PROMPT

PRactical Obstetric Multi-Professional Training

T0276165

Course Manual

Third Edition

Edited by

Cathy Winter, Joanna Crofts, Timothy Draycott
and Neil Muchatuta

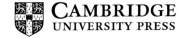

CAMBRIDGE
UNIVERSITY PRESS

CAMBRIDGE
UNIVERSITY PRESS

University Printing House, Cambridge CB2 8BS, United Kingdom

One Liberty Plaza, 20th Floor, New York, NY 10006, USA

477 Williamstown Road, Port Melbourne, VIC 3207, Australia

4843/24, 2nd Floor, Ansari Road, Daryaganj, Delhi – 110002, India

79 Anson Road, #06–04/06, Singapore 079906

Cambridge University Press is part of the University of Cambridge.

It furthers the University's mission by disseminating knowledge in the pursuit of education, learning, and research at the highest international levels of excellence.

www.cambridge.org
Information on this title: www.cambridge.org/9781108430296
DOI: 10.1017/9781108333627

© 2017 PROMPT Maternity Foundation

Registered Charity in England and Wales No. 1140557
Registered Company No. 7506593
Registered Office: Stone King LLP, 13 Queen Square, Bath, BA1 2HJ
www.promptmaternity.org

PROMPT Training Permissions and Licences

Units or institutions paying for a multi-professional team to attend an authorised PROMPT Train the Trainers (T3) day are only permitted to run PROMPT multi-professional obstetric emergencies training courses, using PROMPT course materials, within their own unit or institution.

Any PROMPT training conducted outside the unit or institution that has permission (see above) requires a licence from the PROMPT Maternity Foundation (PMF), e.g. a professional organisation or body wishing to roll out PROMPT training within a region or country, or a unit wishing to run PROMPT training at other hospitals outside of their own hospital group.

PMF is happy to discuss licensing arrangements or answer any questions relating to training permissions at any time. Please contact info@promptmaternity.org giving details of the training that is proposed.

Any training tools within this manual are based on national guidance where available, but PMF is not a national body. Therefore, we would advise that to use these tools locally, they should be approved by your governance structures after adapting for local use.

Registered names: The use of registered names, trademarks, etc. in this publication does not imply, even in the absence of a specific statement, that such names are exempt from the relevant laws and regulations and therefore free for general use.

The rights of Cathy Winter, Joanna Crofts, Timothy Draycott and Neil Muchatuta to be identified as Authors of this work on behalf of the PROMPT Maternity Foundation have been asserted by them in accordance with the Copyright, Designs and Patents Act, 1988.

This publication is in copyright. Subject to statutory exception and to the provisions of relevant collective licensing agreements, no reproduction of any part may take place without the written permission of Cambridge University Press.

First edition published by the Royal College of Obstetricians and Gynaecologists 2008
Second edition published 2012
Third edition published by Cambridge University Press 2017

A catalogue record for this publication is available from the British Library.

Library of Congress Cataloging-in-Publication Data
Names: Winter, Cathy, editor.
Title: PROMPT course manual / edited by Cathy Winter, PROMPT Maternity
    Foundation, Joanna Crofts, University of Bristol, Timothy
    Draycott, University of Bristol, Neil Muchatuta, University of Bristol.
Description: Third edition. | Cambridge, United Kingdom ; New York, NY :
    Cambridge University Press, 2017. | Revised edition of: PROMPT : Practical
    Obstetric Multi-Professional Training : course manual / edited by Cathy
    Winter, Jo Crofts, Chris laxton, Sonia Barnfield and Tim Draycott. Second
    edition. 2013. | Includes bibliographical references and index.
Identifiers: LCCN 2017023994 | ISBN 9781108430296 (paperback)
Subjects: LCSH: Pregnancy – Complications – Handbooks, manual, etc. |
    Obstetrical emergencies – Handbooks, manual, etc.
Classification: LCC RG571 .P72 2017 | DDC 618.2–dc23
LC record available at https://lccn.loc.gov/2017023994

ISBN 978-1-108-43029-6 Paperback

Cambridge University Press has no responsibility for the persistence or accuracy of URLs for external or third-party internet websites referred to in this publication and does not guarantee that any content on such websites is, or will remain, accurate or appropriate.

Every effort has been made in preparing this book to provide accurate and up-to-date information that is in accord with accepted standards and practice at the time of publication. Although case histories are drawn from actual cases, every effort has been made to disguise the identities of the individuals involved. Nevertheless, the authors, editors, and publishers can make no warranties that the information contained herein is totally free from error, not least because clinical standards are constantly changing through research and regulation. The authors, editors, and publishers therefore disclaim all liability for direct or consequential damages resulting from the use of material contained in this book. Readers are strongly advised to pay careful attention to information provided by the manufacturer of any drugs or equipment that they plan to use.

Contents

Editorial team and contributors   *page* v

Acknowledgements   viii

List of abbreviations and terms   x

Foreword   xv

Module 1 Team working   1

Module 2 Basic life support and maternal collapse   13

Module 3 Maternal cardiac arrest and advanced life support   29

Module 4 Maternal anaesthetic emergencies   47

Module 5 Fetal monitoring in labour   65

Module 6 Pre-eclampsia and eclampsia   99

Module 7 Maternal sepsis   119

Module 8 Major obstetric haemorrhage   135

Module 9 Maternal critical care   173

Module 10 Shoulder dystocia   189

Module 11 Cord prolapse   217

Module 12 Vaginal breech birth   229

Module 13 Twin birth   245

Module 14 Acute uterine inversion   259

Module 15 Newborn resuscitation and support of transition   269

Module 16 Measuring quality in maternity care   291

Index   303

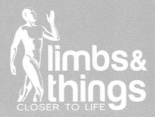

limbs&things
CLOSER TO LIFE

Advancing technical skills for better outcomes

PROMPT Flex + **PROMPT 3**

Multiple Training Scenarios

Shoulder Dystocia

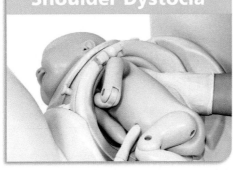

Impacted Fetal Head

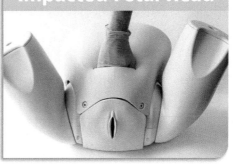

Scenario Management

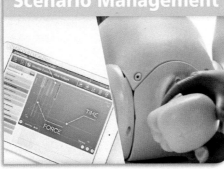

Cervical Assessment

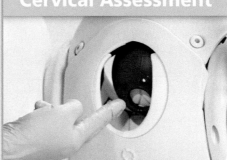

limbsandthings.com

E: sales@limbsandthings.com   T: +44 (0)117 311 0500

Editorial team and contributors

PROMPT Editorial Team

Joanna Crofts	Consultant Obstetrician, Bristol
Timothy Draycott	Consultant Obstetrician, Bristol
Neil Muchatuta	Consultant Anaesthetist, Bristol
Cathy Winter	Senior Research Midwife, Bristol

Contributors

Ms Mary Alvarez	Senior Research Midwife, Bristol
Lt-Col Tracy-Louise Appleyard	Consultant Obstetrician and Gynaecologist, Bristol/RAMC
Dr Sonia Barnfield	Consultant Obstetrician, Bristol
Ms Andrea Blotkamp	Clinical Fellow in Midwifery, RCOG
Dr Christy Burden	NIHR Academic Clinical Lecturer, University of Bristol
Dr Yealin Chung	Academic Research Fellow, Bristol
Dr Kate Collins	PMF Research Fellow, Bristol
Dr Katie Cornthwaite	NIHR Academic Clinical Fellow, Bristol
Dr Joanna Crofts	Consultant Obstetrician, Bristol
Mr Max Crofts	PMF Volunteer, Bath
Dr Ishita Das	Specialty Trainee in Obstetrics and Gynaecology, Bristol
Dr Fiona Donald	Consultant Anaesthetist, Bristol

Professor Timothy Draycott	Consultant Obstetrician, Bristol
Dr Sian Edwards	Specialty Trainee in Obstetrics and Gynaecology, Gloucester
Dr Islam Gamaleldin	NIHR Academic Clinical Lecturer, University of Bristol
Dr Kiren Ghag	PMF Research Fellow, Bristol
Ms Susan Hughes	Senior Midwife, Bristol
Dr Judith Hyde	Consultant Obstetrician, Bristol
Mr Mark James	Consultant Obstetrician and Gynaecologist, Gloucester
Ms Sharon Jordan	Senior Midwife, Bristol
Dr Christina Laxton	Consultant Anaesthetist, Bristol
Dr Erik Lenguerrand	Medical Statistician, University of Bristol
Ms Mary Lynch	Senior Midwife, Bristol
Ms Lisa Marshall	PMF Midwife Project Manager, Bristol
Dr Neil Muchatuta	Consultant Anaesthetist, Bristol
Dr Helen van der Nelson	Specialty Trainee in Obstetrics and Gynaecology, Gloucester
Dr Stephen O'Brien	PMF Research Fellow, Bristol
Dr Kate O'Connor	Consultant Anaesthetist, Bristol
Dr David Odd	Consultant Neonatologist, Bristol
Ms Beverley Osborne	Senior Midwife, Bristol
Dr Mark Scrutton	Consultant Anaesthetist, Bristol
Ms Debbie Senior	Practice Development Midwife, Bristol
Dr Dimitrios Siassakos	Clinical Lecturer in Obstetrics, University of Bristol
Dr Thabani Sibanda	Consultant Obstetrician, New Zealand
Dr Rebecca Simms	Consultant Obstetrician, Bristol
Ms Debbie Sirett	PMF Support Manager

Ms Angie Sledge   Senior Midwife, Bristol

Ms Ellie Sonmezer   Senior Midwife, Gloucester

Dr Maria Tsakmakis   Consultant Neonatologist, Bristol

Dr Tim Walker   Specialty Doctor in Anaesthetics, Bristol

Dr Nicky Weale   Consultant Anaesthetist, Bristol

Ms Heather Wilcox   Senior Midwife, Bristol

Mr Nigel Williams   PMF Voluntary Legal Advisor, Wales

Ms Cathy Winter   PMF Senior Research Midwife, Bristol

Ms Meg Winter   PMF Volunteer, Bristol

Ms Stephanie Withers   Practice Development Midwife, Bristol

Ms Elaine Yard   Senior Midwife, Bristol

Dr Christopher Yau   PMF Research Fellow, Bristol

Acknowledgements

The PROMPT Maternity Foundation (PMF) is a registered charity in England and Wales (Charity No. 1140557). The aim of the charity is to improve awareness and facilitate the distribution of effective, multi-professional, obstetric emergencies training as widely as possible to areas of the world requesting access to an economical and sustainable training model.

Over the past 5 years, there has been increasing evidence that the PROMPT method of training for maternity emergencies is having a significant impact, not only in the UK but internationally. In 2016, PROMPT training was recognised in the NHS England National Maternity Review, *Better Births*.

The growth and increasing recognition of PROMPT training is underpinned by robust research, collecting further evidence to support the improvements in outcomes seen in some maternity units in the UK and across the globe. PMF research projects are funded through fundraising, corporate partnerships and research grants from both UK and international bodies.

Internationally, PROMPT is now being taught in the USA, Australia, New Zealand, Zimbabwe, Laos, Abu Dhabi and UAE, Singapore, Hong Kong, Philippines, Switzerland, France, Germany, Spain and the West Indies.

This is the third edition of the PROMPT *Course Manual*, and it has been developed and produced with the help of:

- Maternity staff of North Bristol NHS Trust
- The PROMPT Maternity Foundation trustees, members, researchers and facilitators
- Maternity teams that attended the PROMPT 3 Pilot T3 training from the South West Obstetric Network, Bolton NHS Trust and St Thomas' Hospital, London
- Limbs & Things
- Laerdal Medical
- The Health Foundation

The final production of the third edition of the PROMPT *Course in a Box* would not have been possible without the invaluable commitment and support of:

- The Louise Stratton Memorial Fund – whose fundraising projects enabled the very first PROMPT training package to be produced.

- All the volunteers and supporters who have held fundraising activities on behalf of the PROMPT Maternity Foundation.

- Christopher Eskell – Chief Executive Officer (CEO) of the PROMPT Maternity Foundation (2011–2016), who sadly died in October 2016 after a short illness. He was the CEO of PMF for 5 years, and thanks to his skills and dedication, PROMPT has grown from a small Bristol project into an international gold standard for training. Thank you to Christopher for his contribution to creating our charity, and for his meticulous work underpinning all of our successes.

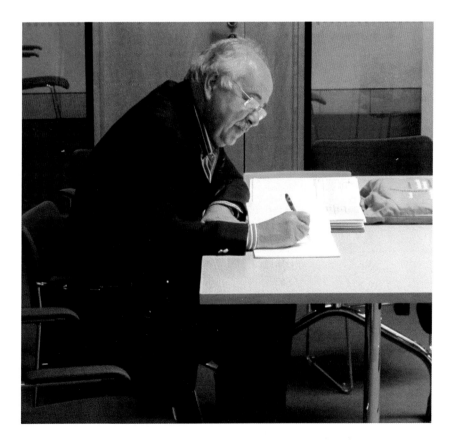

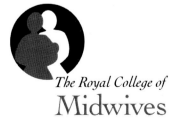

The Royal College of Midwives

Royal College of Obstetricians and Gynaecologists

Bringing to life the best in women's health care

Obstetric Anaesthetists' Association

Abbreviations and terms

ABC .... airway, breathing, circulation

AED .... automated external defibrillator

AFE .... amniotic fluid embolism

ALS .... advanced life support

ALT .... alanine aminotransferase

AOI .... Adverse Outcome Index

APH .... antepartum haemorrhage

APTT .... activated partial thromboplastin time

AST .... aspartate aminotransferase

AVPU .... alert, responsive to voice, responsive to painful stimuli, unresponsive

bd........................ twice daily

BE........................ base excess

BIPAP .... bi-level positive airway pressure

BLS .... basic life support

BMI .... body mass index

BP .... blood pressure

BPI .... brachial plexus injury

bpm .... beats per minute

Ca^{2+} .... calcium

CMACE .... Centre for Maternal and Child Enquiries

CNST .... Clinical Negligence Scheme for Trusts

CO_2 .... carbon dioxide

CPAP .... continuous positive airway pressure

CPR .... cardiopulmonary resuscitation

CQC .... Care Quality Commission

CRM .... crew resource management

CRP .... C-reactive protein

CT .... computed tomography

CTG .... cardiotocograph

CTPA .... computed tomography pulmonary angiography

CUSUM .... cumulative sum control chart

CVE .... cerebrovascular event

CVP .... central venous pressure

DAS .... Difficult Airway Society

DIC .... disseminated intravascular coagulation

DVT .... deep vein thrombosis

ECG .... electrocardiogram

ECV .... external cephalic version

EFM .... electronic fetal heart rate monitoring

eGFR .... estimated glomerular filtration rate

EUA .... examination under anaesthetic

FBC .... full blood count

EUA .... examination under anaethetic

FBS .... fetal blood sample

FFP .... fresh frozen plasma

FH .... fetal heart

FHR .... fetal heart rate

FIGO .... International Federation of Gynecology and Obstetrics

FSE .... fetal scalp electrode

FSS .... fetal scalp stimulation

GA .... general anaesthesia

GAS .... group A *Streptococcus*

GDG .... guideline development group

GI .... gastrointestinal

GMC .... General Medical Council

GTN .... glyceryl trinitrate

HELLP syndrome ... haemolysis, elevated liver enzymes and low platelets

HELP .... Head Elevating Laryngoscopy Pillow

HES .... Hospital Episode Statistics

HIE .... hypoxic–ischaemic encephalopathy

HIV .... human immunodeficiency virus

HVS .... high vaginal swab

IA .... intermittent auscultation

ICU .... intensive care unit

IM .... intramuscular

IMox Study .... Intramuscular Oxytocics Study

IO .... intraosseous

IOL .... induction of labour

IPPV .... intermittent positive pressure ventilation

IV .... intravenous

IVF .... in-vitro fertilisation

J .... joules

K$^+$ .... potassium

LCAs .... legal claim analyses

LFT .... liver function test

LMA .... laryngeal mask airway

MBRRACE-UK ...... Mothers and Babies: Reducing Risk through Audits and Confidential Enquiries across the UK

MLU .... midwife-led unit

MOEWS .... modified obstetric early warning score

MRI .... magnetic resonance imaging

Na⁺ .... sodium

NEWS .... neonatal early warning score

NHS .... National Health Service

NHSLA .... NHS Litigation Authority (known as NHS Resolution from 2017)

NICE .... National Institute for Health and Care Excellence

NIHR .... National Institute for Health Research

NMC .... Nursing and Midwifery Council

NPSA .... National Patient Safety Agency

OAA .... Obstetric Anaesthetists' Association

ODP .... operating department practitioner

OVB .... operative vaginal birth

PaCO₂ .... arterial partial pressure of carbon dioxide

PACS .... picture archiving and communication system

PaO₂ .... arterial partial pressure of oxygen

PCI .... percutaneous coronary intervention

PEA .... pulseless electrical activity

PEEP .... positive end-expiratory pressure

PO .... by mouth (per os)

PPH .... postpartum haemorrhage

PPROM .... preterm pre-labour rupture of membranes

PR .... per rectum

PROMs .... patient-reported outcome measures

PV .... per vaginam

qds .... four times daily

QI .... quality indicator

RAG .... red / amber / green

RCM .... Royal College of Midwives

RCOG .... Royal College of Obstetricians and Gynaecologists

RCT .... randomised controlled trial

RDS .... respiratory distress syndrome

rFVIIa .... recombinant factor VIIa

RR .... respiratory rate or relative risk

SI .... Severity Index

SBAR .... situation, background, assessment and recommendation/response

SC .... subcutaneous

SRM .... spontaneous rupture of membranes

tds .... three times daily

TXA .... tranexamic acid

U&Es .... urea and electrolytes

UKOSS .... United Kingdom Obstetric Surveillance System

VBAC .... vaginal birth after caesarean

VE .... vaginal examination

VF .... ventricular fibrillation

V/Q scan .... ventilation/perfusion scan

VT .... ventricular tachycardia

VTE .... venous thromboembolism

WAOS .... Weighted Adverse Outcome Score

WBC .... white blood cell count

WHO .... World Health Organization

WOMAN trial .... World Maternal Antifibrinolytic trial

Foreword

Nine years after the first edition, this is the third and expanded edition of the PROMPT *Course Manual*. It is part of the PROMPT multi-professional obstetric emergencies training package, and it will be useful in all areas of the world requesting access to an economical and sustainable training model.

Training in obstetric emergencies and obtaining appropriate knowledge and skills has to be multi-professional, since cooperation between maternity caregivers is essential, and the weakest part of the chain may determine maternal and perinatal outcomes. That is why the first module of this *Course Manual* is dedicated to team working. The next 14 modules cover a large range of maternal emergencies, as well as fetal monitoring in labour, complicated births and basic newborn resuscitation.

The PROMPT training package consists of a 'Course in a Box' which includes a *Course Manual*, a *Trainer's Manual* and additional downloadable lectures, videos and algorithms. It provides course materials to enable local staff to run in-house multi-professional obstetric emergencies courses in their own maternity units or other local settings.

The training package is written by a team of expert clinical researchers who have many years of experience of conducting PROMPT training, both locally and around the world. PROMPT has been implemented across the UK and also in North America, Australasia, parts of Africa, Asia and Europe. The training materials are adaptable to low- and high-resource settings.

The evaluation of the effectiveness of the training with regard to its associated improvements in clinical outcomes is a priority of the PROMPT team. The final chapter of this manual emphasises the importance of measuring and monitoring outcomes to ensure the provision of the best-quality care.

Improving safety and quality by better knowledge, skills, teamwork and leadership is our responsibility. Worldwide, there is still much to improve.

I am sure that the PROMPT training programme and materials will serve such a purpose.

Gerard H. A. Visser

Emeritus Professor of Obstetrics, Utrecht, the Netherlands

Chair of the FIGO Committee for Safe Motherhood and Newborn Health

Module 1
Team working

Key learning points

- Good team working is important, because poorly functioning teams are associated with preventable harm.
- More efficient teams state the emergency earlier and use closed-loop communication.
- Teamwork training may improve clinical outcomes when incorporated into clinical training.
- Effective teams appreciate the different roles and responsibilities of team members and the importance of shared decision making. They are also able 'stand back and take a broader view' in an emergency situation.
- Multi-professional training locally for all staff has been associated with improved teamwork, improved safety attitudes and, most importantly, improved perinatal outcomes.
- Recent national reports recommend that teams that work together should also train together.

Problems identified with local training

- Not training all groups and grades of staff together
- Not incorporating teamwork training into clinical training
- Staff working in 'silos' and not understanding the value of shared decision making

Introduction

Poor teamwork is directly associated with preventable morbidity and mortality for mothers and babies, with communication, ownership, leadership and teamwork all being identified as problematic areas in the 2009–12 MBRRACE-UK report.[1] There have been repeated recommendations for more and better teamwork training in these national reports,[1,2,3] and in recent years a groundswell of endorsements for 'human factors training'.[4] However, there are a number of studies that have demonstrated that isolated teamwork, clinical resource management (CRM) training, and/or human factors training do not appear to be associated with improvements in clinical[5,6] or process[7] outcomes. Therefore, teamwork training and human factors training should not, by themselves, be regarded as panaceas for all current ills.

Nevertheless, some teamwork training, including elements of human factors training, does appear to be clinically effective.[8] It is therefore important to understand the differences between team training interventions that were associated with improvements in outcome and those that were not. Moreover, it is also important to understand the barriers that prevent teams from working together effectively, so that useful interventions and solutions can be identified.

Teamwork training

Team working, including obstetric teamwork training, is complex and more than merely a summation of knowledge or skill.[9] In one study of simulated eclampsia, the more efficient teams were likely to have stated (recognised and verbally declared) the emergency earlier (e.g. 'this is eclampsia' and used closed-loop communication (with each task clearly delegated, accepted and executed, and completion acknowledged).[10]

Integrating and teaching these simple team behaviours within simulated emergency drills appears to be clinically effective.[8,11] This has been reiterated in a US study, which reported a statistically significant and persistent improvement in perinatal morbidity in a hospital which was exposed to a programme combining team training and clinical drills, whereas another study identified no improvements in a hospital exposed to team training alone, nor in the control.[12]

Improving team working is important, and the current evidence base supports local, multi-professional training for all staff annually, with teamwork training integrated within the clinical training.[13]

Definition

Teamwork is the combined effective action of a group working towards a common goal. It requires individuals with different roles to communicate effectively and work together in a coordinated manner to achieve a successful outcome.

Local training

As previously mentioned, current evidence supports training for obstetric emergencies in multi-professional teams, locally within the hospital unit.[14]

The key features of training programmes associated with improvements in perinatal outcomes are:[13,15]

- ■ Training is conducted in-house.
- ■ 100% of maternity staff are trained regularly.
- ■ All maternity staff are trained together, incorporating teamwork principles into clinical training scenarios.
- ■ System changes are introduced, often suggested by staff participating in the training.
- ■ Financial incentives for the provision of local training.

In-house training appears to be the most efficient, and cost-effective, means of training all staff in an institution. In-house training can also address specific local issues and can be used as a driver for system changes.[16,17]

Local training may also carry additional benefits, by creating a means through which an organisation can identify inherent risks that occur as a result of clinical unpredictability, and harnessing expertise capable of providing solutions to them.[18]

Local simulation of unpredictable intrapartum emergencies acts as a source of organisational stability and organisational adaptation, i.e. standardising practice wherever possible, while simultaneously retaining sufficient flexibility for clinical teams to be able to adapt to different clinical presentations.

High reliability and resilience

An independent researcher identified three core processes that are supported by PROMPT and that underpin high reliability and resilience: relational rehearsal, systems structuring, and practice elaboration:[19]

3

- **Relational rehearsal** represents the social processes that are involved in building shared expectations, establishing patterns of collective working and maintaining trust amongst the many diverse professionals who must rapidly come together to respond to an obstetric emergency.

- **Systems structuring** concerns the processes that are involved in testing and improving the organisational systems that support rapid and adaptive responses to emergency situations.

- **Practice elaboration** is when clinical practices are examined, refined, improved and embedded, to allow timely and effective responses to a wide variety of emergencies.

Costs of effective local training

Local training in clinical units is also likely to be cheaper, as well as more effective, than training in simulation centres.[20] However, local training is not without cost. Although there are expenses associated with training materials, training models and venues, the main costs of local training are release of staff to provide both the trainers and the staff to be trained. Few programmes have been costed formally, but one UK training programme associated with improvements in outcomes required more than 400 multi-professional (midwife, anaesthetist, obstetrician and healthcare assistant) staff days to train all staff in a large UK maternity department, at an estimated cost of £120,000 per year.[21,22]

Effective training is not cheap. Furthermore, the costs of training are usually borne locally by the obstetric department, whereas the benefits of improved intrapartum outcomes are felt in areas of the health system outside of maternity care. Therefore, a whole-system approach is required to incentivise effective training using existing financial levers.

However, a word of caution: unannounced simulation in local clinical settings has also been proposed, with suggested advantages of decreasing required resources and increasing realism, as well as widening multi-professional team participation.[2,23,24,25,26,27,28] However, these benefits appear to be based on comparing training in simulation centres with local, multi-professional training models, rather than with any 'ad hoc' local training schedules. Moreover, when unannounced simulation has been evaluated in an obstetric setting, a significant minority of staff considered it to be stressful and unpleasant, with midwives expressing these feelings more frequently. Furthermore, the planning and implementation of unannounced simulations was deemed time-consuming and challenging.[29,30,31]

The recent NHS England National Maternity Review, *Better Births*, recognises the benefits of local multi-professional training, recommending that 'those who work together should train together'.[32] Furthermore, multi-professional training should be a standard part of continuous professional development, both in routine situations and in emergencies.

Communication

Communication is the transfer of information and the sharing of meaning. Often, the purpose of communication is to clarify or acknowledge the receipt of the information. Communication is often impaired under stress. It is important to learn effective techniques that increase awareness and help overcome these limitations.

In the 2009–12 MBRRACE-UK report, communication problems were identified that directly affected care of women with haemorrhage. These included a lack of communication of concerns regarding the amount of blood loss and not escalating concerns to a senior member of staff when there was a deterioration in the woman's condition. MBRRACE-UK recommends that there should be a named senior doctor allocated to take charge of ongoing care in these circumstances.[1]

The five requirements for effective communication and efficient team performance are:[33,34]

1. **FORMULATED**

    Give a clear message. It should be succinct and not rambling. SBAR (situation, background, assessment, recommendation/response) is a useful acronym for formulating messages and handing over information and has been found to be used almost naturally by the most effective obstetric teams.[9] For example:

    > 'Mary Norton is having an antepartum haemorrhage (S). She is nulliparous and is 30 weeks pregnant (B). She is in severe pain, is hypotensive and tachycardic, and her observations score three red triggers on the MOEWS chart (A). I would like a senior obstetrician and senior midwife to review her immediately (R).'

Figure 1.1 is an example of a maternal SBAR form that can be used when handing over information. MBRRACE-UK recommends that the use of this structured communication tool may be helpful and effective in situations that require prompt decision making and action, such as when there is major haemorrhage or shoulder dystocia.[1]

SBAR obstetric handover sheet for an urgent clinical situation

S

Situation

I am calling about (woman's name): _____ **Ward:** _____ **Hosp No:** _____

The problem I am calling about is: _____

I have just made an assessment:

Her vital signs are: Respirations_____ Blood pressure ____/____ Pulse ____ SPO$_2$ _____% Temperature_____ ^{0}C

I am concerned about:

☐ **Respirations** because they are:
 ☐ less than 10
 ☐ over 30
 ☐ The woman is having oxygen at _____ l/min

☐ **Blood pressure** because it is:
 ☐ systolic over 160
 ☐ diastolic over 100
 ☐ systolic less than 90

☐ **Pulse** because it is:
 ☐ over 120
 ☐ less than 40

☐ **Urine output** because it is:
 ☐ less than 100mls over the last 4 hours
 ☐ significantly proteinuric (+++)

☐ **Haemorrhage:**
 ☐Antepartum
 ☐Postpartum

☐ **Fetal wellbeing:**
 ☐Fetal bradycardia
 ☐Pathological CTG

☐**FBS Result: pH** _____
 Time sample taken: _____ hrs

Obstetric Early Warning Chart Score: [ ] [ ]

B

Background (tick relevant sections)

The woman is:
 ☐ Nulliparous ☐ Multiparous ☐ Grand multparous
 ☐ Gestation: _____ wks ☐ Singleton ☐ Multiple
 ☐ Previous Caesarean section or uterine surgery

☐ **Fetal wellbeing**
 ☐ Abdominal palpation:
 ☐ Fundal height:_____cms ☐ Presentation:_____ Fifths palpable: _____ FH rate:_____bpm
 ☐ Intrapartum CTG: ☐ Normal ☐ Suspicious ☐ Pathological

☐ **Antenatal**
 ☐ A/N Risk sheet (details): _____
 ☐ Antenatal CTG: ☐ Normal ☐ Abnormal

☐ **Labour**
 ☐ Spontaneous onset ☐ Induced
 ☐ IUGR ☐ Pre eclampsia ☐ Reduced Fetal movements ☐ Diabetes ☐ APH
 ☐ Syntocinon infusion
 ☐ Most recent vaginal examination: Time _____hrs
 ☐ Cervical dilatation: _____cms ☐ Station of presenting part: _____ ☐ Position: _____
 ☐ Membranes ruptured ☐ Meconium stained liquor ☐ Fresh red loss PV
 ☐ Third stage complete ☐ Retained placenta

☐ **Birth details/post birth**
 ☐ Date of Birth: _____ Time of Birth:_____hrs
 ☐ Type of birth:_____ ☐ Perineal trauma:_____
 ☐ Blood loss: _____mls ☐ Syntocinon infusion
 ☐ Fundus: ☐ High ☐ Atonic ☐ Uterus tender ☐ Abdominal/perineal wound bleeding

A

Assessment

 The problem seems to be: ☐ red flag sepsis ☐ cardiac ☐ respiratory ☐ haemorrhage
 ☐ severe PET ☐HELLP ☐ pulmonary embolism ☐ pulmonary oedema ☐ severe fetal compromise
 ☐ I am not sure what the problem is, but the woman is deteriorating and we need to do something

 ☐ Treatment given / in progress:_____

R

Recommendation

 Request:
 ☐ **Please come to see the woman immediately**
 ☐ **I think delivering needs to be expedited**
 ☐ **I think the woman needs to be transferred to delivery suite**
 ☐ **I would like advice please**

 Reported to:_____ **Response :**_____

Person completing form (name):_____Date:_____ Time: _____

Figure 1.1 Example of an SBAR handover sheet

2. ADDRESSED TO SPECIFIC INDIVIDUALS (DELEGATED)

Use names of staff, and/or establish visual contact. Allocate appropriate tasks to an identified recipient.

> 'Kate [midwife], please can you get the PPH emergency box.'

> 'Kiren [maternity healthcare assistant], please could you document times and actions as they are called out, on this laminated pro forma. Thanks.'

3. DELIVERED

The problem should be stated clearly, concisely and calmly. When the obstetric emergency team arrives in your room, say:

> 'This is a shoulder dystocia. Please could you call the emergency obstetric team and the neonatologist, immediately.'

Rather than:

> 'Clemmie has been pushing for a long time, and the baby's head has just delivered and it looks like it could be a very large baby and I think I might need some help.'

4. ACKNOWLEDGED

Adequate volume used and repeated back:

> 'OK. You would like me to help Clemmie to get her legs into McRoberts' position.'

5. ACTED UPON

Meaning acknowledged and action performed:

> 'Clemmie is in McRoberts' position at 13.21. Please, Mary [midwife], could you note the time on the laminated pro forma.'

In addition, the use of non-verbal communication, including making eye contact with individuals, helps to prevent ambiguity and promotes a shared knowledge of intention. Improper or imprecise terminology, inaudible communication, many team members talking at the same time and incomplete reports should all be avoided.

Communication with the woman and her birth partner/ relatives

Women and their partners/families also want the same information in an emergency as the rest of the team. In recounted experiences, companions often informed women of the situation and the aims of treatment because they had heard loud and clear messages from small yet effective teams.[35] When extra staff are available, it is a good idea to allocate a designated team member to communicate with the woman and her relatives. More important than *who* communicates with the woman and her birth partner is the *content* of the messages being delivered: the cause of the emergency, the condition of the baby, and the aims of immediate and ultimate treatment.[35]

It would appear that using an SBAR-style structure during the emergency can be useful not only for teams but also for parents, and furthermore, it is likely to result in a patient perception of safety and good communication.[33]

Leadership: roles and responsibilities

Good leadership is often recommended in reports, but it can be hard to define in practice. However, there is some recent work that has analysed the characteristics of good leaders in simulated and recounted actual emergencies. These studies demonstrate that leadership is best established by the person who has the most experience of the emergency.[35] Leadership may also be more effective when the leader knows all members of the multi-professional maternity team and their relevant roles, before the emergency happens (from previously working together or from handover). The leader should be mindful of the same three components of the situation as the rest of the team (team, situation, patient focus), establish the situation (SBAR), allocate critical tasks with closed-loop communication (directed–acknowledged–confirmed) and, if necessary, pass leadership to other team members more experienced in the specific emergency at hand.[35]

Other members of the team should have their individual roles identified and agreed as early as possible. The leader should allocate critical tasks to the team members, including a designated person to talk to the woman and her partner/relatives.[33,34] Team members should be mutually supportive, communicate clearly and give regular updates. They should also avoid becoming fixated on minutiae or running around aimlessly.[35,36]

Key qualities of a good team member
■ Good communicator
■ Good understanding and acceptance of own limitations
■ Awareness of environment and limitations of others
■ Assertive
■ Non-confrontational but willing to challenge if necessary
■ Receptive to the suggestions of all other team members
■ Thinks clearly

Situational awareness: 'standing back and taking a broader view'

Situational awareness is how we notice, understand and think ahead in a fast-paced, constantly changing situation. It is that 'gut instinct' or 'sixth sense' that makes an expert midwife, obstetrician or anaesthetist. It involves recognising and understanding important cues, anticipating problems and sharing them with the team so that shared decision making and goals are achieved.

A lack of situational awareness was highlighted in the 2009–12 MBRRACE-UK report as the main human factor that contributed to some of the deaths from haemorrhage. The report identified delays in recognising the severity of the problem, and also staff persisting with ineffective or inappropriate care owing to a failure to continually re-evaluate the condition of the woman and her treatment.[1]

Three levels of situational awareness have been suggested. These levels are as follows:

1. **NOTICE**
   Be aware of the woman's status, the team members' status and all available resources. Anticipate potential errors by noticing cues and sharing decision making.

2. **UNDERSTAND**
   Share information with the team, think what these cues and clues may mean, be aware of common pitfalls, re-evaluate/stand back and take

a broader view at regular intervals, and seek to engage other team members in decisions.

3. **THINK AHEAD**

Anticipate, plan and prioritise. Situational awareness allows individuals to be 'ahead of the game'. Experienced clinicians usually have good situational awareness; they often pick up subtle cues, understand their significance and use them to anticipate and pre-empt problems.[10,35]

Recognising cues for a loss of situational awareness

In extreme situations, people can sometimes enter 'fast time', whereby their capacity to reason is so severely impaired by the stress of the workload that they are no longer able to function interactively with the rest of the team. Characteristic signs of 'fast time' include:

■ Poor communication

■ Inability to plan ahead

■ Tunnel vision

■ Fixation on irrelevant issues (such as less than ideal equipment) or displacement activities such as unnecessary disputes with colleagues

'Fast time' at its worst can cause even good team players to completely 'freeze up'.

Maintaining/regaining situational awareness

One suggested way of maintaining situational awareness is to adopt the philosophy of the 'non-participant' leader: try not to become engaged in practical tasks that can be undertaken by others. This allows the leader to take a step back and maintain a broader view of the unfolding crisis. Team leaders sometimes have difficulty doing this in practice, because they often have the particular 'hands-on' skills required to deal with the problem.

To regain control of a situation, the following strategies can be tried by the team leader:[10,33,35]

■ Take the 'helicopter view': stand back to get the broader picture.

■ Declare an emergency early: you will engage everyone's attention and boost the available human resources. Early declaration is associated with improved clinical team performance and efficiency, but also with improved patient perception of care.

■ Communicate clearly and simply, starting with the critical tasks for each emergency.

■ Plan ahead: for example, prepare for a perimortem caesarean section early (well within the first 5 minutes) in cases of maternal collapse.

■ Delegate the critical tasks appropriately.

Team working under pressure

Streesful situations give us the feeling that everything needs to be done immediately, and so the tendency to rush increases. Rushing tasks while under pressure increases the potential for making errors. Therefore, a good team leader should try to manage the emergency at a steady but efficient pace.

References

1. Knight M, Kenyon S, Brocklehurst P, *et al.*; MBRRACE-UK. *Saving Lives, Improving Mothers' Care: Lessons Learned to Inform Future Maternity Care from the UK and Ireland Confidential Enquiries into Maternal Deaths and Morbidity 2009–12.* Oxford: National Perinatal Epidemiology Unit, University of Oxford, 2014.

2. Cantwell R, Clutton-Brock T, Cooper G, *et al.* Saving Mothers' Lives: reviewing maternal deaths to make motherhood safer: 2006–2008. The Eighth Report of the Confidential Enquiries into Maternal Deaths in the United Kingdom. *BJOG* 2011; 118 (Suppl. 1): 1–203.

3. Institute of Medicine Committee on Quality of Health Care in America. *Crossing the Quality Chasm: A New Health System for the 21st Century.* Washington, DC: National Academies Press, 2001.

4. Carthey J, Clarke J. *The 'How to Guide' for Implementing Human Factors in Healthcare.* London: Patient Safety First, 2009.

5. Nielsen PE, Goldman MB, Mann S, *et al.* Effects of teamwork training on adverse outcomes and process of care in labor and delivery: a randomized controlled trial. *Obstet Gynecol* 2007; 109: 48–55.

6. Timmons S, Baxendale B, Buttery A, *et al.* Implementing human factors in clinical practice. *Emerg Med J* 2015; 32: 368–72.

7. Wears RL. Improvement and evaluation. *BMJ Qual Saf* 2015; 24: 92–4.

8. Siassakos D, Hasafa Z, Sibanda T, *et al.* Retrospective cohort study of diagnosis–delivery interval with umbilical cord prolapse: the effect of team training. *BJOG* 2009; 116: 1089–96.

9. Siassakos D, Draycott T, Crofts J. More to teamwork than knowledge, skill and attitude. *BJOG* 2010; 117: 1262–9.

10. Siassakos D, Bristowe K, Draycott T, *et al.* Clinical efficiency in a simulated emergency and relationship to team behaviours: a multisite cross-sectional study. *BJOG* 2011; 118: 596–607.

11. Mann S, Pratt S. Role of clinician involvement in patient safety in obstetrics and gynecology. *Clin Obstet Gynecol* 2010; 53: 559–75.

12. Riley W, Davis S, Miller K, et al. Didactic and simulation nontechnical skills team training to improve perinatal patient outcomes in a community hospital. *Jt Comm J Qual Patient Saf* 2011; 37: 357–64.

13. Draycott TJ, Collins KJ, Crofts JF, *et al.* Myths and realities of training in obstetric emergencies. *Best Pract Res Clin Obstet Gynaecol* 2015; 29: 1067–76.

14. Bergh AM, Baloyi S, Pattinson RC. What is the impact of multi-professional emergency obstetric and neonatal care training? *Best Pract Res Clin Obstet Gynaecol* 2015; 29: 1028–43.

15. Siassakos D, Crofts JF, Winter C, Weiner CP, Draycott TJ. The active components of effective training in obstetric emergencies. *BJOG* 2009; 116: 1028–32.

16. Thompson S. Clinical risk management in obstetrics: eclampsia drills. *BMJ* 2004; 328: 269–71.

17. Sutcliffe KM, Paine L, Pronovost PJ. Re-examining high reliability: actively organising for safety. *BMJ Qual Saf* 2017; 26: 248–51.

18. Hollnagel E, Wears RL, Braithwaite J. *From Safety-I to Safety-II: A White Paper*. Resilient Health Care Net, 2015. www.england.nhs.uk/signuptosafety/wp-content/uploads/sites/16/2015/10/safety-1-safety-2-whte-papr.pdf (accessed June 2017).

19. MacRae C, Draycott T. Delivering high reliability in maternity care: in situ simulation as a source of organisational resilience. *Saf Sci* 2016 Nov. https://doi.org/10.1016/j.ssci.2016.10.019 (accessed June 2017).

20. Ellis D, Crofts J, Hunt LP, *et al.* Hospital, simulation center, and teamwork training for eclampsia management: a randomized controlled trial. *Obstet Gynecol* 2008; 111: 723–31.

21. Draycott T, Sibanda T, Owen L, *et al.* Does training in obstetric emergencies improve neonatal outcome? *BJOG* 2006; 113: 177–82.

22. Yau CW, Pizzo E, Morris S, *et al.* The cost of local, multi-professional obstetric emergencies training. *Acta Obstet Gynecol Scand* 2016; 95: 1111–19.

23. Walker ST, Sevdalis N, McKay A, *et al.* Unannounced in situ simulations: integrating training and clinical practice. *BMJ Qual Saf* 2013; 22: 453–8.

24. Hankins GD, Clark SL, Pacheco LD, O'Keeffe D, D'Alton M, Saade GR. Maternal mortality, near misses, and severe morbidity. *Obstet Gynecol* 2012; 120: 929–34.

25. Saucedo M, Deneux-Tharaux C, Bouvier-Colle MH. Ten years of confidential inquiries into maternal deaths in France, 1998–2007. *Obstet Gynecol* 2013; 122: 752–60.

26. MRC Research Unit for Maternal and Infant Health Care Strategies. *Saving Babies 2003–2005: Fifth Perinatal Care Survey of South Africa*. Pretoria: South African Medical Research Council, 2006.

27. Mavalankar D, Singh A, Patel SR, Desai A, Singh PV. Saving mothers and newborns through an innovative partnership with private sector obstetricians: Chiranjeevi scheme of Gujarat, India. *Int J Gynaecol Obstet* 2009; 107: 271–6.

28. Nossal Institute for Global Health, World Vision. *Reducing Maternal, Newborn and Child Deaths in the Asia Pacific: Strategies that Work*. Melbourne: Nossal Institute and World Vision, 2008.

29. NHS Litigation Authority. *Ten Years of Maternity Claims: An Analysis of NHS Litigation Authority Data*. London: NHSLA, 2012.

30. Sorensen JL, Lottrup P, van der Vleuten C, *et al.* Unannounced in situ simulation of obstetric emergencies: staff perceptions and organisational impact. *Postgrad Med J* 2014; 90: 622–9.

31. Andreasen S, Backe B, Jørstad RG, Øian P. A nationwide descriptive study of obstetric claims for compensation in Norway. *Acta Obstet Gynecol Scand* 2012; 91: 1191–5.

32. National Maternity Review. *Better Births: Improving Outcomes of Maternity Services in England*. London: NHS England, 2016.

33. Siassakos D, Bristowe K, Hambly H, *et al.* Team communication with patient actors: findings from a multisite simulation study. *Simul Healthc* 2011; 6: 143–9.

34. Siassakos D, Draycott T, Montague I, Harris M. Content analysis of team communication in an obstetric emergency scenario. *J Obstet Gynaecol* 2009; 29: 499–503.

35. Bristowe K, Siassakos D, Hambly H, *et al.* Teamwork for clinical emergencies: interprofessional focus group analysis and triangulation with simulation. *Qual Health Res* 2012; 22: 1383–94.

36. Fox R, Crofts J, Hunt LP, Winter C, Draycott T. The management of a simulated emergency: better teamwork, better performance. *Resuscitation* 2011; 82: 203–6.

Module 2
Basic life support and maternal collapse

Key learning points

- To recognise maternal collapse and call for the clinical emergency team/cardiac arrest team (2222) early for clinical emergencies, peri-arrest and/or cardiac arrest.

- Cardiac disease is the commonest cause of maternal death in the UK.

- Recognition, assessment and resuscitation of maternal collapse:

  - ☐ A B C approach

  - ☐ Manual left uterine displacement (or 15–30° left tilt if on firm tilting surface, e.g. operating table) to reduce aortocaval compression

  - ☐ Use of an automated external defibrillator (AED) if available

- Calling for help: effective communication of the problem to the team.

- Equipment: knowing where to find emergency trolley, defibrillator, anaphylaxis box.

- Appropriate documentation.

Common difficulties observed in training drills

■ Failure to call for senior help in a deteriorating pregnant/postnatal woman

■ Not starting basic life support

■ Forgetting to keep woman supine with manual left uterine displacement during cardiopulmonary resuscitation (CPR)

■ Not administering high-flow oxygen to mother

■ Not using an AED to assess rhythm and defibrillate, if needed

Introduction

Maternal collapse occurs in a variety of circumstances. Presentation may range from an isolated and temporary drop in blood pressure to cardiac arrest and death. It is imperative that all healthcare professionals can provide basic resuscitation, regardless of the cause. In maternal mortality reports, resuscitation skills have been considered poor in an unacceptably high number of the maternal deaths.[1] Recent reports on maternal mortality have continued to recommend that all clinical staff should undertake regular training to improve basic, intermediate and advanced life support skills.[2,3]

Hospital maternity staff should be aware that they can summon the clinical emergencies team (or cardiac arrest team) prior to cardiac arrest, i.e. for a clinical emergency or a peri-arrest situation, by dialling 2222. Community staff should call 999 for a paramedic ambulance team.

Basic life support algorithm

All healthcare professionals should be aware of the principles of basic life support. Early recognition of cardiac arrest and early initiation of basic life support are key steps in the 'chain of survival' from cardiac arrest,[4] as well as early rapid mobilisation of advanced life support teams.[5] The 2009–12 MBRRACE-UK report highlighted that the initiation of life support measures was unacceptably delayed in a number of women.[3] Sudden unexplained loss of consciousness in a mother who is not breathing normally is a good indication of inadequate cardiac output, and basic life support should commence immediately.

An outline of the basic life support (BLS) algorithm is provided in Figure 2.1. This is not intended to be a complete guide, and further information is available from the Resuscitation Council (UK).[4]

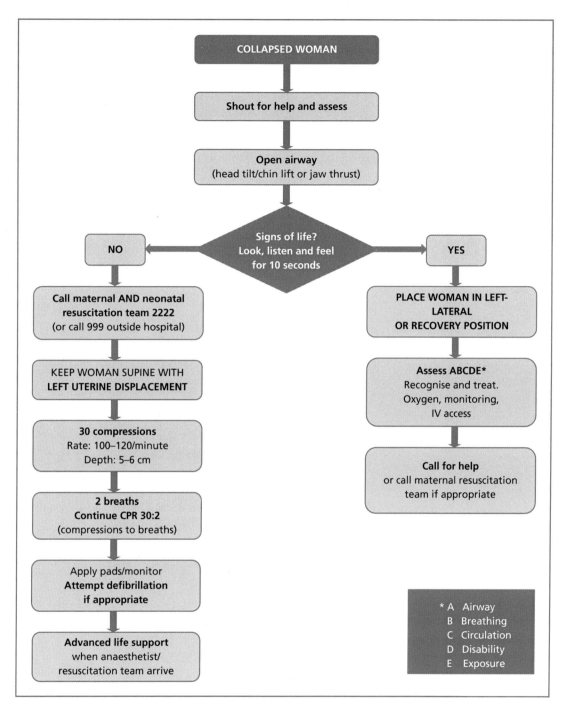

Figure 2.1 Basic life support (BLS) algorithm (based on Resuscitation Council (UK) Guidelines, 2015)

What do we mean by maternal collapse?

Maternal collapse is severe respiratory or circulatory distress that may lead to a sudden change in level of consciousness or cardiac arrest if untreated. Any of the vital observations in Box 2.1 should trigger an emergency response.

Box 2.1 Observations that trigger an emergency response	
Airway	Obstructed and noisy
Breathing	Respiratory rate less than 5 or more than 35 breaths/minute
Circulation	Pulse rate less than 40 or more than 140 beats/minute
	Systolic blood pressure less than 80 or more than 180 mmHg
Neurology	Sudden decrease in level of consciousness
	Unresponsive, or responsive to painful stimuli only
	Seizures

Figure 2.2 illustrates a systematic way of classifying possible causes of maternal collapse. The causes are discussed in more detail in the following sections.

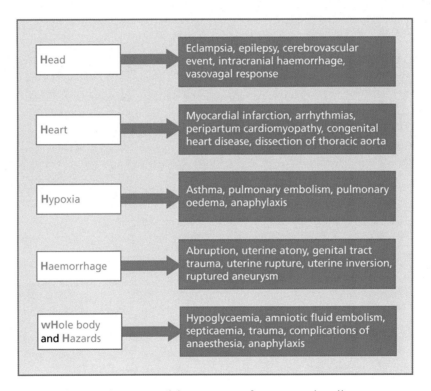

Figure 2.2 Possible causes of maternal collapse

Management of maternal collapse

The key to the effective management of maternal collapse is early recognition, escalation and a simple and structured approach to diagnosis and treatment. The underlying principles of the management of any critically ill pregnant or postnatal woman are the same and are often described through the ABC approach (airway, breathing, circulation). It is recommended that all aspects of basic life support should be initiated simultaneously where possible, and at least four BLS responders are ideally required,[5] which should be achievable when collapse occurs in the hospital setting.

Initial management

■ Assess the responsiveness of the woman by gently shaking her and asking if she is alright. If there is no response, seek immediate help using the emergency bell, dialling 2222 in hospital or 999 if outside hospital.

■ Turn her onto her back and ask an assistant to manually displace the uterus to the left using one or two hands, to reduce aortocaval obstruction (Figure 2.3).[4]

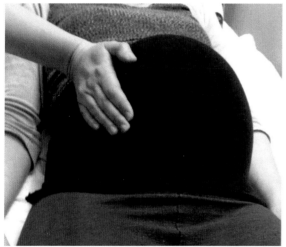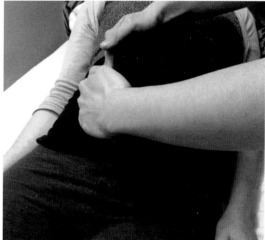

Figure 2.3 Left manual uterine displacement using one-handed and two-handed techniques

■ Open the airway using head tilt/chin lift or jaw thrust manoeuvres.

■ Assess breathing by looking at movement of the chest wall, listening for breath sounds and feeling for air on your cheek (look, listen, feel) for up to 10 seconds. Infrequent, slow or noisy gasps occur commonly in the first few minutes after sudden cardiac arrest; they are an indication for starting CPR immediately and should not be confused with normal breathing.

■ While assessing breathing, observe for other signs of life such as colour and movement.

■ If there are no signs of life, commence basic life support (Figure 2.1) until help arrives (to provide advanced life support) or the woman shows signs of life.

■ Chest compressions should be performed at a rate of at least 100 per minute and to a depth of at least 5–6 cm. A ratio of 30 chest compressions to 2 breaths should be used and attempts made to minimise any interruptions of chest compressions.[4]

■ If in a hospital setting, breaths may be given using a self-inflating bag (e.g. Ambu bag) and 100% oxygen (a two-handed technique is preferred[2]). If outside the hospital setting without equipment available, rescue breaths may be given mouth-to-mouth if safe; if not, compression-only CPR should proceed.[4]

■ The use of an automated external defibrillator (AED) is now recommended as part of basic life support,[4] as there is an immediate need to determine the cardiac rhythm. Following the prompts from the AED, if it is a shockable rhythm, defibrillation should be attempted.[6]

■ If the woman has signs of life, place her in a left-lateral recovery position and give high-flow oxygen via a reservoir mask (NB – a self-inflating bag is not appropriate in the spontaneously breathing patient, as its valve may obstruct and limit airflow). Obtain intravenous access, take blood samples (full blood count, clotting screen, urea and electrolytes, glucose, liver function tests, group and save) and give intravenous fluids. Establish monitoring of vital signs with ECG, respirations, pulse, blood pressure measurement and pulse oximetry. Then perform a primary obstetric survey.

Primary obstetric survey

A primary obstetric survey should be performed in a logical manner, starting at the head and working downwards. This initial management should produce a working diagnosis and should enable treatment of the cause to commence. Box 2.2 shows the questions to be considered when performing the primary obstetric survey. It is important that senior obstetric and anaesthetic support is sought if not already present.

Decide on continuing treatment

After the primary survey, the cause of the collapse and treatment required may be evident; for example, eclampsia or haemorrhage. If the cause is not obvious, only a few key treatment decisions are necessary.

1. Is fluid resuscitation a priority or is it contraindicated? If in doubt, fluid is usually beneficial. The exception is when the woman has, or is at great risk of, pulmonary oedema, as may happen in severe pre-eclampsia or renal failure.

Box 2.2 Primary obstetric survey	
Head	How responsive is the woman? Is she alert, responsive to voice, responsive to painful stimuli, or unresponsive (AVPU)?
Heart	What is the capillary refill like? What is the pulse rate and rhythm? What is the blood pressure? Is there a murmur?
Chest	Is there good bilateral air entry? What is the respiratory rate? What are the oxygen saturations? What are the breath sounds like? Is the trachea central? Is she complaining of chest pain?
Abdomen	Is there an 'acute' abdomen (rebound and guarding)? Is there tenderness (uterine or non-uterine)? Is the fetus alive? Is there a need for a laparotomy or to expedite birth?
Vagina	Is there bleeding? What is the stage of labour? Is there an inverted uterus?
Legs	Is there evidence of deep vein thrombosis (DVT)?

2. Is a laparotomy required for diagnosis or treatment? Is there evidence of an acute abdominal event? Does the birth need to be expedited to aid resuscitation?

3. Is sepsis likely and are antibiotics therefore a priority?

4. Is intensive care needed to provide airway, respiratory or circulatory support?

Secondary obstetric survey

Further management is dependent upon the cause of the collapse. Once the woman has been stabilised, a secondary obstetric survey should be performed (Box 2.3).

Further key treatment decisions

Re-evaluate and continue to support the airway, breathing and circulation of the woman. Do you need intensive care support? Re-evaluate your working diagnosis at intervals to ensure that the pattern still fits and treatment is working.

Box 2.3 Secondary obstetric survey	
ACTION	**DETAIL**
History	Revisit the history of the collapse and the previous history of the woman Read the notes and ask the partner or relatives
Examine	Repeat the examination, going from top to toe
Investigate	Take arterial blood gases, troponins, blood glucose, lactate, blood cultures, ECG, chest x-ray, ultrasound of the abdomen and high vaginal swab
Monitor	Continuous monitoring of ECG, respirations, pulse, blood pressure and pulse oximetry Consider arterial and central venous pressure lines to aid monitoring
Pause and think further	Consider further investigations such as CT/MRI scans and echocardiography Ask relevant experts for their opinions

Specific causes of maternal collapse

Maternal collapse may be a direct result of complications from pregnancy or from deterioration of an existing maternal health condition. MBRRACE-UK reports have identified that 75% of maternal deaths occurred in mothers with pre-existing medical or mental health problems.[3] There is also an association between advancing maternal age and maternal mortality,[2,3] which is relevant as average maternal age continues to rise. Obesity (BMI > 30) is an independent risk factor for maternal morbidity and mortality.[3]

Pulmonary thromboembolism

Pulmonary emboli are more common in pregnancy and the postpartum period, owing to the procoagulant effect of pregnancy and the mechanical obstruction by the abdominal uterus of venous return from the lower body. Pulmonary emboli may be small and non-symptomatic, or large and cause instant collapse and rapid death. Thromboembolism remains a leading common cause of direct maternal death in the UK.[6,7]

Pulmonary emboli may present with shortness of breath, pleuritic chest pain (sharp, and worse on deep breathing or coughing), haemoptysis or sudden collapse in a woman who may or may not have signs of a deep vein thrombosis. Clinical signs may include tachycardia, tachypnoea, hypoxia and evidence of right heart strain on ECG (S1, Q3, T3) with a raised jugular venous pressure. Diagnosis can be difficult. Initial assessment and treatment should be made on symptoms and signs plus arterial blood gases, ECG and chest x-ray.[7]

Treatment should be supportive, using facial oxygen, with ventilatory and cardiovascular support as necessary. Further testing should include duplex ultrasound if there are clinical signs of DVT. If no signs of DVT are present, testing should be either with ventilation/perfusion scanning (V/Q scan) or computed tomography pulmonary angiography (CTPA).[7] In life-threatening pulmonary embolism, portable echocardiography is helpful for diagnosis, and thrombolysis should be considered.[7] In the event of pulmonary embolism leading to cardiac arrest, CPR should be continued for at least 60–90 minutes before abandoning resuscitation efforts if treatment with thrombolytics has been given.[8]

Haemorrhage

Hypovolaemia, usually secondary to haemorrhage, is the most common cause of maternal shock. Signs of hypovolaemia include:

- tachycardia and tachypnoea
- cold, pale skin
- hypotension
- delayed capillary refill (more than 2 seconds)
- reduced urine output
- altered level of consciousness
- narrowed pulse pressure (less than 35 mmHg difference between systolic and diastolic readings)

Prompt resuscitative fluid replacement is essential. If there is significant haemorrhage, arterial ± central venous pressure (CVP) lines are often useful adjuncts for monitoring. The cause is most commonly obstetric in nature (such as uterine atony, vaginal tears/trauma, abruption, ruptured uterus), but non-obstetric causes should also be considered.

Although rare, aneurysm rupture may occur (such as splenic artery, aorta, renal artery, iliac artery). This is often not recognised but is identified as a cause of maternal mortality in the Confidential Enquiries.[3] Urgent laparotomy should be considered when there are signs of an acute abdomen in conjunction with hypovolaemia.

Eclamptic seizures and coma

Eclamptic seizures and coma may resemble seizures related to epilepsy, intracerebral events, syncope/cardiac arrest and metabolic disorders, but a detailed clinical history and the presence of hypertension and proteinuria in the eclamptic woman differentiates these conditions. For more information about diagnosis and treatment refer to **Module 6**.

Cerebrovascular event (CVE)

Cerebrovascular events (CVEs) can present with any manner of neurological signs, but classically present with weakness down one side of the face and/or body, or a drop in consciousness level. CVEs can be embolic or haemorrhagic in origin. Raised blood pressure, for example in severe pre-eclampsia, is a risk factor for haemorrhagic CVE, and any pregnant woman with systolic blood pressure of 160 mmHg or greater requires immediate antihypertensive treatment to reduce the risk of intracerebral bleed.[3] Migraine attacks can mimic CVEs, but on questioning, women will typically report a previous history of migraines, with familiar symptoms. A CT or MRI scan should aid in diagnosis, and direct treatment.

Sepsis

Maternal sepsis remains a leading direct and indirect cause of maternal death.[3] It is crucially important that the symptoms and signs are recognised and acted upon urgently. For more information about diagnosis and treatment refer to **Module 7**.

Disseminated intravascular coagulation

Disseminated intravascular coagulation (DIC) can occur secondary to massive bleeding, severe infection, amniotic fluid embolism or massive abruption. When DIC occurs, there is an excessive consumption of platelets and clotting factors, resulting in a prolonged clotting time, low platelets, low fibrinogen and haemorrhage. Spontaneous bleeding may be noticed from needle puncture, intravenous cannulae or epidural sites. Vaginal haemorrhage may also occur, as may bleeding from the woman's gums.

Early involvement of haematology, senior obstetric and anaesthetic staff, as well as intensive care, is vital if DIC is suspected. Blood should be sent for full blood count, cross-matching, clotting and fibrinogen. Tranexamic acid (TXA) should be considered. Point-of-care coagulation testing can also be helpful in guiding blood product usage. A haematologist can advise on the appropriate blood products required to correct clotting. The cause of DIC should be investigated promptly and treated appropriately.

Hypo- or hyperglycaemia

Women with diabetes may collapse into a hypoglycaemic coma. Although rare, type 1 diabetes mellitus may manifest for the first time in pregnancy. Blood glucose should always be tested in a collapsed or fitting woman if the cause is not obvious. Urine should be tested for the presence of ketones if diabetic ketoacidosis is suspected. Acute fatty liver may also present with maternal hypoglycaemia. If the woman's blood glucose is found to be below 3 mmol/L, then 50 mL of 20% (or 100 mL of 10%) glucose solution should be administered intravenously.

Cardiac disease

Cardiac disease is the leading cause of indirect maternal death in the UK, as well as the most frequent cause of maternal death overall.[3,6] In the most recent MBRRACE-UK report (2016), over 25% of the deaths occurring in pregnancy or postpartum were attributed to a cardiovascular cause.[6] The report identified many circumstances where pregnant or postpartum women had clear symptoms and signs of cardiac disease which were not recognised, often because the diagnosis of heart disease was not considered as a possibility in a young pregnant woman.[6] It is essential that there is early involvement of the senior clinicians from the obstetric and cardiology multi-professional teams, wherever the pregnant or postpartum woman with suspected cardiac symptoms presents, in particular if she is admitted to the emergency department.[6] Some women may have a known history of cardiac disease, chest pain with ECG changes, or a new cardiac murmur which will help to establish the diagnosis. However, any woman presenting with a raised respiratory rate, chest pain, persistent tachycardia and orthopnoea requires investigations, and these should not be delayed just because of pregnancy, as a prompt diagnosis is vital.[6] Investigations should continue until the cause is found.

Risk factors for ischaemic heart disease are listed in Box 2.4. They include increasing maternal age, smoking, and comorbidities such as obesity and diabetes.[6]

Box 2.4 Risk factors for ischaemic heart disease[6]

- Older age
- Smoking
- Obesity
- Diabetes
- Hypertension
- Family history of coronary disease
- Hypercholesterolaemia

Symptoms of chest pain are listed in Box 2.5. Angina in women is more likely to radiate to the throat, into the back and between the shoulder blades. Women and health professionals should be aware of the cardiac symptoms and their importance.[6] If chest pain is a presenting feature, troponin levels should be taken 6 hours after the onset of pain. However, a normal ECG and/or a negative troponin level does not exclude the diagnosis of acute coronary syndrome.[6]

If cardiac ischaemia is suspected, 300 mg aspirin should be given orally, unless contraindicated, and an urgent senior medical review organised, as

---

Box 2.5 Symptoms of chest pain that may be indicative of cardiac ischaemia[6]

- Discomfort developing over minutes in the anterior chest or epigastric area
- Band-like, squeezing, sensation of pressure
- Radiation to the jaw, arms, shoulders
- Radiation into the back
- Associated with breathlessness
- Associated with nausea and/or sweating
- Associated with syncope

---

well as echocardiography and consideration for coronary angiography with percutaneous coronary intervention (PCI), if required.

Pulmonary aspiration of gastric contents

Pregnancy increases the risk of pulmonary aspiration of gastric contents. This is because of progesterone-induced relaxation of the oesophageal sphincter and delayed stomach emptying, a problem that becomes more pronounced during labour. The use of H_2-antagonists such as ranitidine can reduce these risks.

Aspiration is most likely to occur in the unconscious patient (for example, during induction or emergence from general anaesthesia) owing to the loss of the cough reflex. Gastric aspiration may present with coughing, cyanosis, tachypnoea, tachycardia, hypotension or pulmonary oedema. To prevent aspiration, an unconscious woman is likely to require protection of the airway with tracheal intubation.

Anaphylactic or toxic reaction to medications or allergens

Anaphylactic or toxic reaction to drugs or allergens may present as convulsions or collapse. The close timing of administration of the drug or allergen (such as antibiotics, intravenous iron, latex) in relation to the collapse may be indicative of an anaphylactic or toxic reaction.

Severe anaphylaxis should be treated with:

- Removal of the trigger agent.
- Position in full left-lateral position (consider head-down tilt if feasible) or if postnatal lie flat with legs elevated.
- Oxygen 100% via mask with reservoir bag.
- Adrenaline (epinephrine) 500 micrograms (0.5 mL of 1:1000) IM (into side of thigh), repeated every 5 minutes if necessary.
- OR, **if an experienced anaesthetist/specialist is present**, 0.5 mL aliquots of 1:10,000 adrenaline (epinephrine) may be given intravenously if it is safe to do so.
- IV fluid: crystalloid 500–1000 mL bolus.
- Prepare second-line drugs: chlorphenamine 10 mg (IM or slow IV); hydrocortisone 200 mg (IM or slow IV); nebulised salbutamol 2.5–5.0 mg.

An algorithm for the management of anaphylaxis in pregnancy is shown in Figure 2.4.

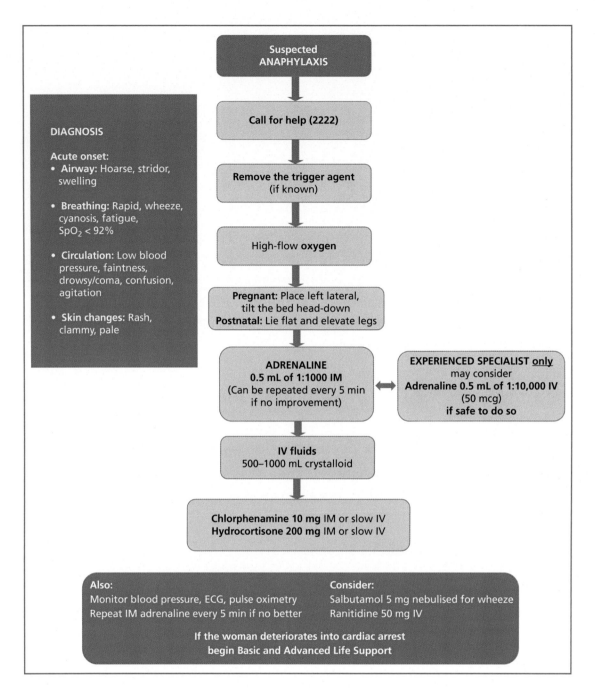

Figure 2.4 Algorithm for management of anaphylaxis (based on Resuscitation Council (UK) Guidelines, 2015)

Amniotic fluid embolism

It is estimated that amniotic fluid embolism (AFE) affects 1 in every 50,000 women giving birth in the UK.[3] It is a serious and unavoidable condition, but fortunately in the UK there has been an improvement in survival rates associated with it. This may be due, in part, to better identification of women who survive AFE, as well as improvements in care.[3] It is thought to occur as a result of an abnormal and exaggerated reaction to amniotic fluid entering the maternal circulation, causing maternal collapse and often cardiac arrest. Six of the 11 women who died from AFE in the UK between 2009 and 2014 underwent induction or augmentation of labour, with 50% of them developing hyperstimulation.[5]

The woman is often conscious at the onset of symptoms. Presentation is acute with anxiety and agitation, coughing, shortness of breath, followed by respiratory distress, cardiovascular collapse (hypotension, tachycardia and possible arrhythmias) and cardiac arrest. DIC can quickly develop, causing massive maternal haemorrhage. The presence of pulmonary hypertension and acute right ventricular failure is common.

Diagnosis must initially be presumptive. Treatment involves support for the respiratory and cardiovascular systems and early correction of clotting abnormalities with blood products. Early liaison with intensive care and haematology staff is vital. The UK Obstetric Surveillance System (UKOSS) data indicate that, in optimal circumstances where excellent resuscitation and ongoing care are provided, many women with AFE do survive.[3]

Air embolism

Air embolism may occur following a ruptured uterus, during administration of intravenous fluids or blood products under pressure, or following manipulation of the placenta at caesarean section. Air embolism is associated with chest pain and collapse. The diagnosis is classically made though the auscultation of a typical waterwheel murmur over the precordium; however, an echocardiogram can also be useful.

Initial management involves preventing further air from entering the circulation (e.g. by stopping any pressurised fluids, tilting the woman head-up to increase venous pressure, flooding a surgical field with saline); thereafter, ongoing treatment is supportive.

References

1. Lewis G (ed.); The Confidential Enquiry into Maternal and Child Health (CEMACH). *Saving Mothers' Lives: Reviewing Maternal Deaths to Make Motherhood Safer 2003–2005. The Seventh Report on Confidential Enquiries into Maternal Deaths in the United Kingdom*. London: CEMACH, 2007.

2. Cantwell R, Clutton-Brock T, Cooper G, *et al*. Saving Mothers' Lives: reviewing maternal deaths to make motherhood safer: 2006–2008. The Eighth Report of the Confidential Enquiries into Maternal Deaths in the United Kingdom. *BJOG* 2011; 118 (Suppl. 1): 1–203.

3. Knight M, Kenyon S, Brocklehurst P, *et al.* (eds.); MBRRACE-UK. *Saving Lives, Improving Mothers' Care: Lessons Learned to Inform Future Maternity Care from the UK and Ireland Confidential Enquiries into Maternal Deaths and Morbidity 2009–12*. Oxford: National Perinatal Epidemiology Unit, University of Oxford, 2014.

4. Resuscitation Council (UK). Adult basic life support and automated external defibrillation. *Resuscitation Guidelines* 2015. www.resus.org.uk/resuscitation-guidelines/adult-basic-life-support-and-automated-external-defibrillation/ (accessed June 2017).

5. Jeejeebhoy FM, Zelop CM, Lipman S, *et al.* Cardiac arrest in pregnancy: a scientific statement from the American Heart Association. *Circulation* 2015; 132: 1747–73.

6. Knight M, Nair M, Tuffnell D, *et al.* (eds.); MBRRACE-UK. *Saving Lives, Improving Mothers' Care: Surveillance of Maternal Deaths in the UK 2012–14 and Lessons Learned to Inform Maternity Care from the UK and Ireland Confidential Enquiries into Maternal Deaths and morbidity 2009–14*. Oxford: National Perinatal Epidemiology Unit, University of Oxford, 2016.

7. Royal College of Obstetricians and Gynaecologists. *Thromboembolic Disease in Pregnancy and the Puerperium: Acute Management*. Green-top Guideline No. 37B. London: RCOG, 2015. www.rcog.org.uk/en/guidelines-research-services/guidelines/gtg37b (accessed June 2017).

8. Truhlář A, Deakin CD, Soar J, *et al.* European Resuscitation Council Guidelines for Resuscitation 2015: Section 4. Cardiac arrest in special circumstances. *Resuscitation* 2015; 95: 148–201.

Module 3
Maternal cardiac arrest and advanced life support

Key learning points

■ Recall the causes of maternal cardiac arrest.

■ Management of maternal cardiac arrest using advanced life support (ALS) algorithm.

■ The importance of left manual uterine displacement to reduce aortocaval compression after 20 weeks' gestation.

■ Performing perimortem caesarean (or operative vaginal birth) immediately if resuscitation is unsuccessful.

■ Document details of management accurately, clearly and legibly.

Common difficulties observed in training drills

■ Failing to recognise cardiac arrest and therefore not starting life support in a timely manner

■ Concentrating on advanced life support (ALS) and neglecting to perform good-quality basic life support (BLS)

■ Not manually displacing the uterus

■ Not connecting the defibrillator

- Unnecessary interruption of cardiac compressions
- Failure to understand that perimortem caesarean section is primarily performed for maternal resuscitation
- Moving the woman to the operating theatre to perform the perimortem caesarean section
- Delaying the commencement of perimortem caesarean section
- Forgetting to call the neonatal team

Introduction

Maternal cardiac arrest is rare. However, over half of victims will survive with good-quality BLS and ALS, adapted for the physiological changes of pregnancy.[1]

This module provides an outline of advanced life support (ALS) in the pregnant woman. More information on advanced resuscitation techniques and specific training is available from the Resuscitation Council (UK)[2] and the European Resuscitation Council.[3]

Obstetric and anaesthetic causes of cardiac arrest during pregnancy and postpartum include:

- haemorrhage
- pre-eclampsia/eclampsia
- pulmonary embolism
- amniotic fluid embolism
- sepsis
- total spinal anaesthesia
- local anaesthetic toxicity
- magnesium toxicity

These pregnancy-related causes should be considered in addition to other more general causes of cardiac arrest in the non-pregnant woman, e.g. cardiac disease, substance abuse, anaphylaxis, trauma. Potentially reversible causes of cardiac arrest (the four Hs and the four Ts) are discussed later in this module.

Cardiorespiratory changes in pregnancy

In the supine position, pressure from the gravid uterus can compress the aorta and vena cava (aortocaval compression). At term, the inferior vena cava is completely occluded in 90% of supine women, decreasing the cardiac stroke volume (the amount of blood pumped out with each contraction of the heart) by up to 70%. This has a significant effect on the cardiac output that can be achieved during cardiopulmonary resuscitation (CPR).

To ensure that aortocaval compression is kept to a minimum while still maintaining good-quality, effective chest compressions, the woman should be kept supine with the uterus manually displaced to the left by an assistant using one or two hands (Figure 3.1).[4,5] Alternatively, if the woman is on an operating table or another firm surface that can be tilted, e.g. a spinal board, then this can be tilted 15–30° to the left.

At term there is a 20% decrease in pulmonary functional residual capacity for pregnant women, with a 20% increase in oxygen consumption. A pregnant woman can therefore become hypoxic more rapidly than a non-pregnant woman.[6] The enlarged uterus, together with the resultant upward displacement of the abdominal organs, decreases lung compliance during ventilation, which makes adequate ventilation during maternal cardiac arrest difficult.

Pregnancy also increases the risk of pulmonary aspiration of gastric contents. Early tracheal intubation reduces this risk. However, oxygenation must always take priority, and prolonged attempts at intubation should be avoided.

If resuscitation has not been immediately successful, plans to expedite the birth (perimortem birth) should be made. Traditional teaching is that

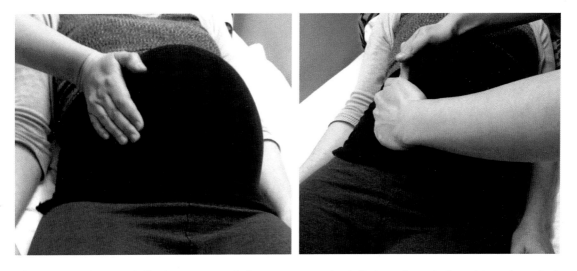

Figure 3.1 Manual displacement of the uterus to the left (one-handed and two-handed)

a perimortem birth should commence at 4 minutes with a view to the baby being born within 5 minutes. However, emerging evidence suggests that collapse-to-birth times of 3 minutes and under are associated with better maternal outcomes. Therefore, attempts to expedite birth should not be delayed once resuscitation efforts have been deemed unsuccessful.[1,5,7]

If the woman is in the second stage of labour and the baby is low enough in the pelvis, then an operative vaginal birth may be performed; otherwise, a perimortem caesarean section should be undertaken. Delivering the baby will immediately relieve the vena caval obstruction caused by the gravid uterus and ensure increased effectiveness of cardiac compressions. It will also improve ventilation attempts. Furthermore, delivery reduces the upward displacement of the lungs and reduces the total oxygen requirements, as fetal oxygenation is no longer required. Perimortem birth is performed to improve the chances of survival of the mother; the baby is more likely to survive too.[8,9,10] In order to expedite birth in a timely fashion, team members must make preparations for birth from the moment that a cardiac arrest is declared.

Maternal cardiac arrest in the community setting

If a maternal cardiac arrest occurs out of hospital, ambulance services and crews need to be aware of the importance of commencing immediate basic life support (BLS) with left manual displacement of the uterus, and rapid transfer of the woman into hospital for perimortem caesarean section. Prolonged resuscitation on the scene – without perimortem birth – reduces the likelihood of success. Equally, emergency department staff, especially those not co-located with an obstetric unit, need to summon staff with surgical training to conduct a perimortem caesarean section as soon as possible after arrival of a pregnant woman in cardiac arrest.[5]

Management of maternal cardiac arrest

An algorithm for the management of maternal cardiac arrest is shown in Figure 3.2. A more detailed list of the actions required in the event of maternal cardiac arrest is given in Box 3.1.

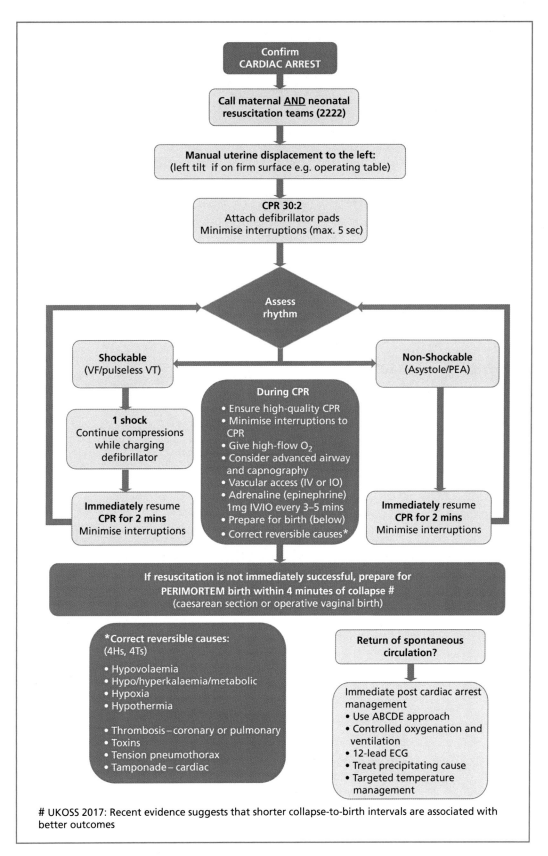

Figure 3.2 Adapted algorithm for the management of maternal cardiac arrest (based on Resuscitation Council (UK) Guidelines, 2015)

Box 3.1 Management of maternal cardiac arrest

EVENT	ACTION
Help	■ Shout for help ■ **Ring 2222** and state '**maternal cardiac arrest**' and location of the incident (adjust to fit local protocol) ■ Ask for the arrest trolley, perimortem caesarean section pack and resuscitaire ■ **Call neonatal team (if antenatal)** ■ Ensure security doors are open so that arrest team can arrive ■ Contact blood bank and ask for emergency blood products (prepare for massive obstetric haemorrhage if mother survives) ■ Phone haematology and biochemistry for urgent blood test requests
Positioning	■ Lay the bed flat ■ Ask assistant to manually displace the uterus to the left (or tilt woman 15–30 degrees to the left if on a firm tilting surface, e.g. operating table) ■ Move the bed into the centre of the room ■ Take head end off the bed
Basic life support	■ Open airway ■ Give 30 chest compressions (at rate of 100–120 compressions per minute) in middle of lower half of sternum to a depth of 5–6 cm: the emphasis is on good-quality chest compressions including all elements – rate, depth and recoil ■ Attempt 2 breaths using a pocket mask or bag-mask ventilation ■ Continue at ratio of 30 chest compressions to 2 breaths (each breath lasting one second)
Equipment	■ **Defibrillator**: apply pads and assess rhythm to decide if a shock should be given (if using an AED, follow instructions). Continue chest compressions while pads are applied ■ Deliver shock if appropriate (or as instructed by AED). Continue chest compressions while defibrillator is charging ■ **Perimortem birth equipment** – open perimortem caesarean pack and disposable scalpel or operative vaginal birth (OVB) set, and be ready to expedite birth if CPR unsuccessful ■ **Resuscitaire** must be obtained and turned on, ready for neonatal resuscitation, and neonatal team should be summoned

Box 3.1 Management of maternal cardiac arrest (continued)

EVENT	ACTION
Investigations	■ **Large-bore IV access** should be obtained as soon as possible. If this is not possible, and the equipment is available, intraosseous (IO) access can be obtained in the proximal humerus (shoulder) or femur ■ **Venous blood** – send urgently for FBC, U&Es, LFTs, clotting screen, cross-matching, calcium and magnesium ■ **Arterial blood gas** – for immediate estimate of haemoglobin, K^+, Na^+, Ca^{2+} and glucose as well as pH, PaO_2 and $PaCO_2$
Advanced life support	■ As soon as the arrest team arrives, a team leader should be appointed. In most hospitals a predetermined member of the arrest team assumes this role. The team leader should coordinate the arrest, including allocating specific tasks to members of the team ■ CPR should be uninterrupted, including during perimortem birth. The only exceptions are to administer shocks and for rhythm checks where appropriate (and any interruption should be for no more than 5 seconds) ■ The anaesthetist will normally manage the airway/ breathing. Once the woman is intubated, chest compressions should be continuous. Capnography should be considered (monitoring of partial pressure of CO_2) ■ **Shocks** – every 2 minutes if VF/pulseless VT (shockable rhythms) ■ **Adrenaline (epinephrine)** – 1 mg IV/IO flushed with at least 20 mL fluid (after 3rd shock if VF/pulseless VT), repeated every 3–5 minutes
Expedite birth of baby	■ As soon as arrest occurs, immediate preparations to expedite birth should be made in case resuscitation efforts are unsuccessful, and certainly within 4 minutes of commencing CPR, preferably earlier, using the fastest means (caesarean section or operative vaginal birth) ■ Continue CPR during birth ■ Ensure the neonatal team are in attendance
Documentation	■ Note the time of the arrest, arrival of staff, timing of defibrillation, timing of medication administered, time of birth of the baby and time cardiac output is regained

Role of the team leader

In the hospital setting, the team leader is usually the lead doctor on the local cardiac arrest team; however, it could be anybody trained in ALS. The team leader should direct the team and ensure everyone's safety. This is best achieved by standing back, delegating specific tasks to members of the team and ensuring that clear commands are given. The team leader must consider any correctable cause of cardiac arrest and decide whether administering any other medication (Table 3.1) may be beneficial.

Table 3.1 Medication to be considered during cardiac arrest

Feature	Medication to be considered
Cardiac arrest	1 mg adrenaline (epinephrine) IV/IO every 3–5 minutes (after 3rd shock if a shockable rhythm)
VF/VT	300 mg amiodarone IV/IO after third shock
Opioid overdose	0.4–0.8 mg naloxone IV/IO
Magnesium toxicity	10 mg calcium gluconate IV/IO
Local anaesthetic toxicity	1.5 mL/kg intralipid 20% IV/IO initially

Medication should be administered via the intravenous or intraosseous route. The tracheal route is no longer recommended.

In a maternal cardiac arrest, it is important for the team leader (or any other members of the team) to state immediately after arrest occurs that a perimortem birth (by caesarean section unless the woman is in the second stage of labour and operative vaginal birth is an option) will need to be performed if resuscitation efforts are unsuccessful, and certainly within 4 minutes of commencing CPR. The perimortem birth should take place where the mother collapses; do not move her to the operating theatre, as this will make effective resuscitation very difficult and delay the birth, both of which will reduce the likelihood of successful resuscitation. The equipment required to assist birth should be immediately available (although a scalpel is the only equipment needed to commence a perimortem caesarean section) (Figure 3.3). A perimortem caesarean pack (contents of pack listed in Table 3.2) should be kept together with the resuscitation equipment in all areas where a pregnant woman may require resuscitation (e.g. antenatal ward, antenatal clinic, labour ward, emergency department).

Table 3.2 Suggested contents of a perimortem caesarean pack

Sterile disposable scalpel (attached to outside of pack to maintain sterility of pack contents)

1 pack of large taped swabs

1 Doyen's retractor

2–3 clamps (Kocher's, Spencer Wells or similar)

1 large dissecting scissors (e.g. Mayo scissors)

1 toothed dissecting forceps

Also: Gloves ± gown for the operator (can be outside the pack)

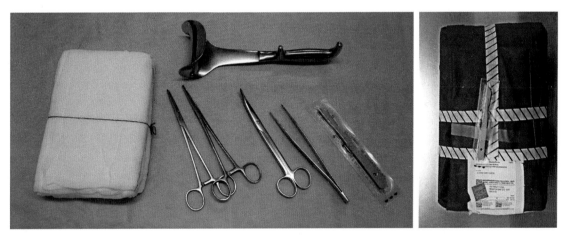

Figure 3.3 Equipment required for perimortem caesarean section, with disposable scalpel attached to outside of pack

If resuscitation is successful post-birth, the abdomen should be packed and the mother moved to the nearest theatre area, where the abdomen can be closed by an obstetrician or a surgeon.

The neonatal team should be called as soon as maternal arrest occurs, so that they have time to prepare the resuscitaire and other equipment needed to aid resuscitation of the baby.

The cardiac arrest team leader should decide, in consultation with the rest of the team, when it is appropriate to abandon maternal resuscitation. The management of the arrest should be fully documented. Staff and relatives must be supported afterwards. It is good practice to ensure that someone remains with the relatives during an arrest to keep them informed.

Recognition of heart rhythms

Resuscitation attempts should follow the predetermined evidence-based algorithms published by the Resuscitation Council (UK).[1] The ALS algorithm (Figure 3.2) has two main pathways: those requiring defibrillation ('shockable rhythms') and those in which this would be inappropriate ('non-shockable rhythms') (Box 3.2). The cardiac rhythm (or the AED) dictates which pathway to follow.

Box 3.2 Heart rhythms found during cardiac arrest	
Shockable rhythms	**Non-shockable rhythms**
Ventricular fibrillation (VF)	Asystole
Pulseless ventricular tachycardia (VT)	Pulseless electrical activity (PEA)

Once cardiac arrest is confirmed, a defibrillator should be used to rapidly assess the cardiac rhythm of the woman. Self-adhesive pads are placed on the woman's chest and may be used for both cardiac monitoring and defibrillation. Do not stop chest compressions to apply the pads. The cardiac rhythm may be determined with the AED, using the self-adhesive defibrillator pads attached to the woman's chest, as illustrated in Figure 3.4.

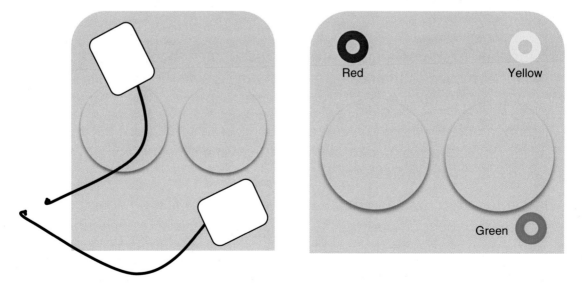

Figure 3.4 Placement of defibrillator pads and ECG electrodes

If defibrillator pads are not available, a 3-lead ECG can be used to monitor the rhythm. The ECG leads are colour coded and should be attached with the red electrode to the right shoulder (Red to Right), the yellow electrode to the left shoulder (yeLLow to Left) and the green electrode below the pectoral muscles (green for spleen) (Figure 3.4). The defibrillator should be set to read the ECG rhythm through lead II.

During cardiac arrest, heart rhythms are categorised as shockable or non-shockable (Box 3.2).

Shockable rhythms

The majority of survivors from cardiac arrests come from the shockable rhythm category (VF and pulseless VT). A typical example of VF is shown in Figure 3.5.

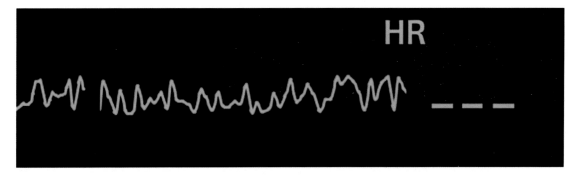

Figure 3.5 An example of ventricular fibrillation

VT is characterised by a broad-complex regular tachycardia (Figure 3.6). VT can cause a profound loss of cardiac output and can suddenly deteriorate into VF. Pulseless VT is treated in the same way as VF.

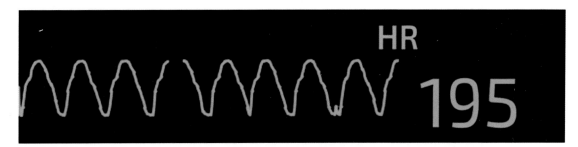

Figure 3.6 An example of ventricular tachycardia

Shockable cardiac rhythms need to be treated by defibrillation. This involves passing an electric current across the heart to simultaneously depolarise a critical mass of the myocardium so that the natural pacemaking tissue of the heart can resume control. Attempted defibrillation is the single most important step in the treatment of VF/VT. The time between the onset of VF/VT and defibrillation is the main determinant of patient survival, as survival falls by 7–10% for each minute following collapse.

Most defibrillators now transmit a biphasic current, which has a higher efficiency, and therefore less energy is required to depolarise the heart. When using a biphasic defibrillator, a current of 150–200 joules (J) should be used for the first shock, and 150–360 J for subsequent shocks; for a monophasic defibrillator, 360 J should be used for the first and subsequent shocks.

> **Know your machine: if unsure, shock at 200 J.**

Remember: only one shock per cycle for shockable rhythms; the shock is then immediately followed by 2 minutes of CPR at a ratio of 30 compressions to 2 ventilations (without checking for a rhythm or a pulse). After 2 minutes, the rhythm should be checked and a second shock delivered, if required. A pulse should be checked only if a non-shockable rhythm is seen.

> **Adrenaline (epinephrine) 1 mg IV/IO should be given after alternate shocks (every 3–5 minutes, starting immediately after the third shock).**
>
> **Amiodarone 300 mg IV/IO should also be given after the third shock.**

Most clinical areas now have automated external defibrillators (AEDs), which are able to analyse the cardiac rhythm and administer appropriate shocks, if indicated.

It is important to continue chest compressions while the defibrillator is charging, prior to administering the shock. If using an AED, follow the machine's instructions. Figure 3.7 shows an example of an AED used for training.

Non-shockable rhythms

Pulseless electrical activity (PEA) is the clinical absence of cardiac output (i.e. no pulse) despite cardiac electrical activity, which may be normal (sinus rhythm or near normal). For example, in exsanguination, the heart's electrical

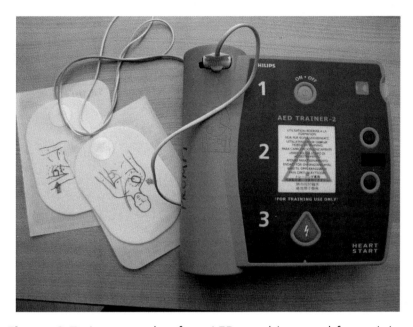

Figure 3.7 An example of an AED machine used for training

activity may continue to show a normal sinus rhythm, as shown in Figure 3.8, but because there is no circulating blood a pulse is not present. PEA is the most common presenting cardiac arrest rhythm in pregnancy.

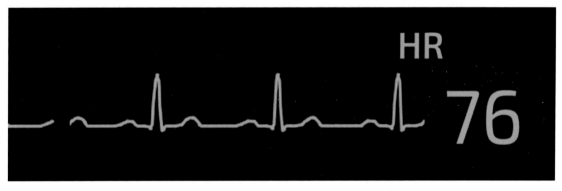

Figure 3.8 An example of normal sinus rhythm, which can also be seen with pulseless electrical activity

Asystole is a slightly wandering flat line. An example is shown in Figure 3.9. Until proven otherwise, a completely flat horizontal line indicates that the monitoring leads are not correctly attached, rather than asystole. Adults in asystole have a very poor prognosis.

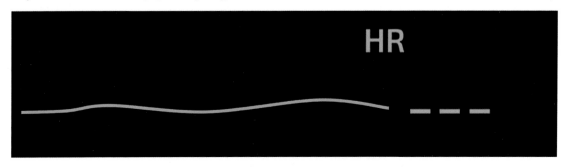

Figure 3.9 An example of asystole

Potentially reversible causes

If the cardiac rhythm is not VF or VT, the outcome will be poor unless a potentially reversible cause can be found and treated. Potentially reversible causes of cardiac arrest can be remembered using the 'four Hs' and 'four Ts'.

The four Hs

1. **Hypoxia** should be minimised by ensuring that the patient is adequately ventilated during the arrest. Basic life support followed by prompt intubation and ventilation using 100% oxygen will maximise oxygen delivery to the woman. She should be examined to check for chest rise and bilateral air entry during ventilation.

2. **Hypovolaemia** in pregnancy is most commonly caused by massive haemorrhage (such as abruption or postpartum haemorrhage). Remember that haemorrhage can be concealed. Intravenous fluids and blood products should be commenced promptly to restore the intravascular volume, and urgent surgery to correct the cause of bleeding should be considered (see **Module 8**).

3. **Hypo/hyperkalaemia/metabolic**

   - **Hypoglycaemia** may occur in a diabetic mother. If the blood glucose measures below 3 mmol/L, give 50 mL of 20% (or 100 mL of 10%) glucose solution IV.

   - **Hyperkalaemia** (high serum potassium) can develop secondary to renal failure.

   - **Hypermagnesaemia** (high serum magnesium) may result from treatment of pre-eclampsia with intravenous magnesium sulfate, especially with concurrent renal impairment.

   - **Hypocalcaemia** (low serum calcium) can result from overdose of calcium channel blocking drugs such as nifedipine.

     High serum levels of potassium or magnesium and low serum levels of calcium should be treated with 10 mL of 10% calcium gluconate (or 10% calcium chloride) IV.

4. **Hypothermia** is an unlikely cause of maternal arrest in hospital, but should be considered with transfers in to hospital. Attempts should be made to keep patients warm in the peri-arrest situation by using warmed intravenous fluids and warming blankets if appropriate. However, once cardiac arrest has occurred, permitting mild hypothermia (**32–36 °C**) and avoiding fever can provide neuroprotection.[4,11]

The four Ts

1. **Thromboemboli** are more common in pregnancy owing to the procoagulant effect of pregnancy and the mechanical obstruction to venous return caused by the gravid uterus. Massive pulmonary embolus can cause sudden collapse and cardiac arrest. Treatment is difficult, but thrombolysis, cardiopulmonary bypass or operative removal of the clot should be considered. Amniotic fluid emboli are also a cause of sudden collapse and cardiac arrest. Treatment remains supportive, and care should be taken to correct clotting abnormalities as disseminated intravascular coagulopathy (DIC) often results. Early liaison with intensive care doctors and haematologist is essential.

2. **Tension pneumothorax** can cause collapse and subsequent PEA. A tension pneumothorax is most likely to occur during attempted central venous line insertion or secondary to trauma (e.g. road traffic accident). Treatment involves acute decompression of the affected side by inserting a large intravenous cannula into the thoracic cavity in the second intercostal space at the midclavicular line, followed by chest drain insertion.

3. **Therapeutic** or **toxic** substances (for example, inadvertent administration of bupivacaine intravenously or opioid overdose) can cause cardiac arrest. Specific antidotes or treatments should be used; for example, for opioid overdose – naloxone 0.4–0.8 mg IV, or for local anaesthetic overdose – IV intralipid (see **Module 4**).

4. Cardiac **tamponade** is an uncommon cause of maternal arrest but should be considered after trauma, especially when there are penetrating chest injuries. Treatment involves relieving the tamponade by resuscitative thoracotomy, or by needle pericardiocentesis.

Medication used during cardiac arrest

Adrenaline (epinephrine) 1 mg should be given IV/IO every 3–5 minutes during a cardiac arrest. Other medications that may be considered are listed in Table 3.1.

All medications should be flushed with at least 20 mL fluid to ensure they enter the central circulation. The most common medications required for a cardiac arrest are kept on the resuscitation trolley in prefilled syringes, so that they can be quickly administered in an emergency. It is important that all staff are aware of the location of the emergency trolley and defibrillator within their own unit. It is also important that staff familiarise themselves with the use of their local emergency equipment and medication, as equipment may vary between locations.

Post-resuscitation care

A comprehensive, structured post-resuscitation protocol is important and would normally include transfer to an intensive care unit:

■ ABCDE approach.

■ Controlled oxygenation and ventilation. Consideration should be given to avoiding hyperoxia. Inspired oxygen should be titrated to maintain arterial oxygen saturations at 94–98% (guided by a pulse oximeter or arterial blood gas).

■ Temperature and glucose control. Consideration should be given to the use of targeted temperature management (32–36 °C). Glucose levels greater than 10 mmol/L should be treated but hypoglycaemia should be avoided.

■ A 12-lead ECG.

■ Treat precipitating causes.

The aftermath

Cardiac arrest in pregnancy can be a traumatic event for all involved; many maternity staff members will not have encountered this situation before. Consideration should be given to the welfare of all involved in the resuscitation. This will include all personnel in the clinical area at the time (even those not directly involved) and may also include ambulance and emergency department personnel, porters, domestic staff and laboratory personnel.

An opportunity should be made, a few days after the event, to allow everyone to contribute to a debriefing session. This should include a factual résumé of the events that occurred, particularly given that misconceptions and misunderstandings are common after such events. An update on the progress of the mother and/or baby can be made if they have survived. Staff should be given an opportunity to share their feelings and thoughts, and to voice any questions in a sympathetic and supportive environment. Furthermore, potential learning points can be discussed in a 'no blame' way, with the aim of addressing any improvements that could be made to the system.

All healthcare trusts have access to professional support services for staff, and access information for these services should be provided.

References

1. Beckett VA, Knight M, Sharpe P. The CAPS study: incidence, management and outcomes of cardiac arrest in pregnancy in the UK: a prospective, descriptive study. *BJOG* 2017 Feb 24. doi: 10.1111/1471-0528.14521. [Epub ahead of print]

2. Resuscitation Council (UK). *Resuscitation Guidelines* 2015. www.resus.org.uk (accessed June 2017).

3. European Resuscitation Council. www.erc.edu (accessed June 2017).

4. Resuscitation Council (UK). Frequently asked questions (FAQs): adult advanced life support. www.resus.org.uk/faqs/faqs-adult-advanced-life-support/ (accessed June 2017).

5. Knight M, Kenyon S, Brocklehurst P, *et al.* (eds.); MBRRACE-UK. *Saving Lives, Improving Mothers' Care: Lessons Learned to Inform Future Maternity Care from the UK and Ireland Confidential Enquiries into Maternal Deaths and Morbidity 2009–12*. Oxford: National Perinatal Epidemiology Unit, University of Oxford, 2014.

6. Zakowski MI, Ramanathan S. CPR in pregnancy. *Curr Rev Clin Anesth* 1990; 10: 106.

7. National Perinatal Epidemiology Unit. UK Obstetric Surveillance System (UKOSS). www.npeu .ox.ac.uk/ukoss (accessed June 2017).

8. Marx G. Cardiopulmonary resuscitation in late-pregnant women. *Anaesthesiology* 1982; 56: 156.

9. Oates S, Williams GL, Res GA. Cardiopulmonary resuscitation in late pregnancy. *Br Med J* 1988; 297: 404–5.

10. Page-Rodriguez A, Gonzalez-Sanchez JA. Perimortem caesarean section of twin pregnancy: case report and review of the literature. *Acad Emerg Med* 1999; 6: 1072–4.

11. Arrich J, Holzer M, Havel C, Müllner M, Herkner H. Hypothermia for neuroprotection in adults after cardiopulmonary resuscitation. *Cochrane Database Syst Rev* 2016; (2): CD004128.

Module 4
Maternal anaesthetic emergencies

Key learning points

- To understand the difficulties of intubating the obstetric patient.
- To understand the management of failed intubation.
- To understand the role of intrauterine fetal resuscitation in potentially avoiding the need for general anaesthesia.
- Recognition and management of high regional block.
- Signs and symptoms of local anaesthetic toxicity.
- Management of cardiac arrest in a patient with local anaesthetic toxicity.

Background

In the Confidential Enquiry into Maternal Deaths in the UK for 2009–12 there were 78 deaths attributable to direct causes: four (5%) of these were attributed to anaesthesia. Direct death rates from anaesthesia was therefore 0.17 per 100,000 maternities, representing a decrease since the 2006–08 triennium. Two of the deaths were associated with hypoventilation after general anaesthesia and two followed complications after inadvertent dural tap.[1] The importance of practising drills for the management of airway crises and the use of capnography were highlighted. Furthermore, anaesthetists must be ready at all times to deal with the adverse effects of local anaesthetics.

Human factors such as communication within/between teams, leadership and fixation error were raised. Ongoing training to include communication, teamwork and reflection, for example using simulation, is considered vital to further a culture of good teamwork within units. The role of the anaesthetist in the multi-professional team involves unique challenges: their specific skills are often required in high-stress situations when time is critical and maternal and/or fetal life is at risk. It is in these circumstances that help from the rest of the maternity team can be invaluable.

Failed tracheal intubation

Introduction

General anaesthesia for caesarean section is now uncommon. Of the 172,594 caesarean sections carried out in England in 2015–16, 6.6% (11,372) were performed under general anaesthesia.[2] The vast majority of general anaesthetics are performed in emergency cases. Box 4.1 outlines the indications for general anaesthesia.

Box 4.1 Indications for general anaesthesia
■ Severe maternal or fetal compromise requiring immediate emergency birth
■ Regional anaesthesia contraindicated (e.g. coagulopathy, haemodynamic instability)
■ Failed or inadequate regional anaesthesia
■ Maternal request

The majority of complications arising from general anaesthesia relate to the airway. When the airway needs to be secured in a pregnant or postpartum woman, it is important that endotracheal intubation (a tube with a cuff placed through, and secured below, the vocal cords to maintain a patent airway) is used, as these women are at increased risk of regurgitation and aspiration of gastric contents.

A failed intubation is an anaesthetic emergency and can be defined in a number of ways. A useful definition for the maternity team is that a failed intubation has occurred when the anaesthetist has been unable to insert the endotracheal tube after two attempts. It is at this point that the failed intubation drill will begin and help will be required from the rest of the team, although it would be prudent to prepare to assist the anaesthetist after the first failed attempt at intubation.

Failed intubation during obstetric general anaesthesia (GA) has an incidence of 2.6 per 1000 GAs, or 1 in 390, with an estimated fatality rate of 1 in 90 failed intubations.[3] Difficult intubation is more common in the obstetric population for several reasons which include: complete dentition (i.e. most pregnant women have a full set of teeth), increased pharyngeal and laryngeal oedema, the larger tongue of pregnancy and the larger breasts associated with pregnancy. In addition, pregnant women rapidly desaturate owing to additional oxygen requirements. Obesity is a risk factor for difficult intubation and postoperative hypoventilation. Both women who died following general anaesthesia in the 2009–12 report on maternal deaths in the UK were obese.[1] A national audit in 2009 found that 5% of pregnant women in the UK had a BMI higher than 35, and 2% had a BMI over 40. Thirty-seven per cent of women with a BMI over 35 had a caesarean section.[4]

Ideally, the majority of difficult intubations would be predicted antenatally so that a plan could be made before the event. An antenatal assessment should aim to identify women who may be at risk of a difficult intubation, and referral to an obstetric anaesthetist should be arranged (Box 4.2).

Box 4.2 Risk factors for difficult intubation

- Known previous difficult intubation
- Obesity
- Pre-eclampsia
- Congenital airway difficulties with restricted neck movement and limited mouth opening (e.g. Klippel–Feil syndrome, Pierre Robin syndrome)
- Acquired airway difficulties with restricted neck movement and limited mouth opening (e.g. rheumatoid arthritis, ankylosing spondylitis, cervical spine fusions)

Unfortunately, most tests used to identify women with potentially difficult airways are unreliable, particularly in the obstetric population. As a result, anaesthetists may be faced with an unexpectedly difficult or impossible intubation. To minimise complications during these infrequent events, it helps to use a clear algorithm. The Obstetric Anaesthetists' Association (OAA) and the Difficult Airway Society (DAS) set up a working group in 2012 to develop some national guidelines on the management of difficult airway in obstetrics.[5] In 2015 they produced a comprehensive guideline and algorithm which provides a useful tool for individual units to follow.[6] The importance of planning with other team members before induction of anaesthesia is emphasised and recommended, and routine and difficult airway equipment for the obstetric theatre is highlighted.

Management and reduction of potential complications

The management of failed intubation in the pregnant woman should involve early recognition of the potentially difficult airway. For example, some recommend inserting an epidural early in labour for morbidly obese mothers.[7] This provides the option of an epidural top-up should an emergency caesarean section be required, as a rapid spinal at this stage would be technically difficult and more likely to fail.

General anaesthesia carries a higher risk to the mother than regional anaesthesia and is most frequently performed when delivery is needed urgently due to fetal compromise. Improving the condition of the fetus prior to emergency birth may allow sufficient time for regional anaesthesia. Intrauterine fetal resuscitation measures such as full left-lateral positioning, fluid bolus and tocolysis (Box 4.3) should be considered and, if appropriate, can be undertaken while the mother is being transferred to theatre. On arrival in theatre, the wellbeing of the fetus can be reassessed to see whether its condition has improved enough to allow time for regional anaesthesia.

Box 4.3 Intrauterine fetal resuscitation for the compromised fetus

S   Stop Syntocinon: stop any oxytocin infusion

P   Position – left-lateral: to minimise aortocaval compression

I   Intravenous fluid bolus: 250–500 mL crystalloid to improve uteroplacental perfusion

L   Low blood pressure: treat (e.g. with fluids, vasopressors) if low

T   Tocolysis: consider tocolytic to stop contractions and thereby improve uteroplacental blood flow

---

Aspiration of gastric contents is more likely during difficult intubation, in emergency cases and in obese pregnant women. For this reason, particular attention should be paid to reducing the volume and acidity of stomach contents in high-risk women during labour. Local guidelines should be in place for the care of women with risk factors in labour (e.g. in cases of obesity) to recommend limiting food intake during labour. Isotonic sports drinks may be encouraged, and regular prophylactic H_2-receptor antagonists given (e.g. oral ranitidine 150 mg 6-hourly). These prophylactic measures provide another safeguard to reduce the potential morbidity and mortality associated with emergency obstetric surgery and anaesthesia.

In the event of an emergency general anaesthetic, preparation can make the difference between success and failure at intubation. It is important to aim for a team discussion before inducing anaesthesia, to plan appropriately for different eventualities. Optimal positioning of the mother is paramount, particularly in the morbidly obese woman. The mother's head should be as near to the anaesthetist as possible, with pillows positioned so that her neck is flexed and her chin is pointing up towards the ceiling (Figure 4.1).

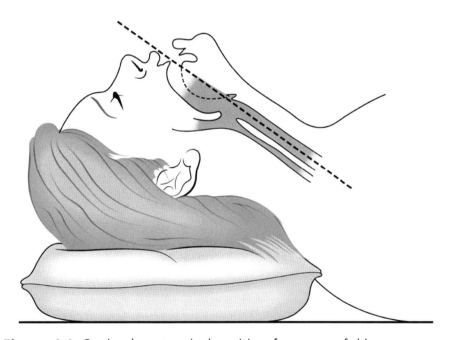

Figure 4.1 Optimal anatomical position for successful laryngoscopy

In pregnant women, and in particular those with large breasts or who are obese, it can be useful to adopt the 'ramped' position. This has been shown to improve the view of the vocal cords at laryngoscopy, making intubation easier.[8] The ramped position aims to create a horizontal line between the sternal notch and the external auditory meatus (ear canal), as shown in Figure 4.2. The position can be achieved using purpose-made pillows such as the Oxford HELP (Head Elevating Laryngoscopy Pillow) or by adjusting the operating table and using extra pillows and wedges.

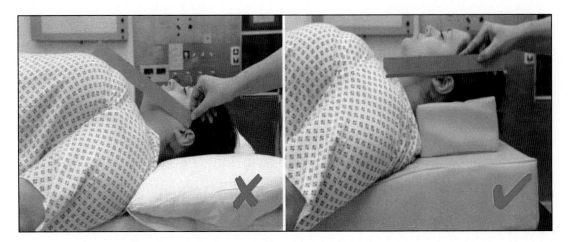

Figure 4.2 Anatomical realignment using the Oxford HELP to improve intubating conditions (© Alma Medical Products 2010, reproduced with permission)

Once the woman is positioned on the operating table, pre-oxygenation will begin. Pre-oxygenation is important to prevent desaturation during intubation, which can occur rapidly in pregnant women. The aim is to fill the lungs with as much oxygen as possible and remove nitrogen so that, when the patient is rendered apnoeic (i.e. has stopped breathing) upon induction of anaesthesia, there is enough oxygen available for gaseous exchange for the period of time it takes to secure the endotracheal tube and commence mechanical ventilation. For effective pre-oxygenation, the facemask must be tightly applied to the woman's face, not leaving any room for air to enter and dilute the oxygen delivered. In an emergency general anaesthetic caesarean section, help from the team at this stage to attach monitoring equipment, cannulate the woman and prepare the abdomen and drapes can maximise time for pre-oxygenation while minimising the time taken to expedite birth.

It is important for members of the theatre team to remain quiet during induction of anaesthesia and to be prepared to help in the event of a failed intubation. If failed intubation has occurred, the anaesthetist should immediately declare the emergency and state 'this is a failed intubation'. Individual roles will vary during the emergency. The anaesthetist and anaesthetic assistant will be unable to leave the woman, so other team members will be needed to provide assistance. All staff in theatre should know where the difficult airway equipment is kept and be able to fetch it if requested. All staff in theatre should also know how to call for additional anaesthetic support. A failed intubation is inevitably a very stressful situation in which clear communication will be essential. The failed intubation algorithm is outlined in Figure 4.3.

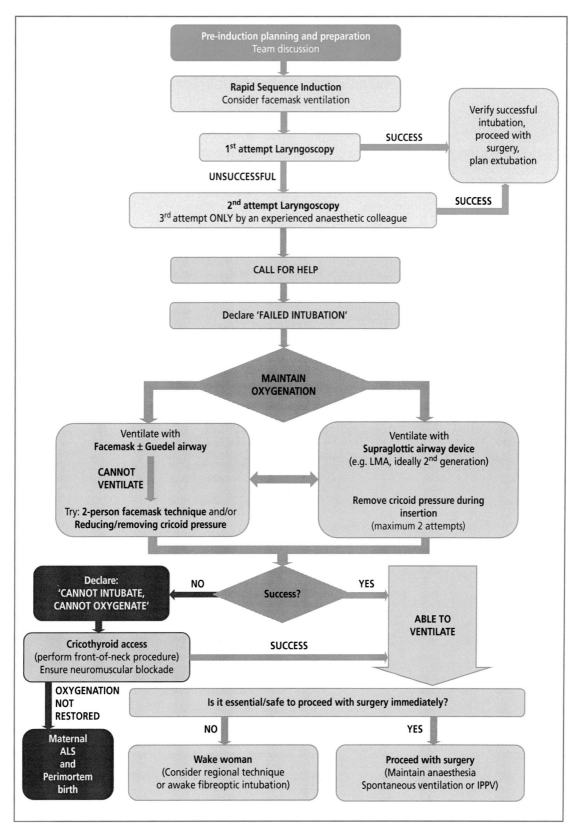

Figure 4.3 Algorithm for management of failed intubation (based on the Obstetric Anaesthetists' Association/Difficult Airway Society guidelines[6])

In the event of a failed intubation, the life of the woman is the anaesthetist's priority. The OAA/DAS 2015 guidance provides a decision tool as to whether the woman is then woken up or whether it is appropriate to continue with surgery if oxygenation and ventilation are possible (Figure 4.4).[6]

Table 1– proceed with surgery?				
Factors to consider	**WAKE** ⟵		⟶	**PROCEED**
Before induction				
Maternal condition	• No compromise	• Mild acute compromise	• Haemorrhage responsive to resuscitation	• Hypovolaemia requiring corrective surgery • Critical cardiac or respiratory compromise, cardiac arrest
Fetal condition	• No compromise	• Compromise corrected with intrauterine resuscitation, pH < 7.2 but > 7.15	• Continuing fetal heart rate abnormality despite intrauterine resuscitation, pH < 7.15	• Sustained bradycardia • Fetal haemorrhage • Suspected uterine rupture
Anaesthetist	• Novice	• Junior trainee	• Senior trainee	• Consultant/specialist
Obesity	• Supermorbid	• Morbid	• Obese	• Normal
Surgical factors	• Complex surgery or major haemorrhage anticipated	• Multiple uterine scars • Some surgical difficulties expected	• Single uterine scar	• No risk factors
Aspiration risk	• Recent food	• No recent food • In labour • Opioids given • Antacids not given	• No recent food • In labour • Opioids not given • Antacids not given	• Fasted • Not in labour • Antacids given
Alternative anaesthesia • regional • securing airway awake	• No anticipated difficulty	• Predicted difficulty	• Relatively contraindicated	• Absolutely contraindicated or has failed • Surgery started
After failed intubation				
Airway device/ventilation	• Difficult facemask ventilation • Front-of-neck	• Adequate facemask ventilation	• First generation supraglottic airway device	• Second generation supraglottic airway device
Airway hazards	• Laryngeal oedema • Stridor	• Bleeding • Trauma	• Secretions	• None evident

Criteria to be used in the decision to wake or proceed following failed tracheal intubation. In any individual patient, some factors may suggest waking and others proceeding. The final decision will depend on the anaesthetist's clinical judgement.
© Obstetric Anaesthetists' Association/Difficult Airway Society 2015)

Figure 4.4 OAA/DAS table to aid in the decision of whether to wake the woman up, or to proceed with surgery in the event of failed intubation at caesarean section (reproduced from Mushambi MC, *et al. Anaesthesia* 2015; 70: 1286–306,[6] with permission from Obstetric Anaesthetists' Association/Difficult Airway Society)

If surgery is allowed to proceed without an endotracheal tube in place, the anaesthetist will decide whether to allow the woman to breathe spontaneously or whether to paralyse (if immediate reversal of neuromuscular block is available). If the woman is spontaneously breathing, the caesarean section may be technically more difficult, as gaining access to the uterus can be problematic and the use of high concentrations of anaesthetic gases may cause uterine relaxation, thus increasing the risk of haemorrhage. Applying uterine fundal pressure during birth increases the risk of regurgitation and aspiration, and should be minimised.[6] The most senior obstetrician available should perform the surgery as quickly as possible to limit the anaesthetic time.

Box 4.4 outlines some best practice points for tracheal intubation.

Box 4.4 Best practice points for tracheal intubation

- Identify women at risk and refer for antenatal anaesthetic assessment
- Assess the airway before induction of anaesthesia
- Anaesthetists and anaesthetic assistants should check all intubation and difficult airway equipment daily, and must be familiar with its use and location
- There should be a team discussion to plan for failed intubation
- Position the patient correctly before induction
- Pre-oxygenate carefully
- Call for help early
- Remember that oxygenation is more important than intubation

---

Extubation and recovery after general anaesthesia

Extubation (the removal of the endotracheal tube, usually at the end of surgery) is another time when airway emergencies can occur. Theatre staff should not leave the operating theatre until the tracheal tube has been safely removed and normal breathing has resumed, as the woman may need re-intubating if problems occur. Extubation should be performed with the woman wide awake, as this minimises the risk of developing airway problems. It is usually done with the woman either sitting up or lying on her side. The anaesthetist may need help to position the woman for extubation.

Women can still be at risk from airway and respiratory complications during their recovery from general anaesthesia. The maternal mortality reports in the UK include women who have died from respiratory failure after general anaesthetic for caesarean section.[1] Pregnant or postpartum women who undergo general anaesthesia require the same standards of staffing and monitoring as for recovery procedures in the non-pregnant population. It is important that the maternity staff caring for women who have undergone a general anaesthetic are trained in theatre recovery, and are able to maintain their competencies through regular sessions in general theatre recovery.[1,5]

High regional block

Introduction

An excessively high block following spinal or epidural anaesthesia that requires a pregnant woman to be intubated has been described as 'the failed intubation of the new millennium'.[9] This is because, as the use of general anaesthesia has decreased, the use of regional anaesthesia is rising, thus increasing the possibility of high regional block.

The height of the block following spinal or epidural anaesthesia varies between women. The term 'high block' encompasses a spectrum of clinical events. At one end of the spectrum a woman may exhibit mild symptoms and only require reassurance with or without supplemental oxygen; at the other end, the woman may stop breathing, which may lead to cardiac arrest.

The term 'total spinal' implies that unconsciousness has also occurred. Total spinal is defined as cardiorespiratory collapse caused by direct action of local anaesthetic on high cervical nerve roots and the brainstem. It is a rare complication of epidural anaesthesia, with an incidence of approximately 1 in 16,000.[10,11]

A high regional block can occur in a number of ways. It can be an exaggerated response to correctly placed and dosed local anaesthetic, or attributable to an inadvertent overdose of local anaesthetic via the spinal or epidural route, or the result of accidental injection of local anaesthetic into the wrong space (e.g. subdural or intrathecal (spinal) injection of an epidural dose).

> **A total spinal or a high block with inadequate breathing requiring intubation are both anaesthetic emergencies.**

Presentation

The presentation of high regional block can vary from rapid loss of consciousness and collapse to a gradual rise in block height with or without eventual loss of consciousness. It is important to monitor women closely after epidural or spinal anaesthesia (including epidural top-ups) and to be alert to warning signs that the block may be extending above the desired height (Box 4.5).

Some women will have a block that reaches the lower cervical nerve roots, especially after spinal anaesthesia. Reassurance is often all that is necessary, but it is important to call for help, observe the woman closely, assess her pulse, blood pressure, respiratory rate and oxygen saturations, and look for the warning signs outlined in Box 4.5.

Box 4.5 Warning signs of rising block

- Nausea
- 'Not feeling right'
- Breathlessness
- Tingling, numbness or weakness in the fingers or arms
- Difficulty speaking
- Difficulty swallowing
- Sedation

If the local anaesthetic reaches the upper cervical nerve roots and blocks the nerves supplying the diaphragm, the woman will have great difficulty breathing and rapidly become hypoxic. In addition, if the brainstem is affected (total spinal) there is also likely to be severe hypotension and bradycardia. Fetal bradycardia may occur as a result of reduced placental blood flow.

There are several risk factors for high regional block, which means that it is not a complication confined to the theatre environment where an anaesthetist would be present (Box 4.6). High regional block should be in the differential diagnosis for maternal collapse in any woman receiving an epidural.

Box 4.6 Risk factors for high regional block

- Accidental dural puncture (recognised or unrecognised) during epidural insertion
- Accidental subdural placement of epidural catheter
- Large or rapid epidural top-ups (e.g. for category 1 caesarean section)
- Spinal injection with epidural in place
- Epidural top-ups after recent spinal injection

Management

In the situation where a woman exhibits warning signs of a high block (Box 4.5), it is imperative to remain with her and to call for help early in case she continues to deteriorate (Figure 4.5).

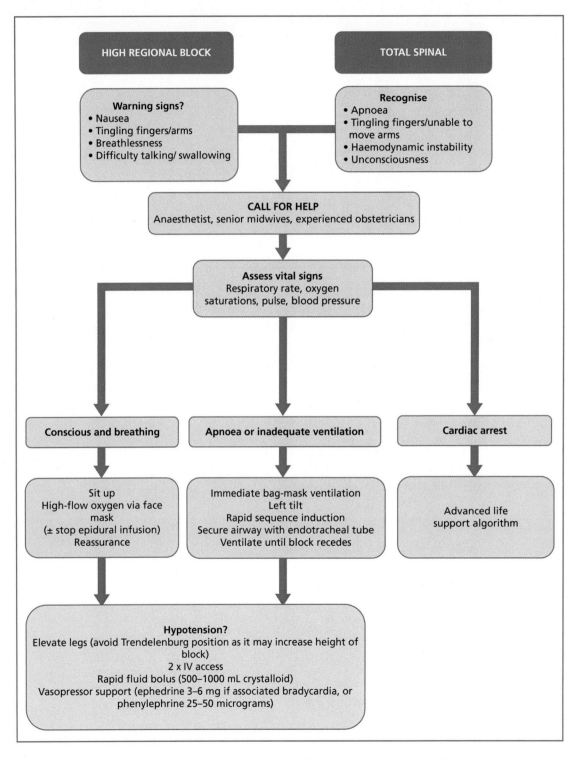

Figure 4.5 Management algorithm for high regional block

In the event of a high block with inadequate ventilation or a total spinal, characterised by cardiorespiratory collapse, the emergency buzzer should be used to summon help immediately. It may be necessary to call the maternal cardiac arrest team to ensure that enough skilled people are present to intubate the woman, manage ventilation and provide circulatory support, expedite the birth of the baby and give advanced life support if cardiac arrest ensues (see **Module 2** and **Module 3**).

> ### Remember: call for help, assess ABC and deliver 100% oxygen.

The woman should be intubated and ventilated. Circulatory support in the form of intravenous fluids, vasopressors and/or inotropes will be necessary, particularly if there is a total spinal. The hypotension and bradycardia may be catastrophic and can result in cardiac arrest, in which case chest compressions should be commenced immediately with manual left uterine displacement (or consider 15–30° left tilt if on an operating table) and advanced life support instituted. Following a total spinal, even without cardiac arrest, the baby is likely to be compromised as a result of maternal hypoxia and hypotension, and this may necessitate urgent birth.

Once the woman has been resuscitated, anaesthetic agents will be needed to keep her asleep, as she may be conscious but, owing to the paralysing effect of the block, unable to move or communicate. The effect of the block may last for less than 1 hour or may take several hours to wear off. It may be possible to manage this situation in the operating theatre, or the woman may require transfer to the intensive care unit.

Local anaesthetic toxicity

Introduction

Local anaesthetics are widely used in obstetric anaesthetic practice. In 2014–15 in England, more than 30% of women had epidural, spinal or caudal anaesthesia for labour or birth.[12] The MBRRACE-UK report *Saving Lives, Improving Mothers' Care* (2014) highlights that every epidural top-up is potentially dangerous if local anaesthetic concentrations greater than 0.1% bupivacaine are given, and all maternity units must have lipid emulsion and a protocol for its administration available.[1]

Wrong-route administration of local anaesthetics can also lead to fatalities. The National Reporting and Learning Service of the National Patient Safety Agency (NPSA) has published several safety alerts since 2009 with the aim that NHS hospitals in the UK should introduce equipment with non-Luer connections to prevent wrong-route errors. However, in anaesthetic practice, full compliance may not be possible currently, as the range of non-Luer and infusion devices for spinal and epidural procedures remains incomplete. Additional safety precautions should be taken in the meantime, with the aim that suitable safer devices (e.g. using NRFit connectors) can be introduced into practice as soon as they are available.[13]

Signs and symptoms of local anaesthetic toxicity

Local anaesthetic toxicity can present in many different ways, making recognition difficult. It is particularly important to remember that, after a bolus dose, toxicity may occur at any point within the next hour. In units where epidural infusions are used during labour, toxicity could happen at any time. The features to look for are shown in Box 4.7.

Box 4.7 Signs and symptoms of toxicity		
Warning signs	Tingling (lips/mouth/tongue)	
	Metallic taste in the mouth	
	Ringing in the ears	
	Light-headedness	
	Agitation ('just not right')	
	Tremor	
Severe toxicity	**Neurological**	**Cardiovascular**
	Severe agitation	Bradycardia
	Convulsions	Heart block
	Loss of consciousness	Ventricular tachyarrhythmias
		Asystole/cardiac arrest

Remember: the first sign of toxicity may be cardiac arrest.

Management

All healthcare professionals caring for women with epidurals should be familiar with the management of severe local anaesthetic toxicity. The Association of Anaesthetists of Great Britain and Ireland published guidelines in 2010, an outline of which is shown in Table 4.1.[14]

Table 4.1 Management of severe local anaesthetic toxicity

Immediate management	■ Stop injecting local anaesthetic ■ Call for help ■ Maintain airway; intubate if necessary ■ Give 100% oxygen and ensure adequate ventilation ■ Confirm/establish IV access ■ Control seizures ■ Assess cardiovascular status throughout	

Treatment	**In cardiac arrest**
	■ Commence advanced life support using standard algorithm with woman supine and uterus manually displaced to the left
	■ Treat arrhythmias using standard protocols
	■ Give intravenous lipid emulsion (follow regimen shown in Figure 4.6)
	■ Continue CPR throughout treatment with lipid emulsion
	■ Recovery may take longer than 1 hour
		Without cardiac arrest
		■ Use conventional therapies to treat:
		  ☐ Hypotension
		  ☐ Bradycardia
		  ☐ Tachyarrhythmias
		■ Consider intravenous lipid emulsion
		■ Keep woman in left-lateral position

Special points	■ Propofol is not a suitable substitute for lipid emulsion ■ Arrhythmias may be very refractory to treatment ■ Lidocaine should not be used as an antiarrhythmic in this setting	

The lipid emulsion regimen is shown in Figure 4.6. Further information can be found at www.aagbi.org and www.lipidrescue.org.

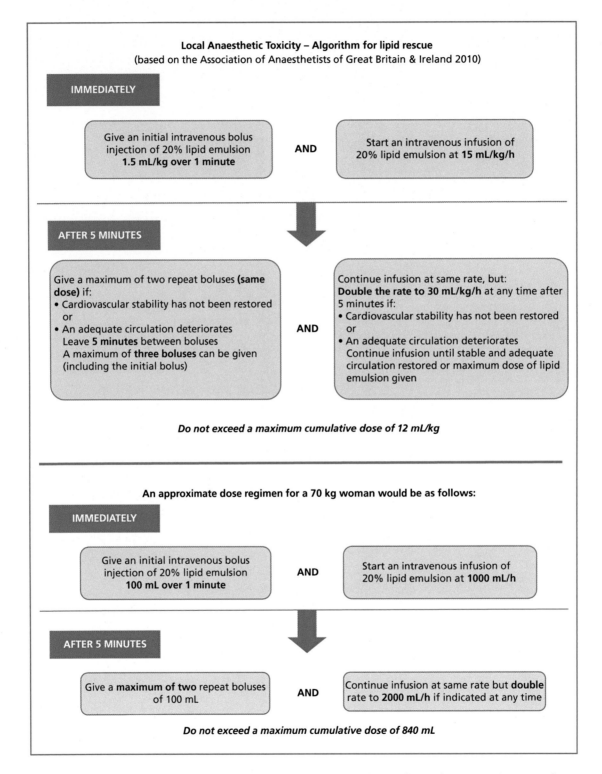

Figure 4.6 Intravenous lipid emulsion regimen (based on the Association of Anaesthetists of Great Britain & Ireland 2010)

Specific treatment for local anaesthetic toxicity

Local anaesthetic toxicity has been successfully treated with an intravenous infusion of lipid emulsion, commercially available in the UK as Intralipid (Baxter Healthcare Corporation, Deerfield, IL, USA). Intralipid has been reported to improve survival from local-anaesthetic-induced cardiac arrest[15,16] and in the treatment of life-threatening toxicity without cardiac arrest.[17] It does not replace the need for CPR, which should continue throughout treatment with lipid emulsion until the return of spontaneous circulation. It should be noted that cardiac arrest secondary to local anaesthetic toxicity can be refractory to treatment, and recovery may take over 1 hour. Thus, the effort of a large number of people is required to ensure that good-quality CPR is maintained throughout.

> **Remember: know where lipid emulsion is kept in your department.**

Severe local anaesthetic toxicity is a rare but very serious complication of local anaesthetic use. Posters can be used in departments to remind staff of the salient points, and, most importantly, where to find treatment guidelines and lipid emulsion should they ever be faced with this emergency.

Follow-up

The management of local-anaesthetic-induced cardiac arrest is very demanding. If successful, transfer to a maternal critical care area will need to be arranged until full recovery is achieved.

Each case should be reported. The lessons learned can potentially prevent other cases from happening and improve our knowledge and treatment of the condition. In the UK, all cases should be reported to NHS Improvement (Patient Safety Alerts), and cases where lipid has been given should be reported to the international registry at www.lipidrescue.org.

References

1. Knight M, Kenyon S, Brocklehurst P, et al. (eds.); MBRRACE-UK. *Saving Lives, Improving Mothers' Care: Lessons Learned to Inform Future Maternity Care from the UK and Ireland Confidential Enquiries into Maternal Deaths and Morbidity 2009–12*. Oxford: National Perinatal Epidemiology Unit, University of Oxford, 2014.

2. NHS Digital. Hospital maternity activity, 2015–16. www.content.digital.nhs.uk/catalogue/PUB22384 (accessed June 2017).

3. Kinsella SM, Winton AL, Mushambi MC, *et al.* Failed intubation during obstetric general anaesthesia: a literature review. *Int J Obstet Anesth* 2015; 24: 356–74.

4. Centre for Maternal and Child Enquiries (CMACE). *Maternal Obesity in the UK: Findings from a National Project.* London: CMACE, 2010.

5. Association of Anaesthetists of Great Britain and Ireland, Obstetric Anaesthetists' Association. *OAA/AAGBI Guidelines for Obstetric Anaesthetic Services 2013.* London: AAGBI & OOA, 2013. www.aagbi.org/sites/default/files/obstetric_anaesthetic_services_2013.pdf (accessed June 2017).

6. Mushambi MC, Kinsella SM, Popat M, *et al.* Obstetric Anaesthetists' Association and Difficult Airway Society guidelines for the management of difficult and failed tracheal intubation in obstetrics. *Anaesthesia* 2015; 70: 1286–306.

7. Centre for Maternal and Child Enquiries, Royal College of Obstetricians and Gynaecologists. *CMACE/RCOG Joint Guideline: Management of Women with Obesity in Pregnancy.* London: CMACE/RCOG, 2010. www.rcog.org.uk/globalassets/documents/guidelines/cmacercogjoint-guidelinemanagementwomenobesitypregnancya.pdf (accessed June 2017).

8. Collins JS, Lemmens HJ, Brodsky JB, Brock-Utne JG, Levitan RM. Laryngoscopy and morbid obesity: a comparison of the 'sniff' and 'ramped' positions. *Obes Surg* 2004; 14: 1171–5.

9. Yentis SM, Dob DP. High regional block: the failed intubation of the new millennium? *Int J Obstet Anaesth* 2001; 10: 159–61.

10. Allman K, McIndoe A, Wilson I (eds.). *Emergencies in Anaesthesia*, 2nd edn. Oxford: Oxford University Press, 2009.

11. Jenkins JG. Some immediate serious complications of obstetric epidural analgesia and anaesthesia: a prospective study of 145,550 epidurals. *Int J Obstet Anesth* 2005; 14: 37–42.

12. Health and Social Care Information Centre. *Hospital Episode Statistics: NHS Maternity Statistics – England 2014–15.* London: HSCIC, 2015. http://content.digital.nhs.uk/catalogue/PUB19127 (accessed June 2017).

13. NHS England. Patient safety alert on non-Luer spinal (intrathecal) devices for chemotherapy, February 2014. www.england.nhs.uk/2014/02/psa-spinal-chemo/ (accessed June 2017).

14. Association of Anaesthetists of Great Britain and Ireland. AAGBI Safety Guideline. Management of severe local anaesthetic toxicity. London: AAGBI, 2010. www.aagbi.org/sites/default/files/la_toxicity_2010_0.pdf (accessed June 2017).

15. Weinberg G, Ripper R, Feinstein DL, Hoffman W. Lipid emulsion infusion rescues dogs from bupivacaine-induced cardiac toxicity. *Reg Anesth Pain Med* 2003; 28: 198–202.

16. Rosenblatt MA, Abel M, Fischer GW, Itzkovich CJ, Eisenkraft JB. Successful use of a 20% lipid emulsion to resuscitate a patient after a presumed bupivacaine-related cardiac arrest. *Anesthesiology* 2006; 105: 217–18.

17. Foxall G, McCahon R, Lamb J, Hardman JG, Bedforth NM. Levobupivacaine-induced seizures and cardiovascular collapse treated with Intralipid. *Anaesthesia* 2007; 62: 516–18.

Module 5
Fetal monitoring in labour

Key learning points

■ On admission in labour, a full clinical and obstetric risk assessment should be undertaken to determine the most appropriate method of fetal monitoring. Risk assessments should continue throughout labour to identify any indications for transferring to continuous electronic fetal monitoring (EFM).

■ Healthy women with an uncomplicated pregnancy should be offered and recommended intermittent auscultation in labour.

■ Continuous EFM should be offered and recommended during labour for women with antenatal and/or intrapartum risk factors.

■ A cardiotocograph (CTG) should always be interpreted holistically, in context with the medical, clinical and obstetric circumstances, as well as the woman's preferences, when determining the appropriate actions to be taken.

■ Excessive uterine activity is the most frequent cause of fetal hypoxia/acidosis.

■ It is best practice for all maternity staff to record their opinion and actions clearly and legibly using a structured pro forma at least hourly, and to obtain a timely 'fresh eyes' review.

Problems identified from case discussions

- Not auscultating the fetal heart rate towards the end of the contraction and continuing for at least 30 seconds after the contraction has ended
- Not documenting a systematic assessment of the CTG at least hourly and at every review
- Interpreting the CTG in isolation and not considering the full clinical picture
- Not seeking help from experienced practitioners from the multi-professional team to assist with decision making when the CTG is difficult to interpret
- Not continuing/recommencing EFM when transferring mother to theatre for birth to be expedited

Introduction

Auscultation of the fetal heart rate has been a key assessment of fetal health in labour for over 200 years, and there are written records as far back as the seventeenth century describing fetal life; a poem written by Phillipe Le Goust in 1650 refers to hearing the fetal heart 'beating like the clapper of a mill'. The Pinard stethoscope was introduced in 1876 for performing intermittent auscultation, and in 1893 Von Winkel established criteria for determining potential 'fetal distress', some of which are still used today, such as fetal tachycardia over 160 beats per minute, fetal bradycardia less than 100 beats per minute, and gross alteration of fetal movements.[1]

Electronic fetal monitoring (EFM) was first introduced at Yale University in 1958. However, in the UK, it was the late 1960s before EFM began to be used clinically.[2,3] Fetal scalp blood sampling was introduced into clinical practice at about the same time as cardiotocographs (CTGs); other forms of intrapartum fetal surveillance such as continuous fetal pH monitoring and ST waveform analysis have subsequently been developed.[4] The original aim of EFM was to prevent intrapartum fetal deaths, and it was later hoped that it would also lead to earlier detection of hypoxia, thus allowing timely intervention to reduce cerebral palsy rates. However, meta-analysis of randomised controlled trials (RCTs) of EFM compared with intermittent auscultation have actually shown no difference in perinatal outcome between the two methods, although this could be attributable to the insufficient sample size of most randomised trials. Continuous CTG was associated with a 63% increase in caesarean births and a 15% increase in operative vaginal births.[5] Very large studies (of at least 35,000 women) would be required to determine the efficacy of EFM. Also, equipment, clinical experience and interpretation criteria for CTGs were all very different in the 1970s and 1980s.[5]

The largest intrapartum fetal monitoring trial, the Dublin trial, was not large enough to detect differences in the rates of cerebral palsy, as perinatal morbidity and mortality were extremely low.[6] In addition, only about 10% of cerebral palsy cases are related to intrapartum events, as occult infection and/or inflammation are increasingly implicated.[7,8]

It is also often forgotten that most randomised trials of EFM and intermittent auscultation have shown that there are important 'human' factors that may affect outcome too. Murphy *et al.* found that of 64 cases of significant birth asphyxia, abnormalities were missed in both the continuously monitored and intermittent auscultation groups.[9]

Inadequate skills in the interpretation of CTGs and failure to take appropriate action once abnormalities have been detected are key problems. These may be vital contributors to the failure of EFM to reduce perinatal mortality, and they have been recurrent themes in many of the Confidential Enquiry reports.[10,11,12]

A Cochrane review published in 2017 identified that CTG interpretation requires a high level of skill and is susceptible to variation in judgement not only between clinicians, but also by the same clinician over time.[13] Variations in skills and judgement can lead to inappropriate care planning and subsequently impact upon perinatal outcomes.[14] The INFANT trial is a National Institute for Health Research (NIHR)-funded randomised controlled trial to determine if a computerised decision support system can improve the management of labour in women requiring continuous CTG, compared with CTG monitoring with no decision support and where the unit adheres to usual guidelines for CTG monitoring and interpretation. The results were published in *The Lancet* in early 2017 and showed that the use of computerised interpretation of cardiotocographs in women who have continuous EFM in labour did not achieve the aim of identifying early signs of fetal hypoxia, and there were no improvements in clinical outcomes for mothers and babies.[15,16]

In 2001, the Royal College of Obstetricians and Gynaecologists (RCOG) produced an evidence-based guideline on fetal monitoring in labour which was subsequently inherited by NICE.[17] The guideline not only aimed to clarify when EFM should be used as an appropriate method for monitoring the fetal heart in labour, but also standardised the classification of CTGs and provided guidance on actions to be taken when abnormalities were detected.

This guidance on fetal monitoring in labour was updated by NICE in 2008 and again in 2014.[18,19] However, in 2016, the RCOG and NICE commenced a further review of the 2014 guidance after stakeholders raised concerns, in particular, with regard to the revised classification of CTGs and implementation feedback.[20] The outcome of this review was released in February 2017 in a revised NICE Clinical Guideline 190.[19]

In 2015, a second body, the International Federation of Gynecology and Obstetrics (FIGO) released a global consensus guideline on intrapartum fetal monitoring, and the FIGO classification system for interpreting CTGs was considered as part of the RCOG/NICE review.[5]

Risk management and intrapartum fetal monitoring

Both intrapartum death and the birth of a baby with severe brain damage are tragedies for the families concerned. Although the evidence for linking brain injury with intrapartum care is inconsistent, it is still a major source of litigation.[21,22,23] The NHS Litigation Authority (NHSLA) report on 10 years of maternity claims identified that the total estimated value of CTG claims was £466 million between 2000 and 2010.[24]

Analysis of the cases identified several themes, including:

- Failure to recognise an abnormal CTG
- Failure to act on an abnormal CTG
- Failure to refer appropriately
- Continuing to prescribe and administer oxytocin in the presence of an abnormal CTG
- Failure to monitor the fetal heart adequately (mistaking maternal pulse for fetal heart, failing to recognise 'doubling' on the CTG)
- Inadequate documentation

If care is found to be suboptimal, this is likely to be indefensible in court, and individual claims can exceed £3 million. Adequate interpretation of CTGs is crucial to quality improvement and the reduction of medicolegal risk. In the UK, claims for damaged babies account for 49% of the NHS litigation bill.[24]

Training for maternity staff

The recent *Saving Babies' Lives* Care Bundle, published in 2016 by NHS England, describes four key elements of evidence-based care that could make an impact on reducing stillbirths and neonatal deaths.[14] One of the elements is 'effective fetal monitoring in labour'. The rationale for including this element is that 'CTG interpretation requires a high level of skill and is susceptible to variation in judgement between clinicians … and can lead to inappropriate care … subsequently impacting on perinatal outcomes.' This element of the Care Bundle recommends that NHS Trusts must demonstrate that all qualified staff who care for women in labour are competent to interpret CTGs, and must identify appropriate training packages to ensure clinical competence.[14]

Draycott *et al.* have demonstrated that mandatory skills training in CTG interpretation and obstetric emergencies has improved neonatal outcomes in one UK maternity unit, and this has been replicated in Kansas, USA, and Victoria, Australia.[25,26,27] The training covered not only CTG interpretation but also the skills required to communicate the interpretation and the actions of the team responding to the emergency, indicating that improving outcomes in labour when EFM is used probably depends on more than CTG interpretation training alone.

A systematic review by Pehrson *et al.* concluded that training can improve CTG competence and clinical practice, but further research is needed to evaluate the type and content of training that is most effective.[28]

Physiology and pathophysiology

The healthy fetus is able to cope with the stresses of labour and adapts appropriately to meet the challenge. The current evidence base supports the use of intermittent auscultation for 'low-risk' pregnancies and continuous CTG monitoring should be considered in all circumstances where there is a high risk of fetal hypoxia/acidosis.[5] These risks include:

- Maternal health conditions (such as antepartum/intrapartum haemorrhage and maternal pyrexia)
- Fetal risk factors: abnormal fetal growth, prematurity, reduced fetal movements, multiple pregnancy, breech presentation
- Epidural anaesthesia
- Significant meconium stained liquor
- Possibility of excessive uterine activity, as occurs with induced or augmented labour
- Fetal heart abnormalities detected during intermittent auscultation

Fetal oxygen supply

In comparison with adults, the fetal partial pressure of oxygen is relatively low. However, the fetus has a remarkable margin of safety. A high concentration of fetal haemoglobin and its greater affinity for absorbing oxygen mean that oxygen saturation is high. The cardiac output of the fetus is also extremely efficient. Consequently, the fetal oxygen supply is usually greater than requirements.

Gas exchange is impaired during contractions, which means that oxygen levels fall and carbon dioxide (CO_2) levels rise. Between contractions the oxygen supply is restored and the accumulated CO_2 is excreted. Conditions that impair gas exchange at the placenta, such as uterine hypercontractility, cord occlusion, maternal hypotension or abruption, will cause retention of CO_2, which lowers the pH of the fetal blood (a respiratory acidosis). This should be resolved when placental perfusion is restored between contractions. However, if gas exchange continues to be impeded, the fetus will rely on the following important defence mechanisms:

■ **Hormonal response**

A reduction in fetal oxygen supply is detected by chemoreceptors in the fetal aorta. This activates a hormonal response with an increase in catecholamines, vasopressin, adenine and adenosine levels. The levels of catecholamines in an asphyxiated infant exceed those of patients with phaeochromocytoma.[29]

■ **Preferential redistribution of blood flow**

There is a decrease in blood flow to 'less essential' organs such as the liver, spleen, gut, kidneys and skin. Blood supply to the 'priority' organs – brain, heart and adrenal glands – is increased. The heart needs to work harder during this time, and myocardial blood flow can increase up to 500% in response to hypoxia. Oxygen requirements for the brain are not as great, and fetal behaviour can adapt to reduce energy requirements.

■ **Glycogenolysis**

When the oxygen supply is no longer sufficient to meet the energy requirements of the fetus, glycogenolysis is activated by the hormonal response. This means that glucose is released from glycogen stores and is metabolised anaerobically (without oxygen) to maintain energy requirements. Release of adrenaline stimulates the activation of glycogenolysis. During anaerobic metabolism, stores of glycogen in the heart, muscle and liver are broken down to provide energy. Lactate, a by-product of anaerobic metabolism, is initially buffered (neutralised) but will eventually cause the pH of the blood to fall further (metabolic acidosis). As the fetus continues to use glycogen stores, the acidosis becomes predominantly metabolic in origin and the pH decreases even further.

Clearly, conditions and events that affect the mother (e.g. pre-eclampsia, diabetes, antepartum haemorrhage) and/or placental function (too frequent or prolonged uterine contractions) and/or the baby's defence mechanisms (growth restriction, infection, chronic hypoxaemia and stress) may make the fetus less able to adapt and more vulnerable to hypoxia (Box 5.1).

Box 5.1 Factors that influence fetal oxygenation

Mother	Uterus/placenta	Fetus
Anaemia	Abruption	Anaemia
Analgesia/anaesthesia	Cord prolapse	Fetal bleeding
Dehydration	Impaired placental function	Infection
Hypertension	Uterine hypercontractility	Growth restriction
Hypotension		
Pyrexia		

Compensatory responses and adaptation to hypoxia can protect the fetus for only a finite amount of time. When the defence mechanisms are blunted, depleted or overwhelmed, the risk of perinatal asphyxia (hypoxia, acidosis and tissue damage) is increased.

Standards and quality

The indications for offering women continuous EFM in labour have been documented in both the NICE intrapartum care guideline and the FIGO consensus guidance for intrapartum fetal monitoring.[5,19] Local guidelines should be developed and approved by in-house multi-professional clinical guideline teams, after consideration and review of the national guidance. Implementation should be supported by local training programmes, as well as management algorithms and documentation tools for use in the clinical areas.

Intrapartum risk assessments

Risk factors should be recorded on the partogram as part of the admission assessment, and there should be continual risk assessments performed and documented throughout labour, together with appropriate action plans (Figure 5.1).[5]

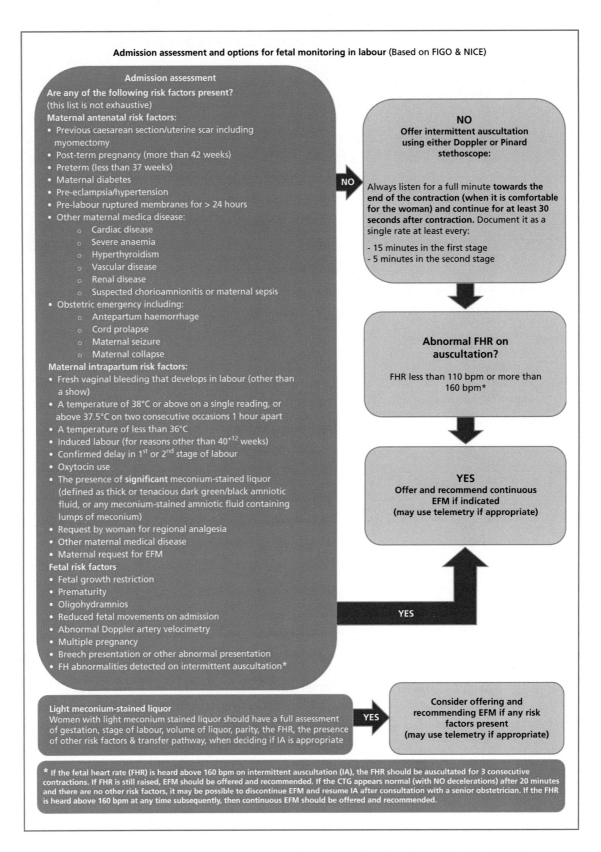

Figure 5.1 Admission assessment and options for fetal monitoring in labour (based on FIGO and NICE)

Informed choice

The assessment of fetal wellbeing is only one aspect of intrapartum care. It is important that the mother makes an informed choice regarding intrapartum fetal monitoring based on the available evidence.[19]

Standards for intermittent auscultation (IA) in labour

For a mother who is healthy and has an uncomplicated pregnancy with no risk factors, intermittent auscultation should be offered and recommended in labour, using either a Doppler ultrasound or a Pinard stethoscope, to monitor fetal wellbeing.[19,30]

There is insufficient evidence to indicate whether an admission CTG as part of the initial assessment for uncomplicated pregnancies either improves outcomes or results in harm for women and their babies, compared with intermittent auscultation alone.[19]

Optimal timing for IA in labour

The ideal timing for conducting IA has not been investigated in a robust way, and clearly there is a balance to be struck between listening at the optimal time for fetal surveillance and not interfering with the mother's neurohormonal responses in labour (which, in turn, might influence the wellbeing of the baby).

The most recent NICE guidelines recommend *listening immediately after a contraction for at least 1 minute and recording it as a single rate*,[19] and the FIGO IA guidelines recommend *listening to the FHR during the contraction and for at least 30 seconds after the contraction and recording it as a single rate*.[30] Some midwives have raised concerns about this recommendation, as it may be uncomfortable for the woman to have any auscultation during a contraction, and it may also affect her positioning when coping with labour.

The PROMPT Maternity Foundation has contacted the authors of the FIGO guidance to ask if they could provide further clarification regarding the meaning of 'during' the contraction. They supplied a very helpful response, indicating that the reason for listening over this suggested time period is based on knowledge of the physiology of the fetal heart rate, in particular, that the infant is most likely to demonstrate auscultatable evidence of acute compromise when responding to or recovering from the effects of a uterine contraction in the period just after the contraction peak. However, they acknowledge that IA should not be so intrusive as to interfere with how the woman copes with her contractions. They also encouraged maternity units to audit this change in practice, and welcomed any additional pragmatic information that units can provide with regard to the optimal timing for IA.

Therefore, based on the above communication, the PROMPT Maternity Foundation has opted for the following approach as the best compromise for the timing of IA: listening to the fetal heart rate towards the end of the contraction (when it is comfortable for the woman) and continuing for at least 30 seconds after a contraction, thus avoiding distracting the mother as she copes with her contractions, while maximising the opportunity of auscultating any signs of fetal compromise.

IA practice recommendations

Intermittent auscultation should be carried out in active labour as per the practice recommendations in Figure 5.2.[30]

Intrapartum intermittent auscultation (IA)
Practice Recommendations (based on FIGO 2015)

Features to evaluate	Action	What to document
Fetal heart rate (FHR) (Normal: 110–160 bpm)	Duration: Listen for at least 60 seconds Timing: Listen towards the end of the contraction (as soon as it is comfortable for mother) and continue for at least 30 seconds after contraction Interval: 1st stage: every 15 minutes 2nd stage: every 5 minutes	• FHR as single number having counted for 60 seconds • Any slowing of FHR that may indicate decelerations or bradycardia • Any increase of FHR that may indicate fetal tachycardia
Uterine contractions	Palpate before and during FHR auscultation	• Number of contractions in 10 minutes
Fetal movements	Palpate at the same time as contractions The fetal heart rate may speed up in association with fetal movement	• Presence or absence of fetal movements • Any speeding up of FHR associated with fetal movement
Maternal pulse rate	At start of IA and at least hourly or if any FHR abnormality	• Maternal pulse as single counted number
If any abnormal features are identified, refer to: 'IA: Guidance and management if abnormal features identified in labour'		
Complete an intermittent auscultation (IA) pro forma on commencement of IA in labour and at handover of care during active labour		
Record FHR and any required actions on the partogram		

Figure 5.2 Practice recommendations for intermittent auscultation (based on FIGO 2015)

Figure 5.3 is an example of an IA pro forma that could be completed and signed by the midwife at the commencement of IA in labour. Thereafter, the midwife need only document the FHR on the partogram, in addition to other features such as the presence of fetal movements and frequency of contractions. Any intrapartum events that may affect FHR should also be documented contemporaneously in the intrapartum notes.[9] It may also be worth the midwife considering obtaining a 'fresh ears' review by a second midwife (or obstetrician) at least 2-hourly in labour.

Intermittent auscultation (IA) in labour

Auscultate the fetal heart rate (FHR) for **at least one full minute, listening towards the end of the contraction (as soon as it is comfortable for mother) and continue for at least 30 seconds after the contraction** using:

Pinard: ☐   Doppler: ☐   **(Normal FHR: 110–160 bpm)**

Listen and document the FHR at least every **15 minutes in 1ˢᵗ stage** and every **5 minutes in 2ⁿᵈ stage**

Palpate for the frequency of contractions and the presence of fetal movements

Consider Fresh Ears 🦻 review of fetal heart rate at least 2-hourly and document on partogram

If any abnormal features are identified, refer to:
'IA: Guidance & management if abnormal features identified in labour'

At the start of IA:

FHR: .... bpm   **Maternal pulse:** .... bpm
                                         (Document maternal pulse **hourly** in established labour)

Date: ....   Time: ....

Signature: ....   Print name: ....

Figure 5.3 An example of an intermittent auscultation documentation pro forma (based on FIGO 2015)

Guidance if an abnormal fetal heart rate is suspected and identified in labour

If an abnormal FHR is suspected in labour, refer to the guidance in Figure 5.4.

IA: Guidance and management if abnormal features identified in labour (based on FIGO 2015)

Features	Abnormal	Action
Fetal heart rate (FHR) (Normal: 110–160 bpm)	FHR less than 110 bpm	• Check maternal pulse rate and listen continuously to FHR. If FH remains at less than 110 bpm for more than 3 minutes, this suggests a prolonged deceleration or bradycardia • Change maternal position, perform VE, commence immediate CTG, (if appropriate) and seek obstetric opinion • If at home, or in midwifery-led unit, arrange for immediate transfer to obstetric unit • In addition: if in the 2nd stage of labour and birth **not** immediately imminent, consider stopping pushing
	FHR less than 110 bpm for more than 5 minutes	• **Expedite birth urgently**
	FHR greater than 160 bpm	• Check maternal pulse rate and listen for 3 consecutive contractions - if still above 160 bpm suggestive of fetal tachycardia (*NB. If fetal heart rate returns to normal range during this period, resume IA as per guidance for 1st or 2nd stage of labour*) • Change maternal position, perform VE, commence continuous CTG, (if appropriate) and seek obstetric opinion • If at home, or in midwifery-led unit, arrange for immediate transfer to obstetric unit • Assess maternal temperature and for signs of infection
Fetal movements	An increasing FHR heard just after a contraction is rarely due to fetal movement	• IA should be carried out over the next 3 contractions to rule out the possibility of decelerations
Uterine contractions	An interval of less than 2 minutes between 2 contractions should trigger palpation over 10 minutes.	• If palpate more than 5 contractions in 10 minutes this indicates tachysystole • If tachysystole is indicated, commence continuous CTG (transfer to obstetric unit if necessary) and seek obstetric opinion • Consider tocolysis

Figure 5.4 Recommended actions if abnormal features are identified in labour (based on FIGO 2015)

Indications for changing from IA to continuous EFM

Electronic fetal monitoring should be offered and recommended to women when:[19,30]

■ There is confirmed evidence on auscultation of an FHR of less than 110 or more than 160 beats per minute (bpm).

■ There is evidence on auscultation of the FHR decreasing after a contraction.

■ Any intrapartum risk factors are present or develop in labour.

This may mean organising for transfer of the woman from home or a birth centre to the nearest consultant-led maternity unit labour ward.

If after a full assessment and review of mother and baby, including a 20-minute CTG, all findings are normal (with *no* decelerations present) and there are no other risk factors identified, then it may be possible to discontinue EFM and resume IA (within the consultant-led maternity unit if the mother has been transferred from home or a standalone birth centre).[5,19]

Presence of meconium-stained liquor

NICE guidance states that EFM should not be offered to women in labour who have non-specific meconium as long as there are no other risk factors. If there is significant meconium present, defined as dark green or black amniotic fluid that is thick or tenacious, or any amniotic fluid containing lumps of meconium, then they recommend that:[19]

■ Continuous EFM should be recommended and commenced.

■ Healthcare professionals trained in fetal blood sampling should be available.

■ Healthcare professionals trained in advanced neonatal life support should be readily available.

■ A woman should be transferred to obstetric-led care provided that it is safe to do so and the birth is unlikely to occur before transfer is completed.

Technical considerations for EFM in labour

It is best to auscultate the fetal heart using a Pinard stethoscope before commencing EFM in labour. In addition, the maternal pulse should be palpated regularly with any form of fetal monitoring, to differentiate between maternal and fetal heart rates. It is possible to generate a signal from a large pulsating maternal vessel, which may be misinterpreted as the fetal heart. Also, the ultrasound may falsely double the rate of the maternal pulse if there is sufficient extended separation between valve movements, generating a rate that would be within the normal range of the fetal heart.

There have been occasional reports of unexpected macerated stillbirths with apparently normal intrapartum CTGs, even with direct fetal scalp clip application.[31,32] It is therefore important that, if fetal death is suspected (despite the presence of an apparently recorded fetal heart rate), fetal viability should be confirmed with real-time ultrasound assessment.[19]

All members of staff should be aware of the technical limitations of EFM and should always read the manufacturer's instructions for each particular monitor.

Standards for electronic fetal monitoring

EFM should not be used as a tool of convenience in place of skilled midwives when monitoring the fetal heart in labour. The unselected use of continuous EFM contributes to unnecessary intervention.

- The date and time clocks on the machine should be correct and the paper speed set to 1 cm per minute (Figure 5.5).

- CTGs should be dated and labelled with the mother's name, date of birth and hospital number as a minimum (Figure 5.5).

- The reason for the CTG should be clearly documented.

- Any intrapartum events that may affect the FHR, such as vaginal examinations, fetal blood sampling, epidural insertion and top-ups, should be noted contemporaneously on the CTG, and signed and dated.

- Mobile fetal monitoring using wireless telemetry has the advantage of allowing the mother to move more freely while ensuring continuous EFM and therefore should be the preferred option for continuous EFM when available.[5]

- If external monitoring is not of sufficient quality for interpretation of the CTG, a fetal scalp electrode should be applied when appropriate.

- Any consultations should be documented in the intrapartum notes and on the CTG, together with a date, time and signature.

- Following the birth, the caregiver should sign and note the date, time and mode of birth on the CTG (Figure 5.5).

- The CTG should be stored securely with the maternal notes or electronically archived.

CTG check list (attach to start of CTG trace)		
Reason for CTG:		
Date:	Date set correctly on CTG? (tick)	
Time:	Time set correctly on CTG? (tick)	
Name:	Paper speed set to 1 cm per min (tick)	
Hospital number:	Centralised monitoring commenced (tick)	
	Gestation:	
	Maternal pulse (rate):	
(or attach addressograph)	FH auscultated prior to CTG (rate):	
Attach to end of CTG trace		
Mode of birth:	Date of birth:	
Signature:	Time of birth:	

Figure 5.5 Example of start and end stickers for attaching to CTG

Features of the intrapartum CTG and terminology

Most clinicians would have no difficulty in recognising the features of a normal intrapartum CTG, as shown in Figure 5.6. When the CTG is normal, we can be confident that the fetus will be normoxic, so the sensitivity of the CTG is high. However, when the CTG is suspicious or pathological there is a limited capacity to predict metabolic acidosis and low Apgar scores; indeed, in a large percentage of cases these outcomes will not be present. Therefore, the specificity of a CTG for detecting intrapartum hypoxia is low, and a pathological CTG has a low positive predictive value for hypoxia. However, it should not be forgotten that the aim of intrapartum fetal monitoring is to avoid fetal injury by pre-emptively taking action before a hypoxic–ischaemic injury occurs.

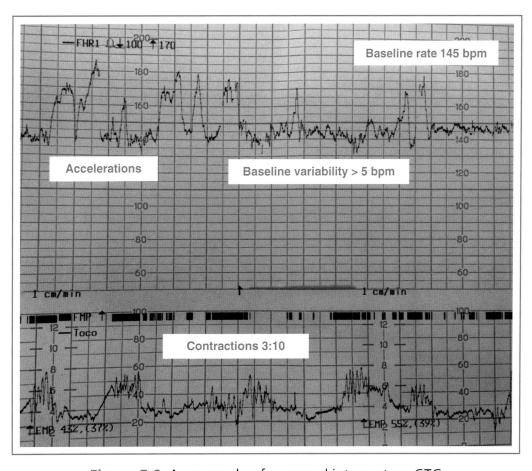

Figure 5.6 An example of a normal intrapartum CTG

In addition, there is no reliable way to determine fetal reserves or, often, the nature or severity of an intrapartum event. The growth-restricted fetus may have a blunted response owing to chronic stress and inadequate glycogen stores. Furthermore, acute catastrophic events may quickly overwhelm the defence mechanisms of even a healthy baby. Therefore, the CTG must always be interpreted in the context of the antepartum and intrapartum clinical history and events.

> **The CTG must always be interpreted in context, taking account of the antepartum and intrapartum clinical history, risk factors and events.**

Clearly, it is important that communication between carers should convey the clinical context using consistent terminology to describe the features of the intrapartum CTG, the level of concern and the urgency of the situation.

There are five main features that should be systematically examined to assist with the interpretation of the CTG:

- baseline rate
- baseline variability
- presence of accelerations
- presence and type of decelerations
- frequency of contractions

These features, **in conjunction with the clinical circumstances**, should all be considered when deciding the action to be taken.[5]

Baseline fetal heart rate

Baseline FHR is the level of the FHR when it is stable, excluding accelerations and decelerations. It is determined over a period of 10 minutes and expressed in beats per minute (see Figure 5.6). The ranges and descriptive terms are shown in Table 5.1.

- It may be necessary to review previous segments of CTG and/or evaluate the rate over a longer period if there are episodes of unstable FHR patterns.

■ *Maternal pyrexia* is the most common cause of fetal tachycardia (FHR more than 160 bpm).

■ A rising baseline rate, even within the normal range, may be of concern if other non-reassuring/abnormal features are present.

Table 5.1 Baseline fetal heart rate ranges (FIGO and NICE)

Level	Rate (beats per minute)
Reassuring	
Normal baseline rate	110–160 bpm Preterm fetuses have a faster heart rate, and term fetuses tend to have a lower heart rate (still within normal range)
Non-reassuring	
Bradycardia	100–109 bpm (lasting more than 10 minutes)
Tachycardia	161–180 bpm (lasting more than 10 minutes)
Abnormal	
Bradycardia	< 100 bpm
Tachycardia	> 180 bpm

Baseline variability

Baseline variability is the minor fluctuation in baseline fetal heart rate occurring at three to five cycles per minute (see Figure 5.6). Details are shown in Table 5.2.

■ Reduced variability can occur due to nervous system hypoxia.

■ During deep fetal sleep, variability is usually in the lower range of normal, but the amplitude is seldom less than 5 bpm.

■ If there is reduced variability following an initially normal CTG, it is unlikely to be due to hypoxia, unless accompanied by decelerations and a rise in the baseline rate.

■ Increased variability (saltatory pattern) of greater than 25 bpm bandwidth for more than 25 minutes may indicate hypoxia. Although the pathophysiology of the pattern is not fully understood, it is thought to be caused by fetal autonomic instability/hyperactivity.[5]

Table 5.2 Fetal heart rate: baseline variability ranges (FIGO and NICE)

Level	Bandwidth amplitude
Reassuring	Normal baseline variability: bandwidth amplitude of 5 bpm or more (but less than 25 bpm)
Non-reassuring	Bandwidth amplitude below 5 bpm for 30–50 minutes Bandwidth amplitude of more than 25 bpm for 15–25 minutes Sinusoidal pattern lasting for less than 30 minutes
Abnormal	Bandwidth amplitude less than 5 bpm for more than 50 minutes Bandwidth amplitude of more than 25 bpm for more than 25 minutes Sinusoidal pattern lasting for more than 30 minutes (usually associated with fetal anaemia)

Accelerations

Accelerations are an abrupt increase in the fetal heart rate of more than 15 bpm in amplitude above the baseline and lasting longer than 15 seconds (but less than 10 minutes) (Figure 5.6).

■ Most accelerations coincide with fetal movement and are a **sign that the fetus is not hypoxic**.

■ The absence of accelerations **within an otherwise normal CTG** is unlikely to indicate hypoxia/acidosis.

Decelerations

Decelerations are a slowing of the fetal heart rate below the baseline level of more than 15 bpm in amplitude for a period of 15 seconds or more.

Early decelerations

Uniform, repetitive, periodic slowing of the fetal heart rate with onset early in the contraction and return to baseline at the end of the contraction. The lowest point of the deceleration will coincide with the highest point of the contraction. There is always normal variability within the deceleration. They are usually associated with fetal head compression and hence tend to occur late in the first stage or during the second stage of labour. True uniform early decelerations are rare and are not indicative of fetal hypoxia/acidosis.

Late decelerations – U-shaped and/or with reduced variability

Uniform, repetitive (present with more than 50% of contractions), periodic slowing of the fetal heart rate with onset mid- to end of the contraction and lowest point more than 20 seconds after the peak of the contraction, **always ending after the contraction** (Figure 5.7). In the presence of a non-accelerative trace with baseline variability less than 5 bpm, the definition would include decelerations with an amplitude of 10–15 bpm. Late decelerations, if present for more than 30 minutes, are indicative of fetal hypoxia and further action is indicated. It may not be appropriate to wait 30 minutes before referral for obstetric review if the CTG is showing late decelerations with more than 50% of contractions from the start of monitoring or if there is reduced variability.

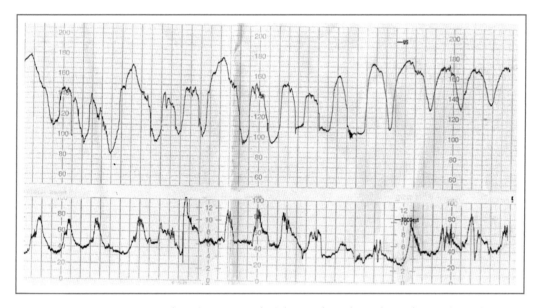

Figure 5.7 Late decelerations (U-shaped with reduced variability)

Variable decelerations – V-shaped (previously called typical)

These are the most common form of deceleration occurring during labour (Figure 5.8). They have a symmetrical rapid drop and rapid recovery to the baseline, with good variability within the deceleration, **and all other features of the CTG are normal**. FIGO describes these as ***V-shaped*** variable decelerations. NICE describes them as variable decelerations *'with no concerning features'*. They are an autonomic nervous system response (triggered by the baroreceptors) to compression of the umbilical cord. If the decelerations remain V-shaped (typical) with good variability and all other features of the CTG are normal, then they are seldom associated with an important degree of hypoxia and are indicative of the fetus coping well with cord compression in labour. They vary in shape, size and relationship to contractions.

However, the fetus may become tired over time, particularly if there is any degree of fetal compromise such as fetal growth restriction.

Variable decelerations – non-V-shaped (U-shaped) with reduced variability (previously called atypical)

Variable decelerations are likely to be associated with hypoxia if they are present with more than 50% of contractions and exhibit any of the following concerning characteristics (Figure 5.8):

■ a non-V-shaped component, i.e. U-shaped or anything other than V-shaped

■ reduced variability within the deceleration

■ Slower recovery back to the baseline

■ individual duration exceeding 3 minutes

Variable decelerations (most common intrapartum decelerations)

Variable decelerations constitute the majority of decelerations during labour. They are an autonomic nervous system response (triggered by the baroreceptors) to compression of the umbilical cord.

Examples of NON-V-Shaped (U-shaped) variable decelerations *(with concerning features)*

V-Shaped variable decelerations
(NO concerning features)

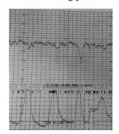

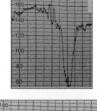

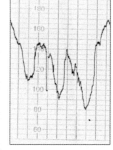

V-shaped variable decelerations (NICE describe these as with **NO concerning features**) typically exhibit a symmetrical rapid drop and rapid recovery back to the baseline, and all other features of the CTG are reassuring.

If variable decelerations remain V-shaped (*and all other FHR features are reassuring*), then they are seldom associated with an important degree of hypoxia/acidosis.

Variable decelerations are likely to be associated with hypoxia if they are present with more than 50% of contractions and they exhibit the following components/*concerning features*:

■ A **NON-V-shaped** component, i.e. **U-shaped** or anything other than V-shaped
■ Reduced variability within deceleration
■ Slower recovery back to the baseline
■ And/or individual duration exceeding 3 minutes

Figure 5.8 Variable decelerations – V-shaped and non-V-shaped (U-shaped)

Prolonged decelerations – lasting more than 3 minutes

Decelerations lasting more than 3 minutes are likely to be indicative of hypoxia, and if a bradycardia persists for 9 minutes, birth should be expedited. Decelerations that exceed 5 minutes, with the FHR maintained at less than 80 bpm and with reduced variability within the deceleration, are frequently associated with acute hypoxia/acidosis and require urgent intervention.

Sinusoidal pattern

This is a regular oscillation of the baseline long-term variability resembling a sine wave (Figure 5.9). This smooth undulating pattern has a relatively fixed period of 3–5 cycles/minute and an amplitude of 5–15 bpm above and below the baseline, and lasts for more than 30 minutes with absent accelerations. A true sinusoidal pattern occurs in association with severe fetal anaemia, as is found in iso-immunisation, fetal–maternal haemorrhage, twin-to-twin transfusion and ruptured vasa praevia.

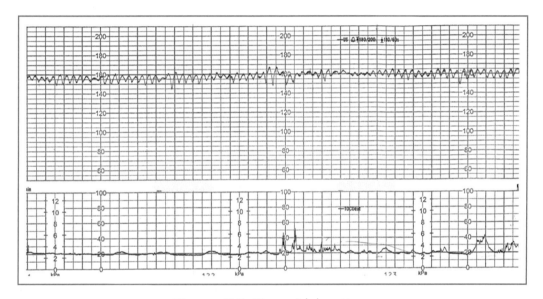

Figure 5.9 Sinusoidal pattern

A pseudo-sinusoidal pattern has a more 'jagged saw-tooth' appearance, rather than a smooth sine-wave form. Its duration seldom exceeds 30 minutes, and there will be normal FHR patterns before and after. This pattern can be seen after analgesic administration to the mother and during periods of fetal thumb sucking and other mouth movements. It can be difficult to distinguish from the true sinusoidal pattern, but the shorter duration of the pseudo-sinusoidal pattern usually helps to discriminate between the two.

Fetal behavioural states

This refers to periods of fetal quiescence reflecting deep sleep (no eye movements), alternating with periods of active sleep (rapid eye movements) and wakefulness. The occurrence of different behavioural states is a hallmark of fetal neurological responsiveness and an absence of hypoxia. Deep sleep can last for up to 50 minutes and is associated with a stable baseline, very rare accelerations and borderline variability. Active sleep is the most frequent behavioural state and is represented by a moderate number of accelerations and normal variability. Active wakefulness is rarer and is represented by a large number of accelerations and normal variability. Sometimes accelerations may be so frequent that it is difficult to determine the baseline fetal heart rate. Transitions between the different patterns become clearer after 32–34 weeks' gestation as the fetal nervous system matures.

Contraction patterns

Always remember to look at the 'bottom line'. Take notice of the duration of contractions (should last between 45 and 120 seconds) and the interval between contractions. They are necessary for progression in labour, but they may transiently decrease placental perfusion as they compress the vessels running inside the myometrium and/or cause umbilical cord compression (especially if membranes are ruptured). With the CTG, only the frequency of the contractions can be observed. The strength and length of contractions is best assessed by the midwife or doctor placing a hand on the fundus of the uterus and feeling the intensity of the contractions over a 10-minute period. It is important to observe for signs of hypercontractility, i.e. excessive frequency of contractions, defined as more than five contractions in 10 minutes in two successive 10-minute periods, or averaged over a 30-minute period. Excessive uterine activity is the most frequent cause of fetal hypoxia/ acidosis. It can usually be reversed by reducing or stopping oxytocin infusions, removing administered prostaglandins if possible, and/or starting acute tocolysis with subcutaneous terbutaline.

During the second stage of labour, maternal pushing efforts can also contribute to fetal hypoxia, and the mother can be asked to stop pushing until the situation is reversed.[5]

Interpretation of the intrapartum CTG

Having systematically examined the five main features of the CTG, the trace should be classified as normal, suspicious or pathological, depending on the presence of any non-reassuring or abnormal features. The clinical circumstances should always be considered when deciding actions to be taken if a CTG is classified as suspicious (low probability of hypoxia) or pathological (high probability of hypoxia) in labour. A structured CTG pro forma (based on the NICE and FIGO consensus guideline), which incorporates relevant guidance on CTG interpretation in a single implementation tool, can be used not only to document the main features and classify the CTG, but also to record actions that should be taken (Figure 5.10).

Documentation pro forma for intrapartum CTG interpretation (based on FIGO 2015 and NICE 2017)			
Feature	**Reassuring (acceptable)**	**Non-reassuring**	**Abnormal**
Baseline rate (bpm)	Baseline 110 – 160 bpm Rate:	Baseline rate 100 – 109 bpm for **more than 10** minutes Rate: Baseline rate **more than 160 bpm for more than 10** minutes Rate:	Baseline **less than 100 bpm** Rate: Baseline rate **more than 180 bpm** Rate:
N.B A rising baseline rate even within the normal range may be of concern if other non-reassuring/abnormal features are present.			
Variability (bpm)	Variability of 5 – 25 bpm	Variability **less than 5 bpm for 30 to 50 minutes**	Variability **less than 5 bpm for more than 50 minutes**
	Comments:	Variability **more than 25 bpm for 15 to 25 minutes**	Variability **more than 25 bpm for more than 25 minutes**
			Sinusoidal pattern **lasting for more than 30 minutes**
Accelerations	Present	Comments:	
Decelerations	None	V-shaped Variable decelerations *(NO concerning features)* with more than 50% of contractions for **more than 90 minutes**	NON V-shaped (U-shaped) Variable decelerations – *(Concerning features present)* **with more than 50%** of contractions and for **more than 30 minutes**
	True early decelerations		
	V-shaped Variable decelerations (NO *concerning features)* **with less than 50%** of contractions	**NON V-shaped (U-shaped) Variable decelerations –** *(Concerning features present)* **with more than 50%** of contractions for **less than 30 minutes**	**Repetitive Late decelerations (U-shaped)** for **more than 30 minutes**
	V-shaped Variable decelerations (NO *concerning features)* **with more than 50%** of contractions for **less than 90 minutes**	**Repetitive Late decelerations (U-shaped)** for **less than 30 minutes**	**Repetitive Late decelerations (U-shaped)** and reduced variability for **more than 20 minutes**
	NON V-shaped (U-shaped) Variable decelerations with less than 50% of contractions *(and all other features of CTG are **Reassuring)***	**Single prolonged deceleration lasting more than 3 minutes, but less than 5 minutes**	Single prolonged deceleration for **more than 5 minutes** *(A prolonged deceleration of less than 80 bpm with reduced variability and lasting more than 5 minutes is often associated with hypoxia)*
Contractions :10 (N.B if more than 5:10 - take action to reduce frequency)	**Dilatation:**	**Liquor colour:**	**Maternal pulse:**
Reason for CTG:		**Gestation:**	
		Other risk factors:	
Opinion (N.B if CTG has any non-reassuring or abnormal features present from the start, it may not be appropriate to wait for specified time limits before requesting review)	**Normal CTG** (All **four** FHR features are reassuring) ***No intervention necessary***	**Suspicious CTG** *(One non-reassuring FHR feature)* ***Low probability of hypoxia*** Correct reversible causes (refer to algorithm & EFM interpretation guidance)	**Pathological CTG** *(Two or more non-reassuring or one or more abnormal FHR features)* **High probability of hypoxia – urgent action required (refer to algorithm & EFM interpretation guidance)**
Action taken: (Always consider the clinical circumstances when reviewing CTG and deciding action)			

Date: .... Time: .... Signature: ....

Fresh Eyes Opinion   *at least 2 hourly*   I agree with opinion? YES / NO   Status: ....   If opinion different complete new pro forma

Date: .... Time: .... Signature: .... Status: ....

NHS North Bristol
NHS Trust

Figure 5.10 Example of an intrapartum CTG documentation pro forma (based on FIGO and NICE)

It is recommended that a clinician asks for a periodic second opinion (e.g. a second midwife or obstetrician) on the assessment of the CTG, to ensure that there is a 'fresh eyes' review regardless of whether the CTG is normal, suspicious or pathological (NICE).

A summary of the guidance for intrapartum CTG classification, interpretation and action is shown in Figure 5.11.

Suspicious or pathological CTGs

When fetal hypoxia/acidosis is anticipated or suspected (suspicious or pathological classification) and action is required to avoid adverse neonatal outcomes, this does not necessarily mean a category 1 caesarean section or operative vaginal birth is indicated. Often, the underlying cause for the appearance of the CTG pattern can be identified, with the possibility that the situation can be reversed, leading to subsequent recovery of fetal oxygenation and a return to a normal CTG. Good clinical judgement is required to diagnose the underlying cause for a suspicious or pathological CTG, and to determine if the problem is reversible. In addition, the clinician needs to consider the timing of the birth, with the aim of avoiding prolonged fetal hypoxia as well as unnecessary intervention. An intrapartum CTG with one non-reassuring feature is classified as suspicious (low probability of hypoxia). Figure 5.12 shows the FIGO and NICE guidelines for suggested actions when the CTG is suspicious.

Excessive uterine activity is the most frequent cause for fetal hypoxia, and can usually be reversed by reducing or stopping oxytocin infusions, removing administered prostaglandins if possible, and/or starting acute tocolysis with subcutaneous terbutaline. During the second stage of labour, because of the additional effect of maternal pushing, fetal hypoxia may develop more rapidly. Urgent action should be taken to relieve the situation, including stopping maternal pushing. If there is no improvement, birth should be expedited.

Pathological CTG and fetal blood sampling

An intrapartum CTG with two or more non-reassuring features or one or more abnormal features is classified as pathological and is indicative of a higher probability of fetal hypoxia. When considering expediting birth because of a pathological CTG, it is recommended that a further assessment of fetal oxygenation is undertaken. Several adjunctive technologies have been developed over the past decades, including fetal blood sampling (FBS), fetal scalp stimulation (FSS), pulse oximetry and ST wave analysis, and some of these have been successfully established. FBS use is limited mainly to the UK and northern Europe, and both FSS and FBS are considered in the NICE and FIGO guidelines.

Intrapartum CTG classification, interpretation and action (based on FIGO 2015 and NICE 2017)

Feature	Information
Baseline rate (bpm) The mean level of the FHR that is estimated over 10 minute periods	• May be necessary to review previous segments of CTG and/or evaluate the baseline over a longer period of time if there are episodes of unstable FHR patterns. Preterm fetuses have a faster heart rate • A bradycardia is a baseline rate below 110 bpm lasting for more than 10 minutes. Values between 100 and 110 bpm may be normal, especially in post term pregnancies, but in this instance, *all other features of the CTG will be reassuring* • Maternal pyrexia is the most common cause of fetal tachycardia (FHR more than 160 bpm)
Variability (bpm) The variability of the FHR signal as displayed via the CTG tracing	• Intermittent periods of reduced variability are normal, especially during periods of quiescence (sleep) • Reduced variability can occur due to central nervous system hypoxia • Increased variability (saltatory pattern) of greater than 25 bpm bandwidth for more than 25 minutes may indicate hypoxia
Sinusoidal pattern Smooth & undulating, resembling a sine wave with amplitude of 5–15 bpm. It lasts for more than 30 minutes and is absent of accelerations	• A sinusoidal pattern occurs in association with fetal anaemia and sometimes acute fetal hypoxia.
Accelerations Abrupt increase in FHR of more than 15 bpm above the baseline, lasting longer than 15 seconds (but less than 10 minutes)	• Most accelerations coincide with fetal movement and are a sign that the fetus **is not hypoxic**. The absence of accelerations in an otherwise normal CTG is unlikely to indicate hypoxia/acidosis

Decelerations
Decrease in the fetal heart rate of more than 15 bpm and lasting for more than 15 seconds
	• **Early decelerations:** Short-lasting and shallow with normal variability within the decelerations, coinciding exactly with contractions – believed to be caused by head compression and does not indicate hypoxia
	• **Variable decelerations:** Varying in shape, size and relationship to contractions. Usually associated with cord compression
	   V-shaped Variable decelerations (NO concerning features) – exhibit a symmetrical rapid drop and rapid recovery to the baseline with good variability within deceleration *and all other features of the CTG are reassuring*. These seldom indicate hypoxia
	   NON-V-shaped/U-shaped Variable decelerations (concerning features present i.e. reduced variability within the deceleration) – *these are highly likely to indicate hypoxia if they occur with more than 50% of contractions and continue for more than 30 minutes*
	• **Late decelerations:** Repetitive, U-shaped and/or with reduced variability within the deceleration and returning to baseline *after the end of the contraction.* Gradual onset and/or gradual return to baseline, starting more than 20 seconds after the onset of a contraction – *these are highly likely to indicate hypoxia*
	• **Prolonged deceleration:** Lasting more than 3 minutes but less than 5 minutes is non-reassuring. It is abnormal if it lasts more that 5 minutes. Expedite birth in shortest possible time if bradycardia persists beyond 5 minutes
	   Decelerations of longer than 5 minutes with a FHR less than 80 bpm and reduced variability are often associated with hypoxia and urgent action is required

Opinion & Actions: Always consider the medical, clinical & obstetric circumstances when interpreting the CTG and determining the actions to be taken If CTG has any non-reassuring or abnormal features present from the start, it may not be appropriate to wait for specified time limits before requesting review	**Normal:** No action required **Suspicious:** Correct reversible causes: Change position, inform midwife coordinator **or obstetrician**, reduce (or STOP) oxytocin infusion, perform VE if appropriate, assess maternal pulse, respiratory rate, BP, temperature, check for signs of infection, continue to monitor FHR closely, consider additional methods to assess fetal oxygenation. **(Refer to Actions for Suspicious CTG algorithm)** **Pathological:** Immediate actions to correct reversible causes, STOP oxytocin infusion, inform midwife coordinator **and senior obstetrician**, perform VE (if appropriate), exclude fetal hypoxia (fetal scalp stimulation (FSS) and/or fetal blood sampling (FBS) if possible & appropriate). If in the 2ⁿᵈ stage of labour and birth is not immediately imminent, consider stopping pushing **If a severe or acute event is suspected, then an FBS is not advised as it may delay action. If fetal hypoxia confirmed or if further assessment of fetal oxygenation is not possible, take action to expedite birth. (Refer to Actions for Pathological CTG algorithm)**

Figure 5.11 Summary of guidance for intrapartum CTG classification, interpretation and action (based on FIGO and NICE)

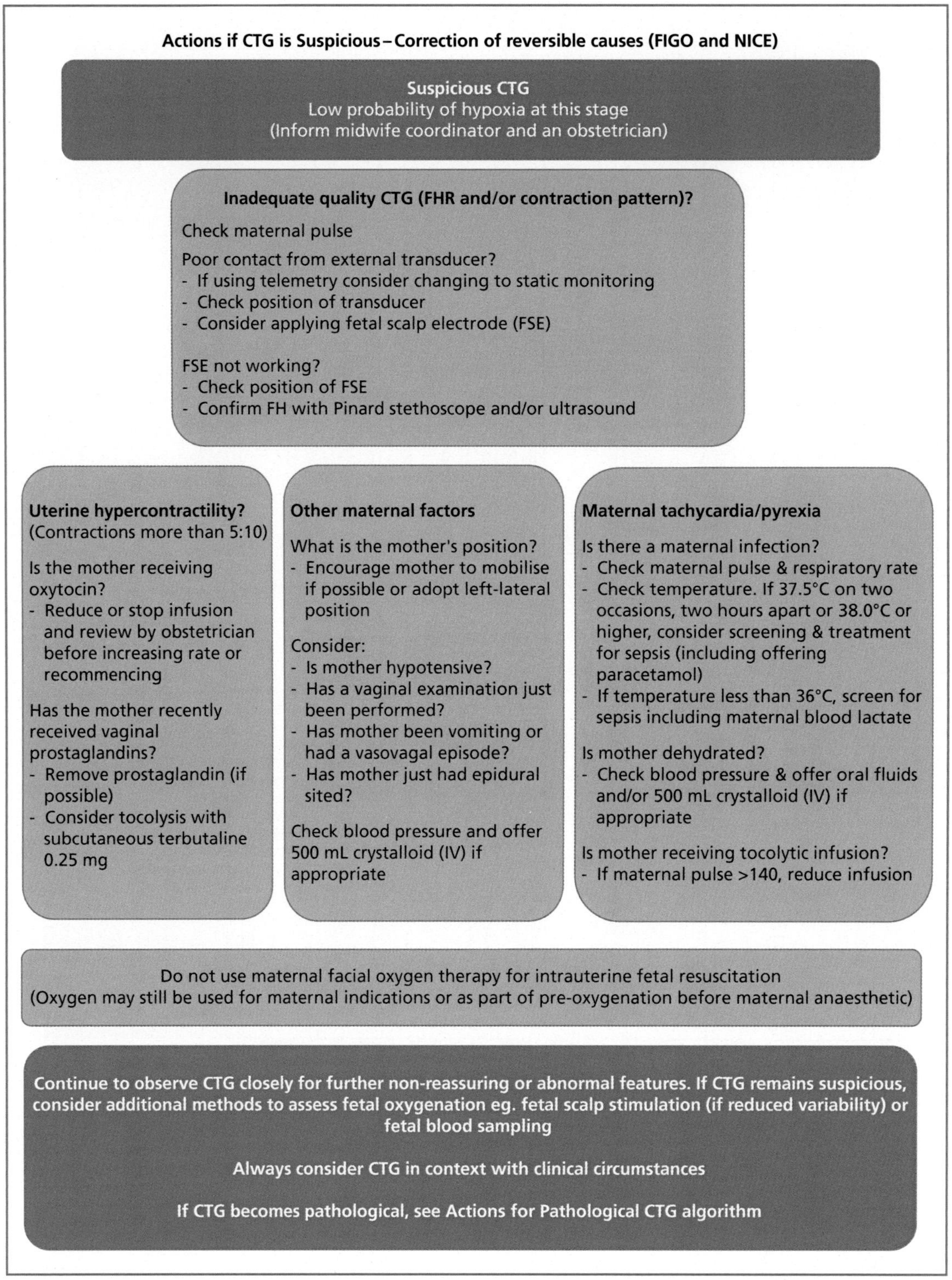

Actions if CTG is Suspicious – Correction of reversible causes (FIGO and NICE)

Suspicious CTG
Low probability of hypoxia at this stage
(Inform midwife coordinator and an obstetrician)

Inadequate quality CTG (FHR and/or contraction pattern)?

Check maternal pulse

Poor contact from external transducer?
- If using telemetry consider changing to static monitoring
- Check position of transducer
- Consider applying fetal scalp electrode (FSE)

FSE not working?
- Check position of FSE
- Confirm FH with Pinard stethoscope and/or ultrasound

Uterine hypercontractility?
(Contractions more than 5:10)

Is the mother receiving oxytocin?
- Reduce or stop infusion and review by obstetrician before increasing rate or recommencing

Has the mother recently received vaginal prostaglandins?
- Remove prostaglandin (if possible)
- Consider tocolysis with subcutaneous terbutaline 0.25 mg

Other maternal factors

What is the mother's position?
- Encourage mother to mobilise if possible or adopt left-lateral position

Consider:
- Is mother hypotensive?
- Has a vaginal examination just been performed?
- Has mother been vomiting or had a vasovagal episode?
- Has mother just had epidural sited?

Check blood pressure and offer 500 mL crystalloid (IV) if appropriate

Maternal tachycardia/pyrexia

Is there a maternal infection?
- Check maternal pulse & respiratory rate
- Check temperature. If 37.5°C on two occasions, two hours apart or 38.0°C or higher, consider screening & treatment for sepsis (including offering paracetamol)
- If temperature less than 36°C, screen for sepsis including maternal blood lactate

Is mother dehydrated?
- Check blood pressure & offer oral fluids and/or 500 mL crystalloid (IV) if appropriate

Is mother receiving tocolytic infusion?
- If maternal pulse >140, reduce infusion

Do not use maternal facial oxygen therapy for intrauterine fetal resuscitation
(Oxygen may still be used for maternal indications or as part of pre-oxygenation before maternal anaesthetic)

Continue to observe CTG closely for further non-reassuring or abnormal features. If CTG remains suspicious, consider additional methods to assess fetal oxygenation eg. fetal scalp stimulation (if reduced variability) or fetal blood sampling

Always consider CTG in context with clinical circumstances

If CTG becomes pathological, see Actions for Pathological CTG algorithm

Figure 5.12 Suggested actions if CTG is suspicious (based on FIGO and NICE)

Fetal scalp stimulation (FSS)

Fetal scalp stimulation (FSS) involves stimulating the fetal scalp by gently rubbing the scalp with the examiner's fingers. The main purpose of FSS is to evaluate fetuses that are showing reduced variability on the CTG to distinguish between deep sleep and hypoxia/acidosis. It has been reported that FSS may reduce the need for FBS in about 50% of cases.[33]

FIGO recommends that when FSS leads to the appearance of **an acceleration <u>and</u> subsequent normalisation of the fetal heart pattern**, this should be regarded as a reassuring feature, with a negative predictive value that is similar to pH > 7.25 on FBS. When FSS **does not** elicit the appearance of accelerations and subsequent normalisation of the CTG, the positive predictive value for fetal hypoxia/acidosis is limited. In these situations, continued monitoring and additional tests are recommended.[33]

Fetal blood sampling (FBS)

FBS as an adjunct to CTG is recommended by NICE and FIGO, although there is continued uncertainty as to whether it improves neonatal outcome and reduces intervention rates, as was originally intended. A recent review of seven trials with FBS as an adjunct and five studies with CTG only concluded that, based on these modest numbers with rather inconsistent results, FBS in addition to CTG can provide additional information on fetal wellbeing and can reduce the risk of operative birth.[34] NICE, therefore, considers that the use of FBS may help to reduce the need for further, more serious interventions.

NICE recommends that when FBS is undertaken, pH or fetal lactate can be measured, as long as the necessary equipment is available and there are suitably trained staff to interpret the results. Fetal lactate and fetal pH results are classified as shown in Table 5.3.

Table 5.3 Fetal lactate and fetal pH cord blood values

Fetal lactate (mmol/L)	Fetal pH	Interpretation
4.1 or below	7.25 or above	Normal
4.2–4.8	7.21–7.24	Borderline
4.9 or above	7.20 or below	Abnormal

FBS is only aimed at identifying fetal hypoxia, and therefore there may be some clinical circumstances, such as maternal sepsis or significant meconium, when a normal FBS result could be misleadingly interpreted as a reassuring result. It is important to remember that the fetus is still at risk due to the maternal sepsis, and further action may be required irrespective of a normal FBS result. The findings in such circumstances should always be discussed with a consultant obstetrician (FIGO and NICE).

FBS should not be undertaken if there is clear evidence of acute fetal compromise (e.g. prolonged deceleration longer than 3 minutes). Birth should then be expedited urgently, accounting for the severity of the FHR abnormality and relevant maternal and clinical factors. Ideally, birth should be expedited within 30 minutes (category 1 caesarean section or operative vaginal birth, dependent on circumstances).

Other contraindications to FBS include:

- maternal infection (e.g. HIV, hepatitis viruses and herpes simplex virus)
- fetal bleeding disorders (e.g. haemophilia)
- prematurity (gestational age < 34 weeks)

FBS should be undertaken with the mother in the left-lateral position. Figure 5.13 shows suggested actions if the CTG is pathological.[5,33]

If there is an abnormal FHR pattern and uterine hypercontractility which is not secondary to the use of an oxytocin infusion, tocolysis should be considered. The suggested regimen is subcutaneous terbutaline 0.25 mg.[5] Its use may also be considered to reduce uterine activity and aid in-utero resuscitation when preparing for a category 1 birth. If terbutaline is used, anticipate the possibility of uterine atony post-birth and treat accordingly.

Newborn assessment

In addition to the Apgar score, paired blood samples from the umbilical artery and umbilical vein should be collected to provide both clinical and biochemical information to differentiate between an asphyxiated infant and one that is depressed for other reasons (infection, congenital abnormalities or maternal analgesia). In the perinatal period, asphyxia is defined as the combination of hypoxia and acidosis with impaired organ function. Thus, the RCOG recommends that paired samples should be obtained in the following circumstances as a minimum:

- Emergency caesarean section
- Operative vaginal birth
- Shoulder dystocia
- Fetal blood sampling has been performed in labour
- CTG is considered suspicious or pathological
- The baby's condition is poor at birth with an Apgar score of 6 or less at 5 minutes

Suggested actions if CTG is pathological (FIGO and NICE)
(in addition to actions to correct reversible causes as listed in Suspicious CTG algorithm)

Pathological CTG
High probability of hypoxia – urgent action required
(Inform midwife coordinator and an obstetrician)

Is there a fetal bradycardia?
- Commence actions to correct reversible causes as listed in Suspicious CTG algorithm
- STOP oxytocin infusion
- Seek obstetric and midwife coordinator support
- Perform vaginal examination to exclude cord prolapse
- Make preparations for urgent birth
- Expedite birth if bradycardia persists for 9 minutes, or sooner if fetal heart rate is less than 80 bpm with reduced variability

Consider fetal scalp stimulation (FSS) if appropriate?
The main purpose of FSS is to evaluate fetuses that are demonstrating **reduced variability on the CTG**, to distinguish between deep sleep and hypoxia/acidosis
When FSS <u>does not</u> elicit the appearance of accelerations <u>and</u> subsequent normalisation of the CTG, continue monitoring and perform fetal blood sampling if possible/appropriate

Fetal blood sampling (FBS) possible and/or appropriate?
Encourage mother to adopt left-lateral position for FBS. Check BP and give 500 mL crystalloid (IV) if appropriate

Fetal blood sample result (pH)	Recommended action
Normal FBS result **7.25 or above**	• If the CTG remains pathological and there are no accelerations in response to fetal scalp stimulation, consider taking a second sample in 1 hour or sooner if there are other new abnormalities • Discuss with a consultant obstetrician if a third fetal blood sample is thought to be needed • If an FBS result is within the normal range, always consider clinical circumstances such as the presence of maternal sepsis or significant meconium, as the fetus may still be at risk
Borderline FBS result **7.21–7.24**	• If CTG remains pathological and there are no accelerations in response to fetal scalp stimulation, consider taking a second fetal blood sample in 30 minutes • Consider expediting birth if there is a rapid fall since the last sample • Discuss with a consultant obstetrician if a third fetal blood sample is thought to be needed
Abnormal FBS result **7.20 or below**	- Inform obstetric consultant and neonatal team - Discuss what is happening with woman and partner - Expedite birth within 30 minutes (category 1)

All FBS results should be interpreted taking into account the previous pH measurement, the rate of progress in labour and the clinical features of mother and fetus.

Fetal blood sampling not possible/inappropriate?
- Encourage mother to adopt left-lateral position. Check BP and give 500 mL crystalloid (IV) if appropriate
- If an FBS cannot be obtained but the associated fetal scalp stimulation results in fetal heart rate accelerations <u>and</u> normalisation of the CTG, decide whether to continue with the labour or to expedite birth considering the clinical circumstances, and after discussion with the consultant obstetrician and the woman

EXPEDITE BIRTH:
- The urgency and mode of birth should take into account the severity of the FHR and the clinical circumstances
- The accepted standard is that birth should be accomplished within 30 minutes
- A caesarean section or operative vaginal birth may be advised, depending on results of FBS and stage of labour

Figure 5.13 Suggested actions if CTG is pathological (based on FIGO and NICE)

If the baby is born in poor condition it may be helpful to process the cord blood samples through a point-of-care blood analyser that includes measurement of haemoglobin and lactate in addition to pH. Early identification of fetal anaemia or lactic acidosis will enable the neonatal team to instigate appropriate treatment in a timely manner. In addition, the umbilical cord acid–base status at time of birth can be important for medicolegal reasons and for risk management strategies.[35]

Antenatal CTG interpretation

Although the evidence for EFM use antenatally is based on only a few small studies (four trials and 1588 women in total) from the 1980s, when CTG monitoring was first being introduced into routine clinical practice, a Cochrane review did not confirm or refute any benefits of routine CTG monitoring of 'at risk' pregnancies.[36]

In clinical practice, there are a variety of antenatal indications for considering and undertaking a CTG from 26 weeks of gestation onwards. The presence of a normal fetal heart rate pattern (i.e. showing accelerations coinciding with fetal movements) is indicative of a healthy fetus with a properly functioning autonomic nervous system. Clinicians should remember that the need to perform an antenatal CTG suggests that the pregnancy is 'high risk' until proven otherwise. The presence of an abnormal FHR pattern in an antenatal CTG is particularly concerning.

The RCOG Green-top Guideline on the management of reduced fetal movements recommends that interpretation of the antenatal CTG fetal heart rate pattern can be assisted by adopting the NICE classification of fetal heart rate features as indicated in their intrapartum care guideline.[37]

Therefore, as is the case when classifying intrapartum CTGs, it would seem reasonable to use a structured pro forma to ensure the use of consistent terminology. However, using an intrapartum pro forma is not appropriate, as it acknowledges that some decelerations are acceptable in labour, which clearly cannot be the case for antenatal CTGs, where there are no contractions.

It is also important to remember that the reason for performing an antenatal CTG is particularly relevant when determining any action to be taken, as is the gestation, the status of the membranes and the findings of a full antenatal assessment.

Figure 5.14 is an example of an antenatal CTG pro forma that may be used for the classification of CTGs in non-labouring women only.

Antenatal CTG Pro forma	Reassuring	Non-reassuring			
Baseline rate (bpm)	110–160	Less than 110 Rate:	Comments:-		
	Rate:	More than 160 Rate:			
N.B Rising baseline rate even within normal range may be a concern if other non-reassuring features present					
Variability (bpm)	5 bpm or more	Less than 5 bpm for 50 minutes or more	Comments:-		
		Sinusoidal pattern for 10 minutes or more			
		Saltatory pattern of more than 25 bpm for 10 minutes or more			
Accelerations	Present	None for 50 minutes	Comments:-		
Decelerations	None	Unprovoked deceleration/s	Comments:-		
		Decelerations related to uterine tightenings (not in labour)			
Opinion	*Normal CTG* (All 4 features reassuring)	*Abnormal CTG* (1 or more non-reassuring features)			
Clinical information	Maternal pulse:	Membranes ruptured: Y/N If yes, date and time:	Liquor colour:		Gestation (wks):
Reason for CTG:					
Action: (An abnormal CTG requires prompt review by experienced obstetrician/senior midwife)					
Date:	Time:	Signature: .... Print: .... Designation:			

Figure 5.14 An example of an antenatal CTG pro forma

Antenatal CTG classification

Normal: A CTG where all four features fall into the 'reassuring' category

Abnormal: A CTG with any non-reassuring features (including any decelerations)

When an abnormal CTG is identified, it should be reviewed by an experienced obstetrician or senior midwife as soon as possible (within 30 minutes), and a clear individualised action plan should be made, to include:

- Other tests to be performed (ultrasound scan for growth, liquor volume, Doppler studies, etc.)
- A specified time for the next obstetric review
- Consideration for expediting birth

References

1. NHS Health Education England, Royal College of Obstetricians and Gynaecologists, Royal College of Midwives. e-Learning for Healthcare. Electronic fetal monitoring. www.e-lfh.org.uk/programmes/electronic-fetal-monitoring/ (accessed June 2017).

2. Hon EH. The electronic evaluation of the fetal heart rate; preliminary report. *Am J Obstet Gynecol* 1958; 75: 1215–30.

3. Beard RW, Filshie GM, Knight CA, Roberts GM. The significance of changes in the continuous fetal heart rate in the first stage of labour. *J Obstet Gynaecol Br Commonw* 1971; 78: 865–81.

4. Ayres-de-Campos D, Arulkumaran S; FIGO Intrapartum Fetal Monitoring Expert Consensus Panel. FIGO consensus guidelines on intrapartum fetal monitoring: introduction. *Int J Gynaecol Obstet* 2015; 131: 3–4.

5. Ayres-de-Campos D, Spong CY, Chandraharan E; FIGO Intrapartum Fetal Monitoring Expert Consensus Panel. FIGO consensus guidelines on intrapartum fetal monitoring: cardiotocography. *Int J Gynaecol Obstet* 2015; 131: 13–24.

6. MacDonald D, Grant A, Sheridan-Pereira M, Boylan P, Chalmers I. The Dublin randomised controlled trial of intrapartum fetal heart rate monitoring. *Am J Obstet Gynecol* 1985; 152: 524–39.

7. Nelson KB. What proportion of cerebral palsy is related to birth asphyxia? *J Pediatr* 1988; 152: 572–4.

8. Nelson KB, Willoughby RE. Infection, inflammation, and the risk of cerebral palsy. *Curr Opin Neurol* 2000; 13: 133–9.

9. Murphy KW, Johnson P, Moorcraft J, *et al.* Birth asphyxia and intrapartum tocograph. *Br J Obstet Gynaecol* 1990; 97: 470–9.

10. Confidential Enquiry into Stillbirths and Deaths in Infancy. *4th Annual Report.* London: Maternal and Child Health Research Consortium, 1997.

11. Confidential Enquiry into Stillbirths and Deaths in Infancy. *5th Annual Report.* London: Maternal and Child Health Research Consortium, 1998.

12. Confidential Enquiry into Stillbirths and Deaths in Infancy. *7th Annual Report.* London: Maternal and Child Health Research Consortium, 2000.

13. Alfirevic Z, Devane D, Gyte GM, Cuthbert A. Continuous cardiotocography (CTG) as a form of electronic fetal monitoring (EFM) for fetal assessment during labour. *Cochrane Database Syst Rev* 2017; (2): CD006066.

14. O'Connor D. *Saving Babies' Lives: A Care Bundle for Reducing Stillbirth.* NHS England, 2016. www.england.nhs.uk/wp-content/uploads/2016/03/saving-babies-lives-car-bundl.pdf (accessed June 2017).

15. Brocklehurst P, INFANT Collaborative Group. A study of an intelligent system to support decision making in the management of labour using the cardiotocograph: the INFANT study protocol. *BMC Pregnancy Childbirth* 2016; 16: 10.

16. INFANT Collaborative Group. Computerised interpretation of fetal heart rate during labour (INFANT): a randomised controlled trial. *Lancet* 2017; 389: 1719–29.

17. Royal College of Obstetricians and Gynaecologists. *Electronic Fetal Monitoring.* National Evidence-based Clinical Guideline. London: RCOG, 2001.

18. National Institute for Health and Care Excellence. *Intrapartum Care: Care of Healthy Women and Their Babies During Childbirth.* NICE Clinical Guideline CG55. London: NICE, 2007.

19. National Institute for Health and Care Excellence. *Intrapartum Care: Care of Healthy Women and Their Babies During Childbirth.* NICE Clinical Guideline CG190. London: NICE, 2014. Updated in 2017. www.nice.org.uk/guidance/cg190 (accessed June 2017).

20. National Institute for Health and Care Excellence. Exceptional review of fetal monitoring recommendations in CG190. www.nice.org.uk/guidance/GID-CGWAVE0613/documents/final-scope (accessed June 2017).

21. Clements RV, Simanowitz A. Cerebral palsy: the international consensus statement. *Clin Risk* 2000; 6: 135–6.

22. Pickering J. Legal comment on the international consensus statement on causation of cerebral palsy. *Clin Risk* 2000; 6: 143–4.

23. Berglund S, Pettersson H, Cnattingius S, Grunewald C. How often is low Apgar score the result of substandard care during labour? *BJOG* 2010; 117: 968–78.

24. NHS Litigation Authority. *Ten Years of Maternity Claims: An Analysis of NHS Litigation Authority Data*. London: NHSLA, 2012.

25. Draycott T, Sibanda T, Owen L, *et al.* Does training in obstetric emergencies improve neonatal outcome? *BJOG* 2006; 113: 177–82.

26. Weiner CP, Collins L, Bentley S, Dong Y, Satterwhite CL. Multi-professional training for obstetric emergencies in a U.S. hospital over a 7-year interval: an observational study. *J Perinatol* 2016; 36: 19–24.

27. Shoushtarian M, Barnett M, McMahon F, Ferris J. Impact of introducing practical obstetric multi-professional training (PROMPT) into maternity units in Victoria, Australia. *BJOG* 2014; 121: 1710–18.

28. Pehrson C, Sorensen J, Amer-Wahlin I. Evaluation and impact of cardiotocography training programmes: a systematic review. *BJOG* 2011; 118: 926–35.

29. Lagercrantz H, Bistoletti P. Catecholamine release in the newborn infant at birth. *Pediatr Res* 1977; 11: 889–93.

30. Lewis D, Downe S; FIGO Intrapartum Fetal Monitoring Expert Consensus Panel. FIGO consensus guidelines on intrapartum fetal monitoring: intermittent auscultation. *Int J Gynaecol Obstet* 2015; 131: 9–12.

31. Herbert WN, Stuart NN, Butler LS. Electronic fetal heart rate monitoring with intrauterine fetal demise. *J Obstet Gynecol Neonatal Nurs* 1987; 16: 249–52.

32. Maeder HP, Lippert TH. Misinterpretation of heart rate recordings in fetal death. *Eur J Obstet Gynecol* 1972; 6: 167–70.

33. Visser GH, Ayres-de-Campos D; FIGO Intrapartum Fetal Monitoring Expert Consensus Panel. FIGO Consensus guidelines on intrapartum fetal monitoring: adjunctive technologies. *Int J Gynaecol Obstet* 2015; 131: 25–9.

34. Jørgensen JS, Weber T. Fetal scalp blood sampling in labor: a review. *Acta Obstet Gynecol Scand* 2014; 93: 548–55.

35. MacLennan A. A template for defining a causal relation between acute intrapartum events and cerebral palsy: international consensus statement. *BMJ* 1999; 319: 1054–9.

36. Pattison N, McCowan L. Cardiotocography for antepartum fetal assessment. *Cochrane Database Syst Rev* 2000; (2): CD001068.

37. Royal College of Obstetricians and Gynaecologists. *Reduced Fetal Movements*. Green-top Guideline No. 57. London: RCOG, 2011. www.rcog.org.uk/womens-health/clinicalguidance/reduced-fetal-movements-green-top-57 (accessed June 2017).

Module 6
Pre-eclampsia and eclampsia

Key learning points

- To understand the risk factors and recognise the signs and symptoms of severe pre-eclampsia.

- To understand the potential complications of severe hypertension (systolic blood pressure ≥ 160 mmHg) and its urgent management.

- To manage an eclamptic fit/seizure effectively.

- To understand the care and monitoring required when a woman is being treated with magnesium sulfate.

- The importance of detailed contemporaneous documentation.

Common difficulties observed in training drills

- Not stating the problem clearly when help arrives
- Not involving a consultant obstetrician and anaesthetist in the management of women with severe pre-eclampsia and eclampsia
- Failure to adequately treat hypertension
- Failure to stabilise the woman, particularly the hypertension, before birth
- Forgetting to perform basic resuscitation during an eclamptic fit/seizure

Introduction

Hypertensive disorders are the second most common cause of maternal death worldwide.[1] In the UK, there has been a significant decrease in the maternal mortality rate from hypertensive disorders of pregnancy in the period between 2009–11 and 2012–14. In this 6-year period, 14 women died in the UK and Ireland; 11 died in 2009–11 (0.42 per 100,000 maternities), whereas only 3 women died in 2012–14 (0.11 per 100,000 maternities). In each of the previous 6-year periods 37 women died.[2,3] This is a very positive reflection on the improvements in the provision of care for women with hypertensive disorders in pregnancy. However, the major failing in clinical care remains inadequate treatment of hypertension resulting in intracranial haemorrhage; severe hypertension (systolic blood pressure above 160 mmHg) is extremely dangerous and must be treated urgently to prevent maternal mortality and morbidity.[4]

Pre-eclampsia

Pre-eclampsia is a multisystem disorder of pregnancy characterised by new hypertension presenting after 20 weeks of gestation with significant proteinuria.[4] Pre-eclampsia is a disorder of the vascular endothelial function specific to pregnancy and is thought to arise in the placenta as a result of ischaemia.

Pre-eclampsia is one of the most common underlying causes of maternal and perinatal mortality (Box 6.1), complicating approximately 3% of pregnancies in the UK.

Box 6.1 Maternal complications of pre-eclampsia

- Intracranial haemorrhage (leading cause of maternal death from severe pre-eclampsia in the UK)
- Placental abruption
- Eclampsia
- HELLP syndrome (characterised by haemolysis, elevated liver enzymes and low platelets)
- Disseminated intravascular coagulation
- Renal failure
- Pulmonary oedema
- Acute respiratory distress syndrome

Pre-eclampsia can affect the fetus and neonate, mediated through poor placental function. Fetal complications are listed in Box 6.2.

Box 6.2 Fetal complications of pre-eclampsia

- Fetal growth restriction
- Oligohydramnios
- Hypoxia from placental insufficiency
- Placental abruption
- Iatrogenic preterm birth

Predisposing risk factors for pre-eclampsia are shown in Box 6.3.

Box 6.3 Predisposing risk factors for pre-eclampsia[4]

- Nulliparity
- Pre-eclampsia during a previous pregnancy
- Hypertensive disease during a previous pregnancy
- Chronic hypertension
- Family history of pre-eclampsia
- Pre-existing diabetes
- Multiple pregnancy
- Obesity
- Extremes of maternal age
- Autoimmune disease (e.g. systemic lupus erythematosus, antiphospholipid syndrome)
- Renal disease
- Interval of 10 years or more since a previous pregnancy

Eclampsia

Eclampsia is defined as one or more seizures in association with pre-eclampsia.[4] Counterintuitively, the majority of women in the UK who have an eclamptic fit/seizure will not be hypertensive and proteinuric prior to their first eclamptic seizure.[5] Furthermore, 44% of seizures occur postpartum, 38% antepartum and 18% intrapartum. The recurrence rate of seizures is 5–30%, even with treatment.

In the UK, the incidence of eclampsia has fallen to 2.7/10,000 maternities (from 4.9/10,000 maternities in 1992).[2] There is a high rate of maternal complications associated with eclampsia, with at least one major morbidity complicating care for 10% of women after a seizure.[5] In the UK, the perinatal mortality associated with eclampsia remains 10 times that of normal pregnancies.[5] Therefore eclampsia, though rare and usually well managed, remains a high-risk condition that requires efficient and accurate management.

Presenting features

Eclampsia presents as generalised seizures, with jerking limb and head movements. The mother may become cyanosed, and tongue biting and/ or urinary incontinence can also occur. Most seizures are single and self-limiting, usually lasting less than 90 seconds. Eclampsia can be a very frightening experience for both family members and staff.

Management of eclampsia

The management of eclampsia should start with basic life support measures, along with direct management of the eclamptic seizures. An outline for the initial management of eclampsia is shown in Figure 6.1.

Call for help

Activate the emergency buzzer to summon help, or call 999 if you are working in the community. Help should ideally include a senior midwife, the most experienced obstetrician and anaesthetist available, and additional midwives and maternity care assistants to provide clinical support and document actions. Contact the consultant obstetrician and consultant anaesthetist as soon as possible.

- Note the time the seizure occurred and its duration.
- Note the time of the emergency call and time of arrival of staff.

Support: airway, breathing, circulation

Remember that most eclamptic seizures are self-limiting. Remain calm. Monitor and maintain airway, breathing and circulation as your first priority. Move the mother into the left-lateral position and protect her from injury.

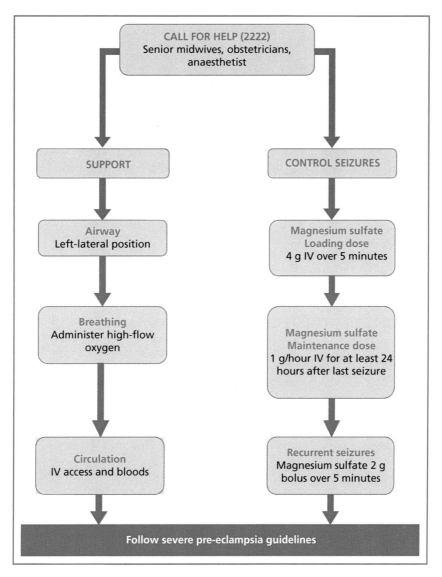

Figure 6.1 Outline of the initial management of eclampsia

Give high-flow facial oxygen using a non-rebreathe mask with a reservoir bag. Do not attempt to restrain the mother or use a tongue depressor during the seizure. Immediately following the eclamptic seizure, ensure that the woman is maintained in the left-lateral position with an open airway.

Eclampsia box

Many units will have an emergency box containing laminated treatment algorithms for eclampsia and severe hypertension as well as the emergency equipment and medication required for the immediate management of eclampsia (Figure 6.2).[7] This should be brought into the room as soon as possible.[8]

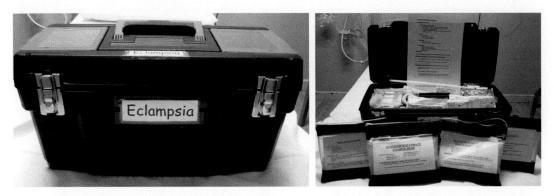

Figure 6.2 Eclampsia box, showing contents and laminated treatment algorithms

Control of seizures

Site a large-bore intravenous cannula and take bloods for: full blood count, urea and electrolytes, liver function tests, clotting, and group and save. Start treatment with magnesium sulfate.

> **Magnesium sulfate is the only medication that should be used to manage eclampsia.**

The results of the Collaborative Eclampsia trial demonstrated that women treated with magnesium sulfate have fewer recurrent seizures than women treated with diazepam or phenytoin.[9] Magnesium sulfate appears to act primarily by reducing cerebral vasospasm.[10] The intravenous route is preferable because intramuscular injections are painful and associated with local abscess formation in 0.5% of cases.

The Magpie trial demonstrated that magnesium sulfate can also prevent eclampsia, although the number of women needing treatment to prevent one woman having an eclamptic fit is high, particularly where the background rate of eclampsia is low.[11] It is therefore more likely to be effective when given to women with severe pre-eclampsia. Additionally, magnesium sulfate given shortly before birth has a neuroprotective effect on the preterm fetus, reducing the risk of cerebral palsy and protecting gross motor function.[12]

Magnesium sulfate emergency regimen

Loading dose: 4 g magnesium sulfate over 5 minutes

■ Draw up 8 mL of 50% magnesium sulfate solution (4 g) followed by 12 mL of 0.9% normal saline into a 20 mL syringe. This will give a total volume of 20 mL.

■ Give manually as an intravenous bolus over 5 minutes (4 mL/ minute).

Maintenance dose: 1 g/hour

■ Draw up 20 mL of 50% magnesium sulfate solution (10 g) followed by 30 mL of 0.9% normal saline into a 50 mL syringe. This will give a total volume of 50 mL. Place the syringe into a syringe driver and set the pump to run intravenously at 5 mL/hour.

■ Continue maintenance infusion for 24 hours following birth or the last seizure, i.e. whichever is the most recent event.

Recurrent seizures while on magnesium sulfate

■ Seek immediate senior help.

■ Draw up 4 mL of 50% magnesium sulfate solution (2 g) followed by 6 mL of 0.9% saline into a 10 mL syringe. This will give a total volume of 10 mL.

■ Give as an intravenous bolus over 5 minutes (2 mL/minute).

■ If possible, take blood for magnesium levels prior to giving the bolus dose.

The maternal condition must be stabilised prior to making plans for birth (if antenatal).

In the event of recurrent or prolonged seizures that are unresponsive to magnesium sulfate, consider other differential diagnoses, including hypoglycaemia or hyponatraemia, intracranial haemorrhage, epilepsy, a space-occupying cerebral lesion or a cerebral vein thrombosis. Organise urgent investigations and imaging (CT, MRI or magnetic resonance venogram) as appropriate. Women with recurrent or prolonged fits may require treatment with IV lorazepam or PR diazepam. Urgent anaesthetic assistance should be sought, as women with prolonged fits may require sedation with thiopentone or propofol.

Magnesium sulfate is excreted in the urine by the kidneys. Magnesium toxicity is unlikely to occur with the above regimen, and routine measurements of magnesium levels are not necessary as long as the woman has a normal urine output. However, if the woman is oliguric (< 100 mL urine over 4 hours) or has renal impairment, the kidneys will not excrete magnesium efficiently and magnesium levels are more likely to become toxic. In such circumstances, it is therefore advisable to administer only the loading dose. If the woman develops oliguria while receiving the maintenance infusion of magnesium sulfate, the infusion should be stopped and blood should be taken to measure the serum magnesium level. The therapeutic range for magnesium sulfate treatment is 2–4 mmol/L.

At toxic levels, magnesium causes a loss of deep tendon reflexes followed by respiratory depression, respiratory arrest and, ultimately, cardiac arrest. If maternal collapse occurs, follow the emergency protocol in Box 6.4. If toxicity is suspected, immediately stop the magnesium sulfate infusion and take blood for magnesium levels.

Box 6.4 Magnesium sulfate emergency protocol

CARDIOPULMONARY ARREST ON MAGNESIUM SULFATE
- Stop magnesium sulfate infusion.
- Start basic life support.
- Give 1 g calcium gluconate (or chloride) IV (10 mL of 10% solution).
- Intubate early and ventilate until respiration resumes.

Documentation

All personnel present at the emergency and all actions and treatment administered should be recorded as contemporaneously as possible. Figure 6.3 gives an example of an eclampsia documentation pro forma that may be used.

Attach Patient ID:

ECLAMPSIA DOCUMENTATION PRO FORMA

DATE: .... TIME OF SEIZURE: .... DURATION OF SEIZURE: ....

PERSONS PRESENT AT ONSET OF SEIZURE...

....

EMERGENCY BELL ACTIVATED   YES / NO   TIME....................................

If emergency bell not activated, please give reason...

	NAME	ALREADY PRESENT (✓)	TIME INFORMED	TIME ARRIVED
EXPERIENCED OBSTETRICIAN				
MIDWIFE COORDINATOR				
ANAESTHETIST				
JUNIOR OBSTETRICIAN				
MATERNITY HEALTHCARE ASSISTANT				
OTHER PERSONS ASSISTING				

CONSULTANT OBSTETRICIAN INFORMED   YES / NO   Name...

If no, give reason...

Time attended (if attended)...

TREATMENT

LEFT-LATERAL POSITION   YES / NO   TIME........................... If no, other position........................

HIGH FLOW O_2 YES / NO   TIME........................... If no, give reason...........................

IV ACCESS   YES / NO   TIME........................... If no, give reason...........................

BLOODS – GROUP + SAVE   YES / NO   TIME........................... If no, give reason...........................
FBC, CLOTTING, U+Es, LFTs
URATE

MAGNESIUM SULFATE INFUSION (see laminated regimen for dosages)	TIME COMMENCED
LOADING DOSE	
MAINTENANCE DOSE	

INITIAL POST SEIZURE OBSERVATIONS   TIME...............................

RESP RATE.................. PULSE RATE.................. BP..................mm/Hg 02 sats...................% TEMP..................°C

URINARY CATHETER INSERTED   YES / NO   TIME................ If no, give reason....................................

(Commence Maternity Critical Care Chart)

HYPERTENSIVE TREATMENT ADMINISTERED   YES/NO   TIME.....................................

If yes, please document medication given and dosage ....

....

FETAL WELLBEING (if appropriate)   FETAL HEART RATE.................bpm   TIME..............

POST SEIZURE CTG PERFORMED   YES / NO   NORMAL / SUSPICIOUS / PATHOLOGICAL

If CTG not performed, give reason...

Please complete Risk Management Reporting Form and attach copy of this pro forma – Thank you.

Figure 6.3 Example of eclampsia documentation pro forma

Severe pre-eclampsia management guidelines

The current NICE hypertension in pregnancy guideline[4] divides pre-eclampsia into different categories:

■ Severe hypertension (BP ≥ 160/110 mmHg) and proteinuria (proteinuria is defined as urinary protein:creatinine ratio > 30 mg/mmol, or > 300 mg protein in a 24-hour urine collection)

   or

■ Mild or moderate hypertension (BP ≥ 140/90 mmHg) and proteinuria with at least one of the following:
   □ Severe headache
   □ Problems with vision such as blurring or flashing
   □ Severe pain just below ribs or vomiting
   □ Papilloedema
   □ Signs of clonus (≥ 3 beats)
   □ Liver tenderness
   □ HELLP syndrome
   □ Platelet count falling to < 100 × 10^9/L
   □ Abnormal liver enzymes (ALT or AST rising to > 70 IU/L)

Clinical discretion should be used to include women who present with atypical symptoms, but where there is a suspicion of pre-eclampsia.[13]

Details of the management principles are outlined in Figure 6.4. These principles are discussed in more detail in the following section.

Management principles

The management of severe pre-eclampsia and eclampsia requires the initiation of complex treatment plans.[4] Local guidelines (based on current national guidance) should be available.

Community setting

If severe pre-eclampsia or eclampsia is diagnosed in the community setting, immediate urgent transfer to an obstetric unit must be arranged. Do not leave the woman unattended. Call 999 to summon an emergency ambulance and establish the estimated time of arrival. Contact the

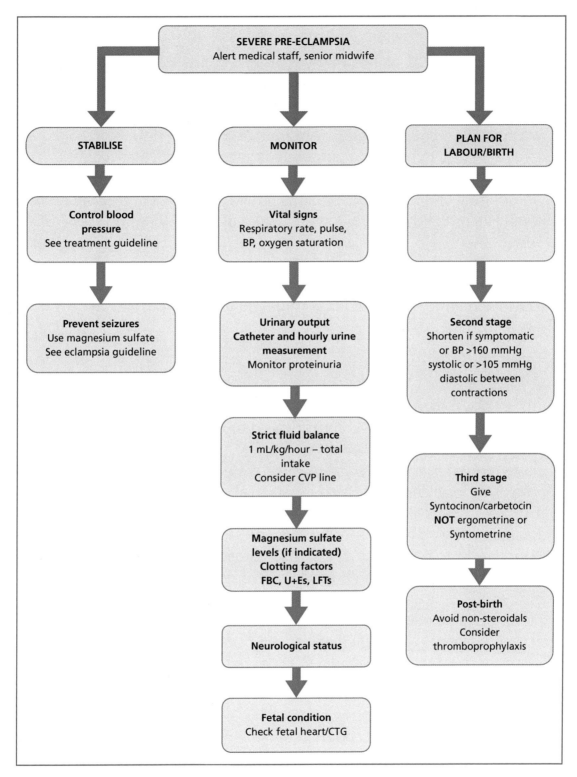

Figure 6.4 Outline management of severe pre-eclampsia

obstetric unit to inform them of the woman's arrival time and clinical status, preferably using an SBAR-like structure. The relevant teams (midwifery, obstetric, anaesthetic, neonatology) should be informed and the necessary emergency equipment should be pre-emptively prepared.

Intrapartum transfer to an obstetric unit from a midwife-led birth environment is recommended for any woman with a systolic blood pressure greater than 140 mmHg, or a diastolic blood pressure greater than 90 mmHg, on two consecutive readings, 30 minutes apart. Immediate transfer to an obstetric unit should be arranged if the systolic blood pressure is above 160 mmHg, or the diastolic blood pressure is above 110 mmHg.[4]

1. STABILISE

Effective and timely antihypertensive treatment is essential and can be life-saving.[2,13]

Control of hypertension

In the 2012–14 triennial report on maternal deaths, intracranial haemorrhage was the most common cause of death in women with eclampsia and pre-eclampsia with inadequate treatment of systolic hypertension contributing to the majority of deaths.[3] The exact causal mechanisms for hypertension and intracranial haemorrhage are still unclear, but **systolic hypertension poses the greatest risk.** Staff can be falsely reassured by relying on the mean arterial pressure or diastolic blood pressure and ignore the real threat of a very high systolic blood pressure. The NICE guideline for hypertension in pregnancy recommends that maternal blood pressure should be maintained below 150/100, with urgent treatment to achieve this in women with severe hypertension.[4] A severe hypertension treatment algorithm is outlined in Figure 6.5.

Antihypertensive medications should be continued in labour and at caesarean section (usually labetalol and/or nifedipine). Anaesthetists and obstetricians should be aware of the hypertensive effects of general anaesthesia during laryngoscopy, intubation and extubation. Hypertension should be controlled before a general anaesthetic is administered.[13]

Automated blood pressure recording devices can significantly underestimate blood pressure in pre-eclampsia. Therefore it is a useful precaution to initially crosscheck the automated blood pressure values with those obtained by a manual device with an appropriately sized cuff.[4] Consideration should also be given to the use of an arterial line for women for whom care is difficult to provide and/or manage.

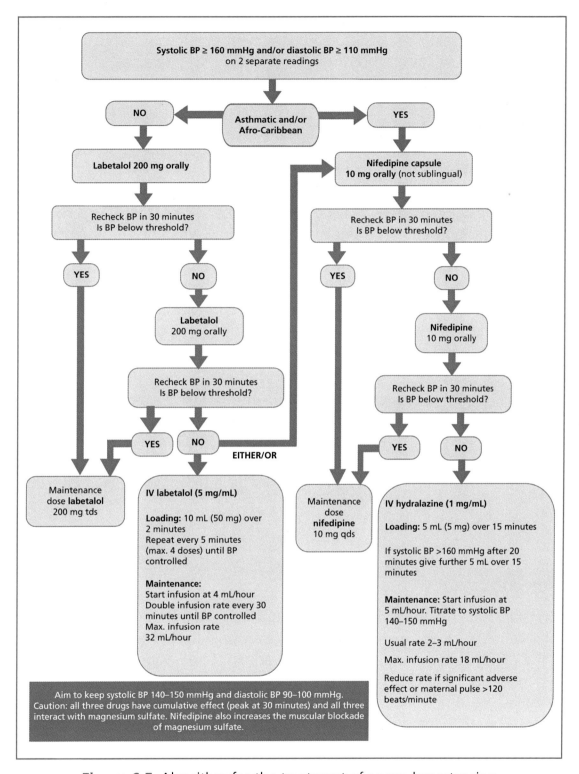

Figure 6.5 Algorithm for the treatment of severe hypertension

Note: All women presenting with new-onset headache or headache with atypical features, particularly focal symptoms, require a neurological examination including assessment for neck stiffness. Between 2009 and 2012, 26 women died (0.75/100,000 maternities) in the UK from intracranial haemorrhage.[2] The majority of women who presented with sudden collapse or severe headache had not expressed any symptoms prior to collapsing. It is important to exclude serious conditions such as intracranial haemorrhage before potentially misdiagnosing these women with migraine.

Choice of antihypertensive

The Guideline Development Group (GDG) for the NICE guideline[4] recognised that there are a number of antihypertensive options, but overall labetalol should be used as first-line treatment. However, there is a caveat that nifedipine can be offered after considering side-effect profiles for the woman, fetus and newborn baby. In making this recommendation, the GDG recognised the potential reduced effectiveness of labetalol in women of Afro-Caribbean origin, and clearly labetalol should be avoided for women with asthma.

Finally, the guideline makes no recommendation for hypertension that is resistant to monotherapy.[4] Many units pragmatically use both oral labetalol and oral nifedipine for some women with resistant hypertension. However, where the systolic BP is > 160 mmHg, parenteral options should be considered.

> **The 2012–14 MBRRACE-UK report identified intracranial haemorrhage as the single largest cause of death from pre-eclampsia in the UK failure to administer effective antihypertensive therapy was implicated in most cases. Systolic hypertension poses the greatest risk and high pressures (> 160 mmHg) should be treated as a medical emergency.**

Prevent seizures

Consider administering intravenous magnesium sulfate to reduce the risk of seizures in women with severe pre-eclampsia if birth is planned within 24 hours. Magnesium sulfate should be administered as per the eclampsia regimen: a loading bolus dose followed by a maintenance infusion. Magnesium sulfate should be continued for 24 hours from birth, or for 24 hours from the time of commencement if the woman is postnatal.

2. Monitor

A woman's condition can deteriorate rapidly. Vigilant observation and assessment is required, and observations should be recorded on a maternity critical care chart (see **Module 9** for more details).

■ Respiratory rate, pulse and blood pressure: every 15 minutes until stabilised, then every 30 minutes

- Hourly urine output: Foley catheter with urometer
- Hourly oxygen saturations
- Routine blood samples 6- to 24-hourly: FBC, clotting screen, U&Es, LFTs

Additional observations and investigation for mothers receiving magnesium sulfate:

- Continuously monitor oxygen saturation
- Hourly respiratory rate
- Hourly deep tendon reflexes
- If loss of reflexes, stop infusion and check magnesium levels:
  - ☐ If level less than 4 mmol/L or reflexes return, recommence infusion at 0.5 g/hour
- If oliguric (less than 100 mL urine in 4 hours), magnesium levels should be taken

Strict fluid balance

Close monitoring of fluid intake and urinary output is essential. Previous Confidential Enquiries have highlighted the risk of fluid overload causing pulmonary oedema in women with severe pre-eclampsia.[14] Reassuringly, between 2012 and 2014 no women died in relation to inappropriate fluid management (pulmonary oedema and renal failure).[3]

The maximum fluid intake (a combination of intravenous and oral intake) should be 1 mL/kg/hour. This is often approximated to 80 mL/hour. Beware of dilute drug administration and of excessive oxytocin, which may inhibit urinary output.

All women with severe pre-eclampsia should have an indwelling urinary catheter, with a urometer for hourly urine measurement. All fluid input and output should be clearly documented on a maternity critical care chart.

The aim is to 'run dry', as women die from fluid overload but rarely from renal failure. The intravenous fluid of choice (if required) for most cases will be a balanced crystalloid solution (e.g. Hartmann's solution – compound sodium lactate) or blood replacement if necessary.

Persistent oliguria (less than 100 mL of urine over 4 hours) requires careful management, as shown in Figure 6.6, and a central line should be considered. A central line may be helpful to aid fluid management when there are added complications such as a postpartum haemorrhage in a woman with severe pre-eclampsia. The aim is to maintain a central venous pressure in the range 0–5 mmHg. Great caution should be exercised with fluid treatment if the central venous pressure is greater than 5 mmHg.

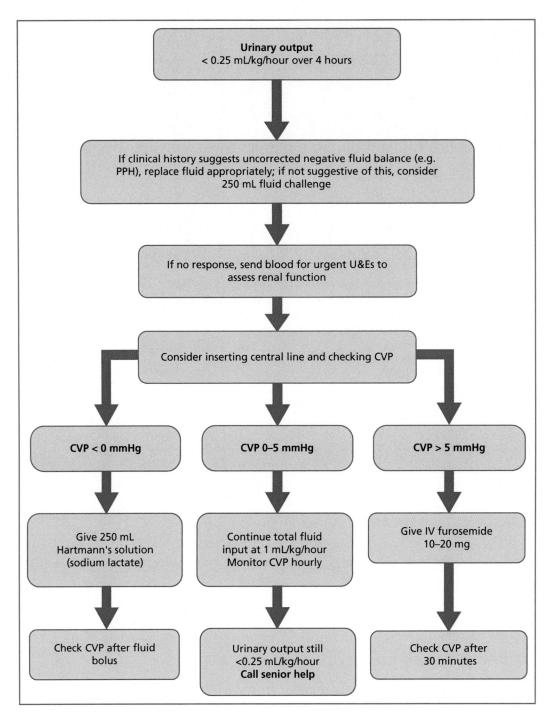

Figure 6.6 Fluid balance in the mother with oliguric pre-eclampsia

Pulmonary oedema

Pulmonary oedema is defined as fluid accumulation in the lungs that leads to impaired gas exchange and may cause respiratory failure. Pulmonary oedema can occur secondary to pre-eclampsia because of hypoalbuminaemia, increased capillary permeability and a high hydrostatic pressure (hypertension). See Box 6.5 for the clinical signs and symptoms of pulmonary oedema.

Box 6.5 Clinical signs and symptoms of pulmonary oedema

Symptoms	Signs
Shortness of breath	Tachypnoea
Unable to lie flat	Crepitations at lung bases
Unable to speak in full sentences	Decreasing oxygen saturations
Confusion/agitation	Positive fluid balance
	Tachycardia
	Frothy sputum (often pink)

The immediate management of pulmonary oedema is shown in Figure 6.7.

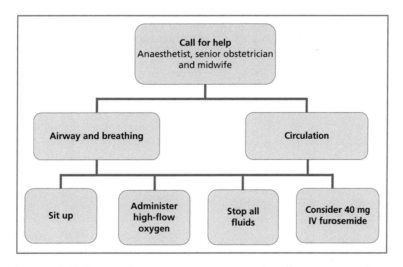

Figure 6.7 Immediate management of pulmonary oedema

Clotting abnormalities

Disseminated intravascular coagulation (DIC) is a potential complication of severe pre-eclampsia. Check activated partial thromboplastin time (APTT), prothrombin time and fibrinogen if platelet levels are less than 100 × 10^9/L. In addition, observe for clinical evidence of undue bleeding/bruises. If any of the investigations are abnormal, consider treatment with platelets, fresh frozen plasma (FFP), cryoprecipitate or fibrinogen concentrate and liaise with the on-call clinical haematologist (more information can be found in **Module 8**).

3. Plan for labour and birth

Make plans for the birth of the baby once the mother's condition is stable. The choice of caesarean section or induction of labour should be made on an individual basis. If the woman is 30 weeks' gestation or less, there are added benefits to administering prophylactic magnesium sulfate for fetal neuroprotection.[12]

First stage of labour

For the first stage of labour, close observation and the continuous attendance of an experienced midwife are required.

■ Continuous electronic fetal monitoring (EFM): there is increased risk of fetal hypoxia and placental abruption.

■ Consider the use of epidural anaesthesia (pain tends to increase blood pressure). Do not preload women with IV fluids prior to epidural or spinal.[4]

■ During labour, measure blood pressure every 15 minutes in women with severe hypertension, or hourly in women with mild or moderate hypertension.

Second stage of labour

It is safe for the mother to have a normal active second stage of labour provided that she does not have a severe headache, visual disturbances, or a systolic blood pressure higher than 160 mmHg. Consider expediting the vaginal birth if:

■ The mother complains of severe headache or visual disturbances.

■ The blood pressure is uncontrolled (higher than 160 mmHg systolic or higher than 105 mmHg diastolic between contractions) despite treatment.

Third stage of labour

The third stage of labour should be managed with oxytocin (Syntocinon; Novartis) 10 units IM or 5 units slow IV infusion or, after a caesarean section, carbetocin 100 micrograms IV given over 1 minute. **Syntometrine (Alliance; Syntocinon and ergometrine) and ergometrine should not be given to women with pre-eclampsia or eclampsia, as ergometrine exacerbates hypertension.**

Postnatal care

The mother will require continuous maternal critical care after birth. This may be for several hours or several days, depending on the circumstances. Remember that most eclamptic seizures occur in the postnatal period and pre-eclampsia can worsen several days after birth. If symptoms arise, monitor and investigate. Women may require transfer back to the labour ward for clinical monitoring.

Blood pressure should be checked at least four times a day while the woman is an inpatient. Antihypertensive treatment should be continued, but reduced if the blood pressure falls below 130/80 mmHg. Platelet count, renal and liver function should be tested as clinically indicated until they are improving, and again at the 6–8-week postnatal review. If the blood tests are normal at 48–72 hours post-birth, they do not need to be repeated. Observations should be plotted on a MOEWS chart, ideally incorporated into the maternal critical care chart (**Module 9**).

Ensure adequate analgesia, but note that non-steroidal anti-inflammatory drugs such as diclofenac *must not be given*, as they can precipitate renal failure.

Consider the need for thromboprophylaxis, because severe pre-eclampsia is a risk factor for thromboembolism. Apply thromboembolic deterrent stockings, for example TED (Covidien), as soon as possible and consider the use of pneumatic compression devices, for example Flowtron (ArjoHuntleigh). Commence low-molecular-weight heparin post-birth provided that the mother's platelet count is greater than 100×10^9/L.

The mother should be counselled regarding the long-term health risks following severe pre-eclampsia, HELLP syndrome or eclampsia.[4]

- Increased risk of pre-eclampsia in a future pregnancy:
    - 1 in 4 (25%) if pre-eclampsia led to birth at less than 34 weeks
    - 1 in 2 (55%) if pre-eclampsia led to birth at less than 28 weeks
- Increased lifetime risk of hypertension and cardiovascular disease
- Increased relative risk of end-stage kidney disease, although the absolute risk is low if proteinuria and hypertension are not present at 6–8 weeks postnatally

Prior to discharge, a care plan should be written outlining management in the community, including:[4]

- Frequency of blood pressure monitoring
- Thresholds for reducing or stopping antihypertensive medication
- Indications for referral for a medical review

References

1. Kassebaum NJ, Bertozzi-Villa A, Coggeshall MS, *et al.* Global, regional, and national levels and causes of maternal mortality during 1990–2013: a systematic analysis for the Global Burden of Disease Study 2013. *Lancet* 2014; 384: 980–1004.

2. Knight M, Kenyon S, Brocklehurst P, *et al.* (eds.); MBRRACE-UK. *Saving Lives, Improving Mothers' Care: Lessons Learned to Inform Future Maternity Care from the UK and Ireland Confidential Enquiries into Maternal Deaths and Morbidity 2009–12*. Oxford: National Perinatal Epidemiology Unit, University of Oxford, 2014.

3. Knight M, Nair M, Tuffnell D, *et al.* (eds.); MBRRACE-UK. *Saving Lives, Improving Mothers' Care: Surveillance of Maternal Deaths in the UK 2012–14 and Lessons Learned to Inform Maternity Care from the UK and Ireland Confidential Enquiries into Maternal Deaths and Morbidity 2009–14*. Oxford: National Perinatal Epidemiology Unit, University of Oxford, 2016.

4. National Institute for Health and Care Excellence. *Hypertension in Pregnancy: the Management of Hypertensive Disorders During Pregnancy*. NICE Clinical Guideline CG107. London: NICE, 2010. www.nice.org.uk/guidance/cg107 (accessed June 2017).

5. Knight M. Eclampsia in the United Kingdom 2005. *BJOG* 2007; 114: 1072–8.

6. Douglas KA, Redman CW. Eclampsia in the United Kingdom. *BMJ* 1994; 309: 1395–400.

7. Draycott T, Broad G, Chidley K. The development of an eclampsia box and fire drill. *Br J Midwifery* 2000; 8: 26–30.

8. Thompson S, Neal S, Clark V. Clinical risk management in obstetrics: eclampsia drills. *BMJ* 2004; 328: 269–71.

9. Duley L. Magnesium and eclampsia. *Lancet* 1995; 346: 1365.

10. Naidu S, Payne AJ, Moodley J, Hoffmann M, Gouws E. Randomised study assessing the effect of phenytoin and magnesium sulphate on maternal cerebral circulation in eclampsia using transcranial Doppler ultrasound. *Br J Obstet Gynaecol* 1996; 103: 111–16.

11. Altman D, Carroli G, Duley L, *et al.* Do women with pre-eclampsia, and their babies, benefit from magnesium sulphate? The Magpie Trial: a randomised placebo-controlled trial. *Lancet* 2002; 359: 1877–90.

12. Royal College of Obstetricians and Gynaecologists. *Perinatal Management of Pregnant Women at the Threshold of Infant Viability: the Obstetric Perspective*. Scientific Impact Paper No. 41. London: RCOG, 2014. www.rcog.org.uk/en/guidelines-research-services/guidelines/sip41/ (accessed June 2017).

13. Lewis G (ed.); Confidential Enquiry into Maternal and Child Health (CEMACH). *Saving Mothers' Lives: Reviewing Maternal Deaths to Make Motherhood Safer 2003–2005. The Seventh Report on Confidential Enquiries into Maternal Deaths in the United Kingdom*. London: CEMACH, 2007.

14. Confidential Enquiry into Stillbirths and Deaths in Infancy. *5th Annual Report*. London: Maternal and Child Health Research Consortium, 1998.

Module 7
Maternal sepsis

Key learning points

- Recognise maternal sepsis.
- Importance of using modified obstetric early warning score (MOEWS) charts.
- Importance of senior, multi-professional clinician involvement.
- Use of serum lactate to triage sepsis severity.
- Need for early intravenous antibiotics and fluids.
- Knowledge of the emergency management of sepsis and septic shock.
- Understand the role of the Sepsis Six.

Common difficulties observed in training drills

- Not stating the problem or the possibility of maternal sepsis
- Failure to measure the woman's respiratory rate
- Not plotting clinical observations correctly on a MOEWS chart
- Failure to recognise clinical features of sepsis, especially non-obstetric causes
- Delayed administration of antibiotics
- Failure to treat sepsis with a fluid bolus
- Failure to take microbiology cultures and serum lactate
- Failure to summon appropriate senior support early
- Failure to liaise with critical care if woman is unresponsive to Sepsis Six, or if lactate is greater than 4 mmol/L

Introduction

Before the introduction of antibiotics in the 1940s, genital tract sepsis was the leading cause of maternal death in the UK, accounting for over one-third of direct deaths occurring in pregnancy and childbirth. Since then, the number of maternal deaths attributable to sepsis has fallen dramatically.

In more recent years, there has been a concerning increase in maternal deaths due to sepsis. In the 2006–08 Confidential Enquiry into Maternal Deaths, almost a quarter of all maternal deaths were due to sepsis: the highest reported mortality rate due to genital tract sepsis for 20 years (Table 7.1).[1] Thankfully, death rates from maternal sepsis have reduced since then, although sepsis overall remains a leading contributor to maternal mortality and is also responsible for significant maternal morbidity. During 2009–12, 83 women died from sepsis; 20 of these deaths were related to infections of the genital tract, while 63 women died from sepsis associated with other infections not directly linked to pregnancy. Influenza was a significant contributor to deaths from sepsis, with 36 maternal deaths associated with the H1N1 influenza pandemic in 2009–10, but a range of other infections including meningitis, pneumonia, urinary tract infections and breast abscess all resulted in maternal deaths during this period.[2]

Table 7.1 Number and proportion of maternal deaths from genital tract sepsis in the UK

	1952–54	1985–87	2000–02	2003–05	2006–08	2009–12[a]
Rate/100,000 maternities	7.8	0.40	0.65	0.85	1.13	0.5
Number (all organisms)	—	9	13	21	26	20
Number (GAS)*	—	—	3	8	13	12

[a] Note 4-year period reported for MBRRACE-UK compared to triennial reporting in previous reports, such that case numbers cannot be compared directly

*GAS, group A *Streptococcus*.

Despite the observed increase in sepsis overall, life-threatening maternal sepsis remains a rare obstetric emergency in the UK, and many doctors and midwives may have never had to manage such a case. Worldwide, sepsis remains a very important cause of maternal death: in 2005, over 80,000 women across the world died from pregnancy-related sepsis.[3]

The immune suppression associated with normal pregnancy means that pregnant women are uniquely susceptible to developing sepsis.[2] Pregnant or postpartum women are usually relatively young and fit and can often withstand the effects of sepsis until it is life-threatening, and they often appear relatively well up until the point of sudden collapse. Women with medical comorbidities and those who have undergone surgical interventions are at increased risk of acquiring sepsis; however, previously fit and healthy women with normal pregnancies and straightforward vaginal births also continue to die from sepsis.[2]

What is sepsis?

Sepsis is a life-threatening condition that arises when the body's response to an infection injures its own tissues and organs.[4] The source of the infection may be found in a particular body region (e.g. chorioamnionitis) or may be widespread in the bloodstream, resulting in septicaemia. Sepsis is a medical emergency because it can result in an interruption to the supply of oxygen and nutrients to vital organs such as the brain, heart, liver, kidneys, lungs and intestines, resulting in acidosis, organ failure and death.

Prevention of sepsis

The importance of hand washing, hygiene and antisepsis is well established in maternity care.

In Vienna in the mid-nineteenth century, Dr Ignaz Semmelweis observed a marked increase in maternal mortality rates in patients under the care of doctors compared with those under the care of midwives. He also noted that doctors coming straight from the autopsy room to the delivery room had a disagreeable smell on their hands. He postulated that puerperal fever was caused by particles transmitted via the hands of the doctors. Semmelweis ordered a mandatory hand-washing policy for doctors, requiring them to use a chlorinated solution before they examined women in labour. This intervention resulted in a dramatic fall in maternal mortality.[5]

More recent techniques to reduce the incidence of maternal sepsis include barrier nursing, the use of antibiotic prophylaxis for preterm and prolonged rupture of membranes, and the use of perioperative antibiotics for caesarean births, manual removal of placenta and anal sphincter tear repairs.

Recognition of sepsis

The onset of life-threatening sepsis in pregnancy or the puerperium can be insidious or may show extremely rapid clinical deterioration, particularly when it is the result of streptococcal infection. In many of the sepsis-related maternal deaths reviewed by the Confidential Enquires in the UK, women had a short duration of illness and in some cases were moribund by the time they presented to hospital. It is therefore essential that all staff, including community midwives, maternity care assistants, health visitors, emergency department staff and general practitioners, are aware of the signs and symptoms of sepsis. The potential severity of illness in women presenting with signs and symptoms of sepsis is often unrecognised or underestimated, resulting in delays in referral to hospital, delays in administration of appropriate antibiotic treatment, and late involvement of senior medical staff.[6]

Women themselves should also be informed of the risks, signs and symptoms of genital tract infection and the need for them to seek early advice if they are concerned.[1]

Signs and symptoms

Genital tract sepsis

Common signs and symptoms of obstetric sepsis are shown in Box 7.1. Women with genital tract sepsis may present with abdominal pain, diarrhoea and vomiting. Some, but not all, will have a raised temperature. It can be very difficult to differentiate such symptoms from gastroenteritis, and therefore all pregnant or postnatal women presenting with such symptoms should be carefully examined. Women may also present antenatally with offensive vaginal discharge or with increased and/or offensive lochia in the puerperium. Antenatally, the combination of abdominal pain and an abnormal or absent fetal heart rate may signify sepsis rather than placental abruption.

Many of the deaths from genital tract sepsis in the Confidential Enquiries were caused by group A *Streptococcus* (GAS). This bacterium is commonly carried on the skin and in nasal passages, particularly in young children. It can cause localised upper respiratory tract (tonsillitis, pharyngitis) or skin infections (impetigo), but pregnant and postpartum women seem

---

Box 7.1 Signs and symptoms of genital tract sepsis

Symptoms	Signs
Fever	Tachypnoea/raised respiratory rate (respiratory rate greater than 24 breaths/minute)
Diarrhoea	
Vomiting	Hypotension (systolic blood pressure less than 90 mmHg)
Abdominal pain	
Sore throat	Tachycardia (heart rate greater than 100 bpm)
Upper respiratory tract infection	Pyrexia (higher than 38 °C) or hypothermia (lower than 36 °C)
Vaginal discharge	Rash (scarlet patches over generalised redness or petechial)
Wound infection	
	Low oxygen saturations (less than 95% on air)
	Poor peripheral perfusion (capillary refill of more than 2 seconds)
	Pallor
	Clamminess
	Anxiousness, confusion, feeling of 'impending doom'
	Mottled skin
	Low urine output (less than 0.5 mL/kg/hour)

---

to be particularly vulnerable to invasive infection, which can rapidly lead to overwhelming sepsis.[7] The Confidential Enquiries show that puerperal sepsis caused by GAS is commonly preceded by a sore throat or other upper respiratory tract infection, and most of the women who died from GAS had either worked with, or had their own, young children.[1]

Women may also present with a rash. The typical rash of GAS (Figure 7.1) develops over 12–48 hours, first appearing as erythematous (red) patches on the chest and axillae which spread to the trunk and extremities. Typically, the rash consists of scarlet patches over generalised redness (a patchy sunburnt appearance). This rash will momentarily disappear with pressure, unlike the petechial rash typical of meningococcal septicaemia.

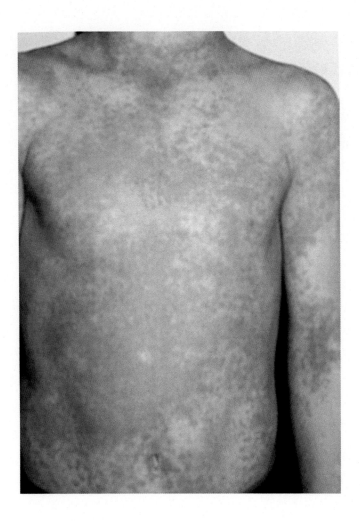

Figure 7.1 Group A
Streptococcus rash

Non-obstetric sepsis

Sepsis can develop from bacterial or viral infections occurring at any site. Certain infections are more common during pregnancy, e.g. urinary tract infections or pyelonephritis, and pregnancy can make the diagnosis of some infections, e.g. appendicitis, more difficult. A careful history and thorough examination are required to identify the most likely source of infection in women presenting with sepsis. As mentioned previously, 43% of women (n = 36) who died from sepsis in the 2009–12 MBRRACE-UK report were suffering from influenza, and a further nine died from pneumococcal disease.[2] Irrespective of the cause of infection, women with sepsis can initially appear deceptively well. They may maintain their blood pressure and conceal serious illness for a prolonged period before sudden cardiovascular decompensation. It is therefore vital that basic clinical observations (respiratory rate, heart rate, blood pressure, temperature and, if available, oxygen saturations) are monitored for every woman who presents with any risk factors or symptoms suggestive of infection, or who simply 'just feels unwell'.

People with sepsis often have non-specific, non-localised presentations, and survivors often report having felt extremely unwell, with a sense of 'impending doom'. These presentations, as well as concerns of changes in usual behaviour, as is often reported by family members, should be taken seriously.[8] Box 7.1 lists some of the signs and symptoms.

Risk factors

Many women who present with sepsis will have no risk factors. Risk factors for sepsis are listed in Box 7.2 and potential causes of sepsis are listed in Box 7.3. In a postpartum woman with possible sepsis, any history of ragged membranes or possible incomplete placenta should be noted, and the woman should be examined for the presence of uterine tenderness or enlargement.

Box 7.2 Risk factors for maternal sepsis

- Retained products of conception (following miscarriage, termination of pregnancy or birth)
- Caesarean birth (an emergency caesarean birth carries a greater risk than an elective or planned procedure)
- Operative vaginal birth
- Prolonged ruptured membranes
- Preterm labour
- Wound haematoma
- Invasive intrauterine procedure (e.g. removal of retained products, amniocentesis, chorionic villus sampling)
- Cervical suture
- Obesity
- Impaired immunity (e.g. immunosuppressants, high-dose steroids, HIV infection)
- Diabetes mellitus
- Working with, or having, young children
- Close contact with people with group A streptococcal infection (e.g. scarlet fever)

> **Box 7.3 Potential causes of maternal sepsis**
>
> **Pregnancy-related**
>
> Chorioamnionitis following:
> - Retained products of conception
> - Prolonged ruptured membranes
> - Caesarean birth
> - Invasive procedures
>
> Postoperative causes:
> - Caesarean birth
> - Cervical suture
> - Haematoma
> - Amniocentesis
>
> Breast abscess or mastitis
>
> **Non-pregnancy-related**
>
> Pneumonia
>
> Influenza
>
> Meningitis
>
> Appendicitis (may present atypically in pregnancy)
>
> Pyelonephritis (more common in pregnancy)
>
> Cholecystitis
>
> Bowel perforation (more common with inflammatory bowel disease)
>
> Cellulitis

Management

Maternal sepsis can be challenging to manage, but better training, a structured approach, earlier recognition and good care in both community and hospital settings may help to save lives. Prompt investigation and treatment, particularly immediate intravenous antibiotic treatment, intravenous fluids and early involvement of senior clinical staff, is crucial. Recently in the UK, the National Institute for Health and Care Excellence (NICE) has published guidance on the identification and management of sepsis, including maternal sepsis.[8] This guidance uses the identification of sepsis risk factors to guide appropriate investigations and management, based on completing all 'Sepsis Six' actions within 1 hour.

'Sepsis Six' – actions within 1 hour

The management of maternal sepsis requires the rapid initiation of multiple overlapping actions. The exact sequence will be dictated by the needs of the individual mother and the resources available. To avoid unnecessary delays in treatment, it is important that the clinicians who document an action plan in the maternal notes should also initiate the actions required, such as administering the antibiotics and commencing fluids.[2] An outline of the risk assessment to aid in the identification of maternal sepsis is shown in Figure 7.2, and the initial actions when there is a high risk of maternal sepsis are listed in Figure 7.3.

Risk assessment and action for suspected maternal sepsis
(adapted from UK Sepsis Trust Inpatient Maternal Sepsis Tool – 2016)

1. Has MOEWS been triggered?
2. Does the woman look sick?
3. Is the fetal heart rate ≥ 160 bpm?
4. Could this woman have an infection?
   Common infections include:
   - Chorioamnionitis/endometritis
   - Urinary tract infection
   - Wound infection
   - Influenza/pneumonia
   - Mastitis/breast abscess

Affix Patient ID

If YES to any of the above, complete risk assessment

High-risk criteria (tick all those that are appropriate)	Moderate-risk criteria (tick all those that are appropriate)	Low-risk criteria (tick all those that are appropriate)
• Respiratory rate ≥ 25 ☐ • SpO$_2$ < 92% without O$_2$ ☐ • Heart rate > 130 ☐ • Systolic BP ≤ 90 ☐ • Altered mental status/ responds only to voice, pain or unresponsive ☐ • Blood Lactate ≥ 2.0* ☐ • Non-blanching rash/mottled/ cyanotic ☐ • Urine < 0.5 mL/kg/hr ☐ • No urine for 18 hours ☐	• Respiratory rate 21–24 ☐ • Heart rate 100–130 ☐ • Systolic BP 91–100 ☐ • Temperature < 36°C ☐ • No urine output for 12–18 hours ☐ • Fetal heart > 160bpm/pathological CTG ☐ • Prolonged ruptured membranes ☐ • Recent invasive procedure ☐ • Bleeding/wound infection/vaginal discharge/abdominal pain ☐ • Close contact with Group A Strep ☐ • Relatives concerned about mental/ functional status ☐ • Diabetes/ gestational diabetes/ immunosuppressed ☐	• Respiratory rates ≤ 20 ☐ • Heart rate < 100 ☐ • Systolic BP > 100 ☐ • Normal mental status ☐ • Temperature: 36–37.3°C ☐ • Looks well ☐ • Normal CTG ☐ • Normal urine output ☐
If ONE criterion is present:		**If ALL criteria are present:**
Commence 'Sepsis Six' NOW • **Immediate obstetric review ST3 or higher** (transfer to Obstetric Unit if in the community) • **Inform consultant obstetrician & consultant anaesthetist** • **Commence Maternal Critical Care Chart** • **Commence 'High Risk of Maternal Sepsis' Pro forma**	**If TWO criteria are present (also consider if only ONE criterion):** **Send bloods:** FBC, lactate, CRP, U+Es, LFTs, clotting **OBSTETRIC REVIEW (ST3 or higher) within one hour** **Consider 'Sepsis Six'** Review Bloods: If lactate ≥ 2 or acute kidney injury present, follow HIGH risk pathway	**LOW RISK OF SEPSIS** Review and monitor for improvement or deterioration Consider obstetric needs and full clinical picture

* NB: Lactate measurement may be transiently elevated during and immediately after normal labour and birth. If unsure, repeat sample.

Completed by:
Name: Designation: Time:
Signature: Date:

Figure 7.2 Risk assessment for suspected maternal sepsis
(adapted from UK Sepsis Trust)

High Risk of Maternal Sepsis Pro forma

(adapted from the UK Sepsis Trust

Inpatient Maternal Sepsis Tool - 2016)

Affix Patient ID

CALL FOR HELP and complete ALL 'SEPSIS SIX' ACTIONS within ONE HOUR		Time zero:

Action	Time completed & initials	Reason not done/ variance/comments
1. Administer 100% OXYGEN ○ 15 L/min via non-rebreathe mask ○ Aim to keep saturations > 94%		
2. Take BLOOD CULTURES *(but do not delay administering antibiotics)* ○ Also consider sputum/urine/high vaginal swab/throat swab/breast milk sample/wound swab/stool sample, etc		
3. Take bloods – CHECK SERUM LACTATE ○ If venous lactate raised, recheck with arterial sample ○ Discuss with critical care if lactate ≥ 4 mmol/L ○ Continue to check serial serum lactates to monitor response to treatment (& FBC, CRP, U+Es, LFTs, clotting)		
4. Give IV BROAD SPECTRUM ANTIBIOTICS (as Trust protocol) ○ Administer urgently, consider allergies ○ Aim to take blood culture first but do not delay antibiotics if culture bottles not available		
5. Give IV FLUID THERAPY ○ If lactate 2 mmol/L give 500 mL stat ○ If hypotensive or lactate 4 mmol/L can repeat boluses up to 30 mL/kg (e.g. 2 L for a 70 kg woman) ○ Extreme caution if woman has pre-eclampsia: discuss with anaesthetist		
6. Accurate MEASUREMENT OF URINE OUTPUT ○ Urinary catheter & hourly measurement ○ Document fluid balance record		

If after 'Sepsis Six': systolic BP remains < 90 mmHg, level of consciousness remains altered, respiratory rate > 25, lactate not reducing (or was previously ≥ 4 mmol/L), refer IMMEDIATELY to critical care team

Also consider: ○ If antenatal – monitor fetal heart rate/commence CTG ○ Remove the source of infection e.g. retained products, expedite birth ○ Refer to Critical Care Team	**Document actions taken:**

Maternal sepsis requires multi-professional team input from: (tick staff contacted)

• Midwife coordinator	☐	• Microbiologist	☐
• Senior/consultant obstetrician	☐	• Intensive/critical care team	☐
• Senior obstetric anaesthetist	☐		

Figure 7.3 Maternal sepsis documentation pro forma (adapted from UK Sepsis Trust)

This set of interventions, adapted from the UK Sepsis Trust and the Sepsis Six principles, was introduced in the UK to simplify the initial management of women with maternal sepsis.[9] One prospective observational study has shown that using the Sepsis Six increases the uptake of other, more complex, interventions in sepsis.[10] The use of the Sepsis Six is only the first stage of management, and is described in more detail in the next section.

Call for help and complete ALL 'Sepsis Six' actions within 1 hour

Early involvement of senior midwives, obstetricians, anaesthetists and critical care consultants is crucial. Then consider the need for referral to critical care.

1. Administer 100% oxygen: support airway, breathing, circulation

Monitor and maintain airway, breathing and circulation as your first priority. If the woman has collapsed, check that her airway is patent and that she is breathing. Give high-flow oxygen by facemask with a reservoir bag at 15 L/minute, and ensure the woman is maintained in the left-lateral position. Aim to keep oxygen saturations above 94%. Secure intravenous access as soon as possible.

2. Take blood cultures and perform a full clinical examination

A full clinical examination should be performed with the aim of identifying the cause of the sepsis. This should be a top-to-toe examination including a vaginal examination to exclude retained tampons or swabs.

Swabs or cultures should be taken from all potential sources of sepsis. Samples should be sent urgently to the microbiology laboratory, where immediate microscopy should be performed on appropriate samples. The results of microbiology testing should be promptly followed up and antibiotic treatment altered accordingly.

Samples should include:

- Blood cultures (from at least two separate sites and from all intravenous cannulae that have been in place for longer than 48 hours). However, **DO NOT DELAY ADMINISTERING ANTIBIOTICS.**
- Vaginal swabs and wound swabs

- Urine culture
- Throat swab
- Stool sample
- Sputum sample
- Placental swabs (if immediately postpartum)

The most common pathogen associated with death from genital tract sepsis in the UK is group A *Streptococcus*, also known as puerperal sepsis, childbed fever or strep A. Other pathogens which commonly cause genital tract sepsis include *Escherichia coli*, group B beta-haemolytic *Streptococcus, Staphylococcus aureus*, coagulase-negative *Staphylococcus, Pseudomonas* and mixed anaerobes/*Bacteroides* species. Many women with genital tract sepsis will have a mixed infection with two or more organisms.

3. Blood tests

Serum lactate

Women with severe sepsis or septic shock typically have a high serum lactate, which may be secondary to anaerobic metabolism attributable to poor tissue perfusion. A lactate level greater than or equal to 4 mmol/L indicates a poor prognosis[11] and should trigger referral to critical care. Obtaining a lactate level is essential for identifying tissue hypoperfusion in women who are not yet hypotensive but who are at risk of septic shock. An arterial blood gas analyser located on the labour ward or in the neonatal intensive care unit will often be able to measure a serum lactate level. Note that serum lactate can be raised during and immediately following normal labour.[12] If in doubt, seek senior advice and repeat the lactate measurement after birth.

Because of the high risk of septic shock, the UK Sepsis Trust recommends that any woman with reduced tissue perfusion (e.g. with serum lactate ≥ 4 mmol/L) or suspected hypovolaemia due to sepsis is given an initial fluid challenge of 500 mL crystalloid in 15 minutes, regardless of her blood pressure. If there is no improvement in the serum lactate level following treatment with the Sepsis Six, the woman should be referred to intensive care for possible vasopressor support.[9]

Full blood count

The white blood cell count (WBC) is commonly raised (more than 14×10^9/L) with a high neutrophil count in sepsis. However, the WBC can also be low (less than 4×10^9/L), which may indicate an increased severity of illness. The platelet count may be low or raised.

Renal and liver function

Acute tubular necrosis may develop, which can lead to renal failure with raised urea, creatinine and potassium levels. The pro-inflammatory state of sepsis can also lead to hyperbilirubinaemia and jaundice.

C-reactive protein

C-reactive protein, or CRP, is an inflammatory marker that is commonly raised during infection, particularly bacterial infection. Monitoring the trend in CRP can be a useful guide to whether or not a woman is responding to treatment of her infection.

Clotting studies

Disseminated intravascular coagulation (DIC) is a potential complication of severe sepsis. The activated partial thromboplastin time (APTT), prothrombin time and fibrinogen should be checked. In addition, observe for clinical evidence of undue bleeding/bruising. If any of the investigations are abnormal, consider treatment with platelets, fresh frozen plasma (FFP) and/ or cryoprecipitate/fibrinogen concentrate and liaise with the on-call clinical haematologist.

Arterial blood gas

An arterial blood gas is a very useful investigation in any patient who is unwell. It is likely to show acidaemia (arterial pH < 7.35). This is typically a metabolic acidosis secondary to lactate production, as demonstrated by a low serum bicarbonate (normal value 24–33 mmol/L), as bicarbonate is consumed in buffering hydrogen ions, or a base excess below −2.0 mEq/L. Respiratory compensation can occur in the form of hyperventilation leading to a low $PaCO_2$, but this seldom completely corrects the low pH. As septic shock progresses, metabolic acidosis will worsen and compensatory mechanisms are exhausted. As a consequence, the blood pH decreases further (e.g. < 7.20). Early respiratory failure can lead to hypoxia with PaO_2 < 8 kPa on room air.

4. Broad-spectrum intravenous antibiotic treatment

Immediate high-dose broad-spectrum intravenous antibiotic therapy (e.g. 1.5 g cefuroxime and 500 mg metronidazole), in accordance with local prescribing guidelines and known patient allergies, should be commenced as soon as possible. Antibiotic administration should not be delayed to await results of microbiological testing. **If possible, blood cultures should be taken prior to the administration of antibiotics but, again, the commencement of antibiotic treatment should not be delayed.**

A microbiologist should be contacted early for advice. If the woman is already extremely ill, is deteriorating, or does not improve within 24 hours of treatment, additional or alternative intravenous antibiotics such as gentamicin and clindamycin, or piperacillin/tazobactam (Tazocin; Wyeth), should be considered.

5. Intravenous fluid resuscitation

Hypotension and/or an elevated serum lactate level ($\geq$ 2 mmol/L) should be treated with intravenous fluids. The woman should be given an initial fluid challenge of 500 mL crystalloid in 15 minutes, but may require up to 30 mL/kg of intravenous fluids.[5] This means a 70 kg patient with sepsis should be given approximately 2 litres of intravenous crystalloid; however, extreme caution should be exercised in women with pre-eclampsia, who require specialist care. If there is no improvement in the hypotension and/or the serum lactate level following the fluid bolus, the woman should be referred to intensive care where vasopressors can be administered to maintain the mean arterial pressure above 65 mmHg.

6. Monitor – including accurate measurement of urine output

Women with maternal sepsis can deteriorate rapidly. Vigilance in observation and assessment is required, and vital signs should be recorded on a MOEWS chart, ideally as part of a maternal critical care chart. This may aid in the early detection of a deteriorating patient. Monitoring should include:

- Respiratory rate, pulse, blood pressure and oxygen saturations: every 15 minutes until stabilised, then every 30 minutes
- Temperature: at least every 4 hours
- Urine output: hourly, by Foley catheter with urometer
- Blood samples: every 4–12 hours depending on clinical condition: full blood count, clotting screen, urea and electrolytes, liver function tests, bicarbonate, serum lactate, glucose, magnesium, phosphate and calcium
- If the woman is antenatal, then the fetal heart rate should be monitored and a CTG commenced, if appropriate

Removing the source of the infection

If possible, the source of the sepsis should be identified and removed as soon as the mother is stable. Birth should be expedited if there are signs of chorioamnionitis. Severe maternal infection can also affect the fetus, and therefore neonatal advice should be sought.

Any retained products of conception should be removed as soon as the maternal condition is stable. A laparotomy and sometimes hysterectomy may be necessary.

Imaging

Imaging may help to identify the source of the sepsis:

- Abdominal ultrasound for retained products of conception or abdominal collection
- Chest x-ray
- CT of the chest, abdomen and pelvis

Prophylactic treatment

Women with sepsis are at increased risk of venous thromboembolism. Deep vein thrombosis prophylaxis with low-molecular-weight heparin and/or the use of compression stockings should also be considered.

Multi-professional approach

Early advice should be sought from other specialists, such as anaesthetists, intensive care specialists, haematologists and microbiologists as well as obstetricians. Critically ill women should be cared for in maternal critical care (within the labour ward) or, if necessary, the intensive care unit. There is more information on the care of women in maternal critical care in **Module 9**.

References

1. Cantwell R, Clutton-Brock T, Cooper G, *et al.* Saving Mothers' Lives: reviewing maternal deaths to make motherhood safer: 2006–2008. The Eighth Report of the Confidential Enquiries into Maternal Deaths in the United Kingdom. *BJOG* 2011; 118 (Suppl. 1): 1–203.

2. Knight M, Kenyon S, Brocklehurst P, *et al.* (eds.); MBRRACE-UK. *Saving Lives, Improving Mothers' Care: Lessons Learned to Inform Future Maternity Care from the UK and Ireland Confidential Enquiries into Maternal Deaths and Morbidity 2009–12.* Oxford: National Perinatal Epidemiology Unit, University of Oxford, 2014.

3. Betrán A, Wojdyla D, Posner S, Gülmezoglu AM. National estimates for maternal mortality: an analysis based on the WHO systematic review of maternal mortality and morbidity. *BMC Public Health* 2005; 5: 131.

4. Singer M, Deutschman CS, Seymour CW, *et al.* The Third International Consensus Definitions for Sepsis and Septic Shock (Sepsis-3). *JAMA* 2016 315: 801–10.

5. Sumbul M, Parapia LA. Handwashing and hygiene: lessons from history. *J R Coll Physicians Edinb* 2008; 38: 379.

6. Lewis G (ed.); The Confidential Enquiry into Maternal and Child Health (CEMACH). *Saving Mothers' Lives: Reviewing Maternal Deaths to Make Motherhood Safer 2003–2005. The Seventh Report on Confidential Enquiries into Maternal Deaths in the United Kingdom.* London: CEMACH, 2007.

7. NHS Choices. Streptococcal infections. www.nhs.uk/conditions/streptococcal-infections (accessed June 2017).

8. National Institute for Health and Care Excellence. *Sepsis: Recognition, Diagnosis and Early Management.* NICE Guideline 51. London: NICE, 2016. www.nice.org.uk/guidance/ng51 (accessed June 2017).

9. UK Sepsis Trust. Inpatient maternal sepsis tool, 2016. http://sepsistrust.org/wp-content/uploads/2016/07/Inpatient-maternal-NICE-Final-1107-2.pdf (accessed June 2017).

10. Daniels R, Nutbeam T, McNamara G, Galvin C. The sepsis Six and the severe sepsis resuscitation bundle: a prospective observational cohort study. *Emerg Med J* 2011; 28: 507–12.

11. Weil MH, Afifi AA. Experimental and clinical studies on lactate and pyruvate as indicators of the severity of acute circulatory failure (shock). *Circulation* 1970; 41: 989–1001.

12. Nordström L, Achanna S, Naka K, Arulkumaran S. Fetal and maternal lactate increase during active second stage of labour. *BJOG* 2001; 108: 263–8.

Module 8
Major obstetric haemorrhage

Key learning points

- To understand the main risk factors, causes and treatment of major obstetric haemorrhage.

- To consider iron supplementation to optimise haemoglobin concentration before labour and birth.

- To prioritise early fluid resuscitation: intravenous fluid and blood transfusion should not be delayed because of false reassurance from a single haemoglobin result.

- Prompt escalation to senior team members of the multi-professional team.

- For **postpartum haemorrhage (PPH)** – Give tranexamic acid early (alongside uterotonics).

- Consider the use of cell salvage.

- The importance of 'accurately' measuring blood loss, e.g. weigh blood loss.

- Consider giving blood components before coagulation indices deteriorate.

- Consider early hysterectomy, if medical and surgical interventions are ineffective.

- Document details of management accurately, clearly and legibly.

Common difficulties observed in training drills

■ Delay in recognition of the severity of the problem until the woman becomes shocked

■ Underestimation of blood loss, and its significance, particularly in smaller women

■ Failure to promptly recognise and act on signs and symptoms of haemorrhage

■ Delay in commencing adequate fluid resuscitation

■ Delay in obtaining senior support and failing to take a 'broader view' of actions required

■ Uncertainty of how to access blood products rapidly

■ Injudicious use of misoprostol

Introduction

Massive obstetric haemorrhage is the leading cause of maternal death worldwide, accounting for 27% of deaths in the most recent WHO review.[1] In the UK, despite some progress, obstetric haemorrhage remains an important cause of direct maternal deaths; 13 women died from obstetric haemorrhage between 2012 and 2014, a maternal mortality rate of 5.6 per million maternities.[2]

Potential improvements in care were identified in the 2009–12 MBRRACE-UK report, which may have prevented many of the deaths from obstetric haemorrhage. However, there were still delays in recognising the emergency (failure to act on signs and symptoms) and in resuscitation techniques (failure to adequately replace fluids), together with a lack of senior multi-professional involvement and team working. The review also identified that the administration of excessive uterotonics was a key contributory factor in 28% of the deaths from postpartum haemorrhage.[3]

Definitions of maternal haemorrhage

■ **Antepartum haemorrhage** (APH) is bleeding from the genital tract after the 24th week of pregnancy. It can occur at any time until the onset of labour and can be revealed or concealed.

- **Intrapartum haemorrhage** is bleeding from the genital tract at any time during labour until the completion of the second stage of labour.

- **Primary postpartum haemorrhage** (PPH) is traditionally defined as a blood loss of 500 mL or more within the first 24 hours after birth. However, most healthy women can cope with this amount of blood loss without problems. A major PPH is a blood loss greater than 1000 mL.

- **Secondary PPH** is a blood loss of 500 mL or more occurring from 24 hours postpartum until 12 weeks postpartum.

Pathophysiology

The normal adult blood volume is approximately 70 mL/kg, which amounts to a total blood volume of about 5 litres. The circulating blood volume increases in pregnancy to approximately 100 mL/kg, equivalent to a total blood volume of 6–7 litres for a healthy pregnant woman in late pregnancy. This increased blood volume, in conjunction with increased levels of blood coagulation factors such as fibrinogen and clotting factors VII, VIII and X, provides physiological protection against haemorrhage. Young fit pregnant women can compensate extremely well during haemorrhage, and therefore initial normal clinical observations may be falsely reassuring. Tachycardia commonly develops first, but there can also be a paradoxical bradycardia. Hypotension is always a very late sign of hypovolaemia and means that ongoing bleeding should be acted upon without delay.

Blood loss is notoriously difficult to estimate accurately. Furthermore, bleeding may be concealed within the uterus, broad ligament or abdominal cavity. Normal blood loss (< 500 mL) following birth does not usually result in a change in the maternal observations and this is due to the physiological adaptations of pregnancy. However, this can also mean that pregnant and postpartum women are able to mask significant degrees of hypovolaemia before their observations deteriorate. Therefore, if a woman is exhibiting clinical features of hypovolaemia (Table 8.1), these should be taken seriously and rapid resuscitation should be commenced immediately.

Coagulopathy may develop because of severe blood loss, resulting in further heavy bleeding. In disseminated intravascular coagulation (DIC), e.g. after significant placental abruption or amniotic fluid embolism, blood is exposed to high levels of clotting factors, including thromboplastin. Coagulation factors are consumed rapidly and the fibrinolytic system is activated. This causes disruption to the control of coagulation balance and fibrinolysis, resulting in bleeding from wounds and venous puncture sites, which may continue to deteriorate until physiological haemostasis is no longer possible.

137

Table 8.1 Clinical features of shock in pregnancy related to the volume of blood loss

Blood loss	Clinical features	Level of shock
10% blood loss ~500 mL if 50 kg ~800 mL if 80 kg	Mild tachycardia Normal blood pressure	Compensated
15% blood loss ~750 mL if 50 kg ~1200 mL if 80 kg	Tachycardia (> 100 bpm) Hypotension (systolic 90–80 mmHg) Tachypnoea (21–30 breaths/minute) Pallor, sweating Weakness, faintness, thirst	Mild
30% blood loss ~1500 mL if 50 kg ~2400 mL if 80 kg	Rapid, weak pulse (> 120 bpm) Moderate hypotension (systolic 80–60 mmHg) Tachypnoea (> 30 breaths/minute) Pallor, cold clammy skin Poor urinary output (< 30 mL/hour) Restlessness, anxiety, confusion	Moderate
40% blood loss ~2000 mL if 50 kg ~3200 mL if 80 kg	Rapid, weak pulse (> 140 bpm) or bradycardia (< 60 bpm) Severe hypotension (< 70 mmHg) Pallor, cold clammy skin, peripheral cyanosis Air hunger Anuria Confusion or unconsciousness, collapse	Severe

Protocol for major obstetric haemorrhage

All maternity units must have an obstetric haemorrhage protocol for cases of major haemorrhage, and the multi-professional team should update and rehearse their systems and procedures regularly in conjunction with haematology and blood bank staff.[4]

Fluid resuscitation

Fluid resuscitation to restore the circulating volume is a priority in any major obstetric haemorrhage.

Fluid resuscitation and administration of blood products are key elements in the management of any major haemorrhage. Maternal blood loss is notoriously difficult to quantify and is often underestimated. A more accurate estimation can help to initiate earlier recognition of the extent of the problem and earlier fluid resuscitation. Weighing sheets and pads that have been saturated in blood can help to improve estimation of loss (Table 8.2). Pictorial guides can also be helpful in the estimation of blood loss (Figure 8.1).

Table 8.2 Examples of dry weights to aid more accurate estimation of blood loss

Swabs, pads and drapes	Dry weight
Small taped swabs	12 g per swab (5 swabs = 60 g)
Large taped swabs	45 g per swab (5 swabs = 225 g)
Incontinence sheet (60 × 60 cm)	32 g
Theatre incontinence sheet (60 × 90 cm)	50 g
Individual sanitary towels	27 g
Post-birth sanitary towel	42 g
Under buttock drape	230 g
Green paper drape	44 g

Try to remove as much excess liquor as possible before subtracting dry weight from overall wet weight

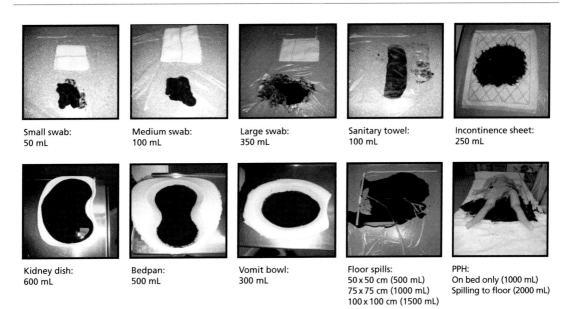

Small swab: 50 mL   Medium swab: 100 mL   Large swab: 350 mL   Sanitary towel: 100 mL   Incontinence sheet: 250 mL

Kidney dish: 600 mL   Bedpan: 500 mL   Vomit bowl: 300 mL   Floor spills: 50 x 50 cm (500 mL) / 75 x 75 cm (1000 mL) / 100 x 100 cm (1500 mL)   PPH: On bed only (1000 mL) / Spilling to floor (2000 mL)

Figure 8.1 An example of a guide to estimating blood loss (adapted from Bose P, et al. BJOG 2006; 113: 919–24[5])

Immediate large intravenous access and fluid replacement

At least two large-bore (14- or 16-gauge, 'orange' or 'grey') intravenous cannulae should be sited as soon as possible. As intravenous access is established, blood should be taken for full blood count, renal function, clotting (including fibrinogen) and cross-matching. Crystalloid solutions (e.g. Hartmann's solution or 0.9% sodium chloride) are the first-line choice for early fluid replacement. Warmed fluids should be available early and infused as rapidly as possible (using pressure bags, a rapid infuser or simply manually squeezing the bag) until the systolic blood pressure has been restored.

Volume to be infused

Aim to maintain normal plasma volume: 2 litres of warmed crystalloid should be administered immediately. If bleeding is ongoing, consider infusing up to a further 1.5 litres of warmed crystalloid if blood products are not available;[6,7,8] however, excessive crystalloid fluid resuscitation can lead to dilutional coagulopathy. Consideration should then be given to replacing blood with the most appropriate product (see below). Recent maternal mortality reports recommend that invasive monitoring (arterial and/or central venous pressure) should be considered at an early stage to guide fluid replacement.[3] Central venous pressure (CVP) monitoring may be particularly useful when major haemorrhage occurs in a woman with pre-eclampsia, where there is a fine balance between adequate fluid replacement and fluid overload.[9]

Give blood products

In massive haemorrhage, both the circulating blood volume and oxygen-carrying capacity need to be restored. While careful consideration is always given before deciding to transfuse when there is major haemorrhage, it is preferable to transfuse fully cross-matched blood (blood of the same group and antibodies as the mother) as soon as possible, using a blood warmer and rapid infuser. However, if fully cross-matched blood is not available after 2–3.5 litres of clear intravenous fluids have been given, or if the bleeding is unrelenting, O-negative or type-specific blood should be given via a fluid warmer without delay.

Transfusing a 'unit of blood' only replaces red blood cells and does not replace clotting factors or platelets. Functioning platelets and clotting factors are necessary for blood to clot, and therefore early consideration should be given to transfusing fresh frozen plasma (FFP), cryoprecipitate and platelets as well (Table 8.3). It is not necessary to wait for the clotting results before transfusing these blood products: the RCOG recommends that up to 15 mL/kg (approx.

1 L or 4 units) of FFP and two packs of cryoprecipitate (10 units) can be given while the clotting results are awaited. The aim is to keep the prothrombin time and activated partial thromboplastin time (APTT) to less than 1.5 × mean control. The dose of FFP is 12–15 mL/kg, which generally equates to giving 4 units of FFP for every 6 units of red blood cells.[4] Fibrinogen is also a vital coagulation factor, and low levels during obstetric haemorrhage are associated with increased bleeding.[10] Recent guidelines recommend replacing fibrinogen with either cryoprecipitate or fibrinogen concentrate during obstetric haemorrhage to maintain maternal plasma levels above 2 g/L.[6]

It is vital that the blood bank is informed early in cases of massive haemorrhage and a haematologist contacted early for advice.[11]

Table 8.3 Transfusion products that aid coagulation[12]

Coagulation product	Comments
Fresh frozen plasma (FFP)	Liquid portion of whole blood. Contains labile as well as stable coagulation products. Not a good source of fibrinogen. FFP at dose of 12–15 mL/kg should be considered for every 6 units of red cells during major haemorrhage. Requires thawing (20–30 minutes).
Cryoprecipitate	More concentrated source of fibrinogen than FFP. Administered at a standard dose of two 5-unit pools early in major obstetric haemorrhage. Requires thawing (20–30 minutes).
Fibrinogen concentrate	Critical protein for haemostasis and clot formation. Not licensed for use in haemorrhage in the UK. Needs reconstituting with water.
Platelet transfusion	To be used when platelet count is low. A platelet transfusion trigger of 75×10^9/L is recommended during active bleeding.
Recombinant factor VIIa (rFVIIa)	Significant risk of arterial thrombosis, and therefore should only be used as part of a trial or after consultation with a consultant haematologist. For rFVIIa to be effective, any surgical bleeding needs to be under control, and acidosis, fibrinogen and platelet counts need to be corrected.
Tranexamic acid (TXA)	Decreases blood loss by preventing the breakdown of fibrin and maintaining blood clots. TXA should be employed early during major haemorrhage.

Point-of-care testing

'Point-of-care' or 'near-patient' tests are increasingly being used to guide transfusion management, as they reduce delay in the results of full blood counts and clotting screens from the laboratory. Examples include haemoglobin assessment with the HemoCue (HemoCue AB, Ängelholm, Sweden), which can provide an estimate of haemoglobin concentration within several seconds. An arterial or venous blood gas sample can provide useful information on the patient status. Moreover, serial measurements of pH, base excess and lactate will assist the anaesthetist in assessing the adequacy of the resuscitation. Some blood gas analysers will also provide a haemoglobin concentration.[13] Real-time coagulation assessment such as with ROTEM (Tem Innovations GmbH, Basel, Switzerland) or TEG (Haemonetics, Braintree, MA, USA) can also be very helpful in guiding treatment of coagulopathies in cases of massive, rapid haemorrhage.

Cell salvage

Intraoperative cell salvage (the process whereby blood lost during an operation is collected, filtered, washed and transfused back into the patient) is commonly used in general surgery and significantly reduces the need for donor blood transfusion. Cell salvage is now increasingly used in obstetrics, especially for women who refuse blood or blood products, or where massive blood loss is anticipated (placenta percreta or accreta).[4]

Previous concerns about the possibility of aspirated amniotic fluid contaminating cell-salvaged blood and causing an amniotic fluid embolus appear to be unfounded. Although aspiration of amniotic fluid should be minimised during surgery, the aspiration of amniotic fluid is not an absolute contraindication to transfusing cell-salvaged red blood cells.[14]

The SALVO study is a randomised controlled trial (RCT) of intraoperative cell salvage during caesarean section in women at risk of haemorrhage. The results, released in January 2017, identified modest evidence of an effect of routine use of cell salvage during caesarean section on donor blood transfusion. In addition, it emphasised the need for adherence to guidance on anti-D prophylaxis due to the increased fetomaternal haemorrhage.[15]

Guidance recommends that women who are rhesus-negative should be given a standard dose of anti-D (minimum 1500 units),[12] and then a Kleihauer test taken 1 hour after cell salvage to determine if further anti-D is required.

Antenatal risk assessment for haemorrhage

Anaemia

Anaemia exaggerates the effect of obstetric haemorrhage, because women who are anaemic are less able to tolerate blood loss. Anaemia may also contribute to uterine atony because of depleted uterine myoglobin levels necessary for muscle action. Haemoglobin levels below the normal UK range for pregnancy (110 g/L at first contact and 105 g/L at 28 weeks) should be investigated and iron supplementation considered to optimise haemoglobin before labour.[16]

Maternal weight

More than half of the women who died of haemorrhage between 2009 and 2012 weighed less than 60 kg.[3] Smaller women have a lower blood volume, and therefore their ability to tolerate blood loss is reduced. Actions in response to the estimated blood loss should also take the woman's stature into account. For example, a woman of 80 kg who loses 1500 mL of blood will have lost about 18% of her circulating volume, while in a woman who weighs 50 kg this would amount to 30% of her total blood volume (Table 8.4).[3]

Conversely, pregnant women who are obese are also at higher risk of an atonic uterus and therefore postpartum haemorrhage.[17]

Table 8.4 Estimated blood volumes and proportionate losses according to body weight[2]

Maternal weight	Estimated total blood volume (mL)	15% blood loss (mL)	30% blood loss (mL)	40% blood loss (mL)
50 kg	5000	750	1500	2000
60 kg	6000	900	1800	2400
70 kg	7000	1050	2100	2800
80 kg	8000	1200	2400	3200

Haemorrhagic disorders

Mothers with inherited haemorrhagic disorders, such as haemophilia and von Willebrand's disease, are at an increased risk of haemorrhage and therefore require specialist care throughout pregnancy. Clear individualised plans for intrapartum and postpartum care should be documented in the woman's notes.

Pre-eclampsia complicated by HELLP syndrome (haemolysis, elevated liver enzymes, low platelets) also increases the mother's vulnerability to bleeding.

Placenta praevia and accreta

Placenta praevia, particularly in women with a previous uterine scar, may be associated with uncontrollable uterine haemorrhage at delivery, sometimes necessitating caesarean hysterectomy. Senior obstetricians and anaesthetists should both plan for, and perform, the caesarean section. Consideration and planning for the use of cell salvage and interventional radiology are also recommended, and referral to a regional centre should be considered.[18]

Women who decline blood products

Women who may decline blood products should be identified in the antenatal period. A clear plan for the management of potential haemorrhage should be documented in the maternal notes. This plan should identify specific blood products and treatments that would be acceptable to the woman (including cell salvage). The principles of the management of haemorrhage in these cases are (1) antenatal optimisation of haemoglobin, (2) securing haemostasis, (3) ensuring senior assistance is summoned early for haemorrhage and (4) having early recourse to pharmacological, radiological and surgical interventions.[9]

The use of modified obstetric early warning score (MOEWS) charts

It is important to recognise signs and symptoms of bleeding as early as possible. All pregnant or recently delivered women are at risk of bleeding, but extra vigilance should be taken in women at high risk (for example prolonged labour). Maternal mortality reports highlight failure to pick up the signs and symptoms of intra-abdominal bleeding, particularly after caesarean section, and recommend the use of MOEWS charts (Figure 8.2) to address this problem.[9]

The use of the MOEWS chart should alert caregivers (including maternity care assistants, who have an increasing role as part of the maternity team) to abnormal trends. However, 'trigger charts' are useful only if measurements are accurately plotted and action is taken appropriately to report any alerts.

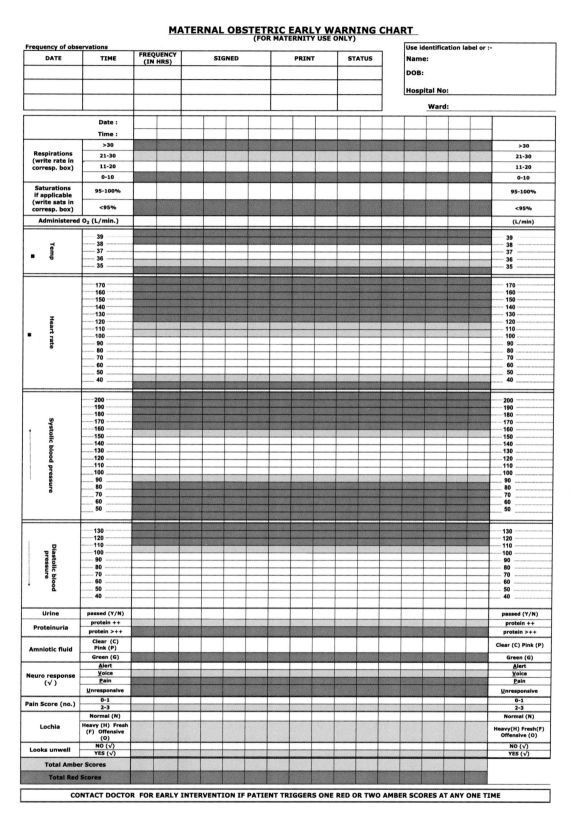

Figure 8.2 An example of a MOEWS chart

Antepartum haemorrhage

Antepartum haemorrhage (APH) complicates 2–5% of all pregnancies. APH is often unpredictable, and the woman's condition may deteriorate rapidly before, during or after there is external evidence of haemorrhage.

Causes of APH

The most common causes of minor APH are marginal placental bleeds, bleeding from a cervical ectropion or a blood-stained 'show'.

The most common causes of major APH are placental abruption and placenta praevia. Uterine rupture (secondary to the forces of labour, or abdominal trauma including road traffic accidents) can also lead to massive haemorrhage.

Ruptured vasa praevia may cause catastrophic APH for the fetus. Although ruptured vasa praevia is not associated with major maternal blood loss, it is an obstetric emergency owing to the rapid development of acute fetal anaemia and risk of fetal death.[18]

Clinical presentation of major APH

A woman with an APH usually presents with obvious vaginal bleeding; however, bleeding may be concealed and therefore haemorrhage must be considered in all pregnant women with signs or symptoms of shock and/or a history of collapse. Table 8.5 lists the presenting features and causes of APH.

Initial management of major APH

Major APH is an obstetric emergency. Blood loss can be torrential, with rapid deterioration in both maternal and fetal condition. Blood loss is often underestimated and may be concealed, especially for cases of uterine rupture or placental abruption.[19]

The management of a major APH requires the rapid initiation of multiple simultaneous actions, including a swift assessment of fetal and maternal wellbeing. The initial management to stabilise the maternal condition will be the same regardless of the cause of bleeding. This should be followed by specific treatment measures dependent on the cause. The exact sequence will be dictated by the needs of the individual mother, the fetal condition and the resources available.

An outline of the initial management for a major APH is shown in Figure 8.3. This is discussed in more detail in the following sections.

Table 8.5 Presenting features and causes of APH

Cause	Possible presenting features	Condition of uterus	Condition of fetus	Risk factors/ contributory factors
Placenta praevia	■ Painless vaginal bleeding ■ High presenting part or transverse lie ■ Shock	■ Non-tender and soft or irritable uterus	■ Dependent on amount of blood loss	■ Low-lying placenta on antenatal ultrasound ■ Previous uterine surgery, e.g. caesarean section ■ IVF
Placental abruption	■ Bleeding (may be concealed) ■ Constant pain ■ Shock ■ Fetal compromise (abnormal/ pathological CTG)	■ Tender, woody, hard uterus ■ Irritable uterus	■ Dependent on blood loss and timing since abruption occurred	■ Previous abruption (up to 25% recurrence rate if two previous abruptions) ■ Pre-eclampsia/hypertension ■ Fetal growth restriction ■ Cocaine use ■ Smoking ■ Abdominal trauma ■ Grand multiparity
Uterine rupture	■ Sudden onset of constant sharp pain ■ Peritonism ■ Abnormal/pathological CTG ■ Very high or unreachable presenting part ■ Bleeding (may be concealed) ■ Shock ■ Haematuria	■ Contractions may cease	■ Likely to have abnormal/ pathological CTG ■ Fetus palpated ex utero	■ Previous uterine surgery (caesarean section, myomectomy, cornual/ectopic pregnancy) ■ Parity ≥ 4 ■ Trauma ■ Oxytocin infusion during labour
Vasa praevia	■ Variable fresh PV blood loss after rupture of membranes ■ Acute fetal compromise ■ No maternal shock	■ Normal	■ Acute fetal compromise (sinusoidal/ bradycardic CTG) ■ Fetal mortality 33–100%	■ Low-lying placenta ■ Succenturiate lobe

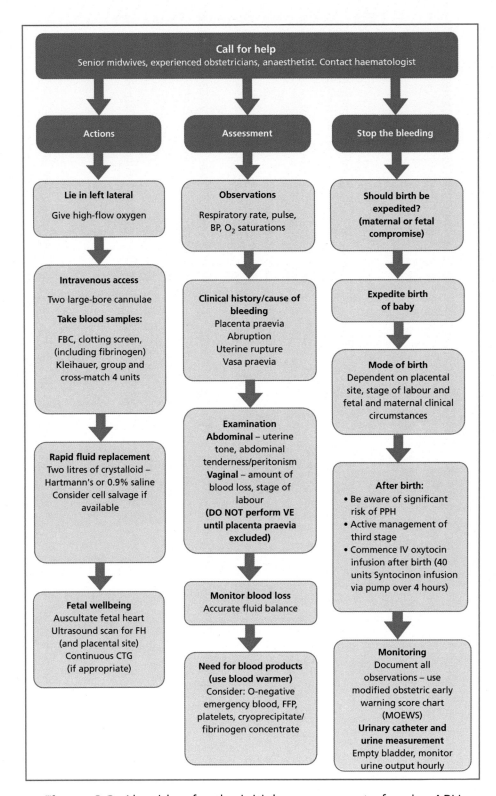

Figure 8.3 Algorithm for the initial management of major APH

Call for help

Activate the emergency buzzer to summon assistance and personnel:

- senior midwife
- experienced obstetrician
- experienced anaesthetist
- experienced neonatologist
- additional support staff

Alert the haematologist, blood bank technician, theatre staff and porter to be on standby, as the major obstetric haemorrhage protocol may be activated and management of the woman in theatre may be required. The consultant obstetrician and anaesthetist should also be informed.

Immediate actions

- Lie the woman in the left-lateral position and give high-flow oxygen with a non-rebreathe mask.
- Clinical observations (pulse, blood pressure, capillary refill, respiratory rate and oxygen saturations).
- Site two large-bore intravenous cannulae.
- Urgent blood samples: full blood count, Kleihauer (even if the woman is rhesus-positive – this will detect a maternofetal haemorrhage), coagulation studies including fibrinogen, cross-match 4 units of blood (consider asking the laboratory to send group-specific blood until cross-matched blood is available), renal and liver function tests.
- Rapid fluid resuscitation with 2 litres of crystalloid (all fluids should ideally be warmed).
- Assess the need for blood products.
- Use O-negative blood (e.g. from labour ward fridge) if there is a life-threatening haemorrhage and consider early use of coagulation products, especially if operative birth is indicated.
- Assess fetal wellbeing – auscultate the fetal heart or commence continuous electronic fetal monitoring if at an appropriate gestation. Ultrasound should not be used as a primary tool to assess fetal wellbeing.
- If there has been fetal demise with an abruption, there is a very high risk of a major APH (possibly at least 1000 mL) and DIC. While the mother will need emotional support due to her bereavement, she will also need close clinical observation and maternal critical care.

> An ultrasound scan will miss up to 75% of cases of abruption, and therefore time should not be wasted attempting to identify a retroplacental clot using ultrasound scanning when there are clinical signs of a placental abruption.[19]

Assessment – rapid evaluation of maternal and fetal condition

Quickly assess the overall condition of the mother and fetus. This includes:

- Ascertain relevant obstetric and clinical history, including:
  - ☐ gestational age
  - ☐ previous uterine surgery/caesarean section
  - ☐ position of placenta (refer to any antenatal scans)
  - ☐ presence of abdominal pain
- Examination:
  - ☐ estimation of blood loss (see Table 8.2 and Figure 8.1)
  - ☐ uterine palpation for tone and tenderness
  - ☐ abdominal palpation for peritonism and ex-utero fetal parts
  - ☐ assess placental site using ultrasound scan
  - ☐ once placenta praevia has been excluded, perform a speculum examination to assess degree of bleeding and possible local causes (trauma, polyps, ectropion)
  - ☐ consider a vaginal examination to ascertain stage of labour

> Remember: do not perform a vaginal examination in the presence of vaginal bleeding without first excluding placenta praevia.

Stop the bleeding – should birth be expedited?

In cases of massive APH, expediting the birth of the baby and placenta is the most effective method of controlling the bleeding, irrespective of the cause, and can be a life-saving intervention.[19]

In cases of major APH it is likely that the birth will be expedited by emergency caesarean section unless the woman is in labour and her cervix is fully dilated. A caesarean section for major APH (whether caused by a placental abruption, praevia or uterine rupture) is likely to be technically challenging and should be performed by the most experienced obstetrician available. If not already present, the consultant obstetrician and anaesthetist should attend as soon as possible.[19]

The choice of anaesthetic for an operative procedure will depend on the clinical circumstances and maternal condition and should be decided by an experienced anaesthetist. Note that coagulopathy may exist in the case of massive abruption. If an APH is related to uterine rupture, the dehiscence should be identified and repaired, and preparations made to perform a hysterectomy if required. An APH is a major risk factor for PPH, so all members of the team should be prepared to pre-empt and manage any subsequent PPH.

Regardless of the suspected fetal compromise, the maternal condition should always take precedence. If birth is indicated (irrespective of the gestation), the mother should be appropriately resuscitated and the birth expedited. Birth should not be delayed for fetal reasons, e.g. waiting for steroids to improve lung maturity at early gestations. The neonatal team should be called early in cases of major APH to ensure adequate time to prepare neonatal resuscitation equipment. APH is associated with neonatal anaemia, particularly when there is vasa praevia or abruption.

Postpartum haemorrhage

Worldwide, major PPH (> 1000 mL) complicates 1.2% of births.[20] The clinical features of shock are the same as previously described in Table 8.1. Major PPH is an obstetric emergency.

Risk factors for major PPH

Pre-labour and intrapartum risk factors for PPH are listed in Box 8.1. Counterintuitively, grand multiparity alone does not appear to be a risk factor for PPH.[20]

Causes of PPH

The four Ts has been used as a tool for the main causes of PPH:

- Tone (uterine atony)
- Tissue (retained products)
- Trauma
- Thrombin (coagulopathy)

Box 8.1 Risk factors for major PPH

Pre-labour

- Previous retained placenta or PPH (recurrence rate of about 8–10%)
- Previous caesarean section (associated with uterine rupture, placenta praevia, percreta and accreta)
- Placenta praevia, accreta or percreta
- Antepartum haemorrhage – especially from placental abruption
- Overdistension of uterus (e.g. multiple pregnancy, polyhydramnios, macrosomia)
- Pre-eclampsia
- Maternal weight below 60 kg (less able to tolerate blood loss due to smaller circulating volume)
- Body mass index above 35
- Increased maternal age (in addition, older women are less tolerant of the effects of a massive bleed)
- Existing uterine abnormalities (e.g. fibroids)
- Maternal haemoglobin below 90 g/L at start of labour (less able to tolerate haemorrhage and increased risk of uterine atony because of depleted uterine myoglobin levels necessary for muscle action)

Intrapartum

- Induction of labour
- Prolonged first, second or third stage of labour
- Use of oxytocin or misoprostol in labour (stimulating or augmenting uterine contractions should be performed in accordance with current guidance and should avoid uterine hyperstimulation)
- Retained placenta
- Precipitate labour
- Operative vaginal birth
- Caesarean section, particularly in the second stage of labour
- Placental abruption
- Pyrexia in labour

Major PPH usually occurs within the first hour after birth, and the most common cause is an atonic uterus (70–90%), with or without retained placental tissue.[21] Genital tract trauma is the second most common cause of PPH. Coagulation defects are rare as a primary cause of PPH, but may occur as a result of significant haemorrhage. Table 8.6 lists some of the presenting features, which may be accompanied by signs and symptoms of shock. It is important to remember that bleeding may also be concealed. Concealed haemorrhage should be suspected when the observations and estimated blood loss do not tally.

Uterine atony should always be anticipated in some common clinical situations, including prolonged labour or second-stage caesarean section.

Uterine rupture typically occurs before or at the time of birth, but the diagnosis may not be made until after birth. Uterine rupture is an increasing cause of maternal death following PPH in the UK. All maternal deaths secondary to uterine rupture in the period 2009–12 occurred in cases of inappropriate, excessive use of uterotonics during induction or augmentation of labour.[3]

Previous maternal mortality reports[9] and the RCOG[18] recommend that there should be a high index of suspicion of placenta accreta for women who have had a previous caesarean section and have a low-lying placenta at the 20-week scan. These women may require MRI and/or ultrasound to attempt to determine whether the placenta is likely to be morbidly adherent, accepting that there is no perfect imaging modality.[18] If a morbidly adherent

Table 8.6 Presenting features and causes of PPH

Presenting feature	Condition of uterus	Possible cause
■ Vaginal bleeding, placenta complete	'Boggy' and high	Uterine atony
■ Vaginal bleeding, placenta incomplete	'Boggy' and high	Retained placental tissue
■ Vaginal bleeding, placenta complete	Well contracted	Vaginal/cervical/perineal trauma
■ Symptoms of shock, severe abdominal pain, fetal compromise immediately prior to birth	Abdominal palpation feels 'unusual'	Uterine rupture
■ Symptoms of shock, often without vaginal bleeding	Seen at vulva/not palpable abdominally	Inverted uterus
■ Continual bleeding, blood not clotting, oozing from wound sites	'Boggy' or contracted	Coagulopathy

placenta is considered likely, forward planning in the antenatal period and the involvement of an experienced multi-professional team during birth are essential to minimise the risk of intrapartum and postpartum haemorrhage.[18]

Morbid adherence of the placenta to the myometrium (placenta percreta or accreta) is usually confirmed when massive haemorrhage occurs following unsuccessful attempts to separate and remove the placenta, although it is often suspected antenatally, particularly for women with a low placenta and previous caesarean section.[18] A case–control study of peripartum hysterectomy carried out by the United Kingdom Obstetric Surveillance System (UKOSS) reported that of the women requiring peripartum hysterectomy because of haemorrhage, 39% had a morbidly adherent placenta.[22]

Prevention of PPH: management of the third stage of labour

Active management

The original active management of labour, administration of a prophylactic uterotonic medication around the time of the baby's birth, early clamping and cutting the umbilical cord, followed by controlled cord traction to expedite delivery of the placenta and membranes,[23] has been superseded by recent evidence.

There are significant advantages to delayed or timely cord clamping for both term[24,25] and preterm infants,[26] including improvements in fine motor skills of children identified at 4 years old.[27] Cord clamping should therefore be delayed for at least 60 seconds at both vaginal and caesarean births for all infants,[25] except those who may require resuscitation.

Furthermore, a recent WHO RCT of controlled cord traction concluded there was no benefit to controlled cord traction, and that the benefits provided by active management of the third stage of labour are likely to be related to the use of oxytocics/uterotonics.[28]

The use of a prophylactic uterotonic as part of active management of the third stage of labour reduces the risk of PPH by 66%.[29] The most commonly used uterotonic agents in the UK are Syntometrine – oxytocin 5 units and ergometrine 500 micrograms – and oxytocin alone (Syntocinon; Novartis). Oxytocin given intramuscularly at a dose of 10 units (or 5 units intravenously) is slightly less effective at reducing blood loss of 500–1000 mL compared to Syntometrine (Alliance) (relative risk (RR) 0.87). However, there is no evidence of a difference in rate of blood loss over 1000 mL.[23] Moreover, the administration of oxytocin alone is not associated with postpartum hypertension, and therefore this should be used instead of

Syntometrine when maternal hypertension is present or if the maternal blood pressure is not known prior to birth.[23]

> **Ergometrine alone or in combination with another drug (e.g. Syntometrine) should not be administered in the presence of known maternal hypertension or if the maternal blood pressure has not been taken during labour.**

Oxytocin is now recommended by UK national bodies to be the agent of choice for active management in women without risk factors for PPH.[3,4,30] Despite this recommendation, a recent survey of obstetric units found that Syntometrine is still the first-line treatment in 71% of units in the UK.[31]

A large randomised controlled trial, IMOX, is due for completion at the end of 2017, and is comparing blood loss and maternal outcomes after vaginal birth when the third stage is managed with intramuscular (1) Syntometrine, (2) Syntocinon or (3) carbetocin (Ferring Pharmaceuticals), a long-acting synthetic oxytocin (https://ukctg.nihr.ac.uk/trials/trial-details/trial-details?trial Number=NCT02216383).

Physiological management

Some women will opt for a physiological management of the third stage, which involves no administration of uterotonics, no clamping and cutting of the cord until the placenta has been delivered, and the promotion of gravity to assist expulsion of the placenta in a timely manner with maternal effort.[29] The NICE intrapartum care guidance recommends that women at low risk of PPH who request a physiological third stage should be supported in their choice,[32] and the Royal College of Midwives (RCM) recommends that women should be given evidence-based information on the benefits and risks of active and physiological management to support them making an informed choice.[33,34] If at any time during physiological management there is excessive blood loss, or the placenta has not been delivered within 1 hour, the midwife should recommend changing to active management.[33]

Initial management of major PPH

The management of a major PPH requires the prompt initiation of multiple simultaneous actions, in a sequence similar to that used for all haemorrhage. The exact sequence will be dictated by the needs of the individual mother and the resources available.

An outline of the initial management for a major PPH is shown in Figure 8.4. This is discussed in more detail in the following sections.

Immediate management of major postpartum haemorrhage (PPH)

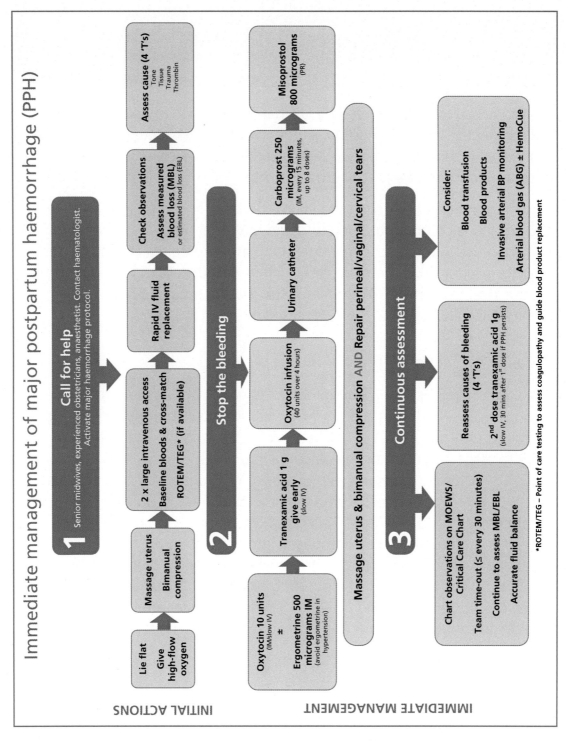

1 Call for help
Senior midwives, experienced obstetricians, anaesthetist. Contact haematologist. Activate major haemorrhage protocol.

INITIAL ACTIONS

Lie flat
Give high-flow oxygen

Massage uterus
Bimanual compression

2 x large intravenous access
Baseline bloods & cross-match
ROTEM/TEG* (if available)

Rapid IV fluid replacement

Check observations
Assess measured blood loss (MBL)
or estimated blood loss (EBL)

Assess cause (4 'T's)
Tone
Tissue
Trauma
Thrombin

2 Stop the bleeding

IMMEDIATE MANAGEMENT

Oxytocin 10 units
(IM/slow IV)
±
Ergometrine 500 micrograms IM
(avoid ergometrine in hypertension)

Tranexamic acid 1 g give early
(slow IV)

Oxytocin infusion
(40 units over 4 hours)

Urinary catheter

Carboprost 250 micrograms
(IM, every 15 minutes, up to 8 doses)

Misoprostol 800 micrograms
(PR)

Massage uterus & bimanual compression AND Repair perineal/vaginal/cervical tears

3 Continuous assessment

Chart observations on MOEWS/ Critical Care Chart
Team time-out (≤ every 30 minutes)
Continue to assess MBL/EBL
Accurate fluid balance

Reassess causes of bleeding (4 'T's)
2nd dose tranexamic acid 1g
(slow IV, 30 mins after 1st dose if PPH persists)

Consider:
Blood transfusion
Blood products
Invasive arterial BP monitoring
Arterial blood gas (ABG) ± HemoCue

*ROTEM/TEG – Point of care testing to assess coagulopathy and guide blood product replacement

Figure 8.4 Algorithm for the initial management of a major PPH

Call for help

Activate the emergency buzzer to summon assistance and emergency call the appropriate personnel:

- senior midwife
- experienced obstetrician
- additional support staff
- consultant obstetrician
- consultant anaesthetist
- porter ready to take urgent samples

Alert the haematologist, blood bank technician and theatre staff to be on standby, as the 'Code Red' major obstetric haemorrhage protocol may be activated.

PPH emergency box/trolley

Many units have found that cognitive aids, including a PPH emergency box or trolley, are extremely helpful. The box/trolley should contain emergency equipment, treatment algorithms and medications required for the immediate management of PPH (Figure 8.5).[35]

Immediate actions – irrespective of cause

- Lie the woman flat and give high-flow facial oxygen through a non-rebreathe mask.

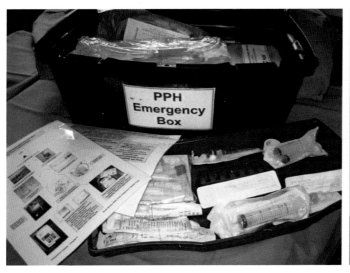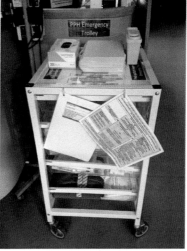

Figure 8.5 Examples of a postpartum haemorrhage emergency box and trolley

- Rub up a contraction, and expel any clots from the uterus.
- Site two large intravenous cannulae and send urgent blood samples: full blood count, coagulation studies including fibrinogen, cross-match 4 units of blood (consider asking haematologist to send group-specific blood until cross-matched blood is available).
- Rapid fluid resuscitation of at least 2 litres of warmed crystalloid (e.g. Hartmann's solution or 0.9% sodium chloride).
- Elevate the mother's legs and/or tilt the mother head-down.
- Use O-negative blood (e.g. from labour-ward fridge), ideally given via a fluid warmer, in cases of life-threatening haemorrhage.

Assessment – rapid evaluation

Quickly assess the overall condition of the mother. This includes:

- pulse, respiratory rate, blood pressure and oxygen saturations
- peripheral perfusion
- check uterine tone
- estimation of blood loss: weigh swabs, incontinence pads, etc.

Observe for signs of shock:

- maternal tachycardia of more than 100 bpm
- respiratory rate of over 30 breaths/minute
- peripheral vasoconstriction – capillary refill greater than 2 seconds

All indicate significant blood loss with initial physiological compensation (see Table 8.1). If the systolic blood pressure falls to less than 100 mmHg, the blood loss is likely to be at least 25% of the maternal blood volume.

Identify the cause:

- Check whether the uterus is well contracted.
- Check that the placenta has been expelled and is complete.
- Examine the cervix, vagina and perineum for tears.
- Observe for signs of clotting disorders, such as oozing from wound and cannula sites.

Stop the bleeding

Remember that there may be more than one cause for the bleeding.

Massage the uterus

The most common cause of PPH is uterine atony. Check that the uterus is well contracted – it should feel firm like a 'cricket ball'. If the uterus is flaccid, 'rub up' a contraction. Expel any blood clots trapped in the uterus, as these inhibit effective uterine contractions. Use bimanual compression if bleeding continues.

First-line medication

If the third stage has not been actively managed give an oxytocic, either 10 units of oxytocin intramuscularly or 1 ampoule of Syntometrine (oxytocin 5 units and ergometrine 500 micrograms) intramuscularly, depending on clinical circumstances and availability.

If an oxytocic has already been given for active management of the third stage but bleeding is continuing, give a second dose of oxytocin as outlined above.

> **Bolus doses of intravenous oxytocin should be used with caution when there is extreme maternal hypotension, as it can cause a further fall in blood pressure.**

If the uterus contracts with the measures outlined above, an oxytocin infusion should be commenced to maintain uterine tone: oxytocin 40 units diluted in 500 mL 0.9% sodium chloride and infused via an infusion pump at 125 mL/hour over 4 hours.

However, if the uterine tone remains poor, other treatments (e.g. further uterotonics, expulsion of blood clots or removal of retained placental tissue) will be required to encourage uterine contraction. Oxytocin infusion is not in itself a primary treatment of PPH.

Tranexamic acid

Tranexamic acid (TXA) is an antifibrinolytic that is used widely to prevent and treat haemorrhage in non-obstetric patients. The results of the World Maternal Antifibrinolytic (WOMAN) trial (published in April 2017) recommend the early use of TXA in the treatment of PPH.[36] The study was a randomised, double-blind, placebo-controlled trial comparing the use of TXA with a placebo; over 20,000 women were randomised into the study after being clinically diagnosed with PPH following vaginal or caesarean birth. The study demonstrated a significant reduction in deaths from haemorrhage and also numbers of laparotomies undertaken to control bleeding when TXA was administered alongside uterotonics, as soon as possible after the onset of primary PPH (and definitely within the first 3 hours), with no increase in vascular occlusive events.

The dosage is 1 g (100 mg/mL) given as a slow IV injection at a rate of 1 mL/minute. If bleeding continues after 30 minutes or re-starts within 24 hours of the first dose, then a second dose of 1 g of TXA may be given.

TXA is an antifibrinolytic that prevents the breakdown of fibrin deposits at bleeding sites in the body. It is important to remember that it will not produce contraction of the uterine muscle, and it should therefore be thought of as an adjunct to the use of uterotonics and surgical control of PPH.

Catheterise the bladder

A full bladder can inhibit effective contraction of the uterus. Insert an indwelling Foley catheter to empty the bladder. Note the amount drained and monitor further urinary output hourly as an indicator of renal function.

Bimanual compression of uterus

If bleeding continues, bimanual compression of the uterus should be performed (Figure 8.6). This may be necessary while the woman is transferred into hospital via ambulance, or transferred to the operating theatre. Bimanual compression is an excellent holding measure and should be continued until the haemorrhage is brought under control.

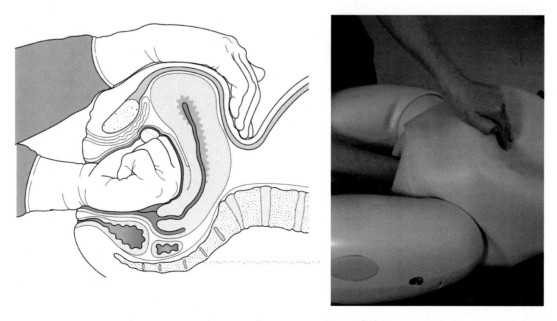

Figure 8.6 Bimanual compression of the uterus

To perform bimanual compression, insert one hand into the vagina and form a fist. Direct your fist into the anterior fornix and apply pressure against the anterior wall of the uterus. With the other hand, press externally on the uterine fundus and compress the uterus between your hands. Maintain compression until bleeding is controlled and the uterus contracts. A device has recently been proposed to help accouchers perform effective compression (https://clinicaltrials.gov/ct2/show/NCT02692287), but there are insufficient data to recommend it currently.

In the community setting or when a woman is on a postnatal ward, bimanual compression provides an effective mechanical holding measure until arrival on the labour ward.

Apply pressure and repair any tears

Tears of the birth canal can be a source of significant blood loss and are the second most frequent cause of PPH.[33] Apply pressure to the area of bleeding as an initial holding measure, using large sterile swabs. Stabilise the mother and repair any tears as soon as possible, ensuring adequate analgesia and good lighting. Consider early transfer to theatre, as a full examination under anaesthesia is often required. Finally, there should be early recourse to seeking extra help.[4]

Examination under anaesthetic

There should be a low threshold for examination under anaesthetic, particularly where there is evidence of haemostatic compromise.

Manual removal of retained products

Persistent uterine atony is often caused by retained placental tissue or blood clots. Exploration and emptying of the uterus should be performed as soon as the mother has been resuscitated. This is best performed in the operating theatre and should be performed as soon as possible. When the uterus has been manually explored and emptied, further oxytocics should be administered to contract the uterus.

Repair of cervical, high vaginal and perineal tears

Adequate analgesia, good lighting and an assistant in theatre make the identification and repair of genital tract tears easier. A systematic approach should be used to ensure that high vaginal and cervical tears are not missed during suturing.

Treatment of unrelenting haemorrhage

In the vast majority of cases of PPH, bleeding will be controlled by giving simple uterotonics and TXA, emptying the uterus and suturing any genital tract trauma. However, if bleeding continues despite these actions, further management will be required, as unrelenting haemorrhage poses a significant threat to the life of the mother.

In cases of unrelenting haemorrhage, both bimanual compression and aortic compression can be used to stem the bleeding until other methods have had time to take effect.

To achieve aortic compression, the aorta must be compressed against the spine. Use a closed fist to apply downward pressure over the abdominal aorta just above and slightly to the left of the umbilicus. The femoral pulse should be obliterated if the compression is adequate. This method is especially useful if the PPH occurs during a caesarean section.

The methods used to stop the bleeding will depend largely on the underlying cause of the haemorrhage, but various techniques that should be considered are outlined below. Hypothermia, coagulopathy and acidosis have been described as a lethal triad in major haemorrhage. Temperature control, volume replacement and coagulation should be aggressively managed.

Keeping the mother warm

When there is major obstetric haemorrhage, the risk of the mother developing a coagulopathy can be reduced by keeping her warm and ensuring that all infused fluids are passed through rapid fluid warming equipment. In addition to impairing clotting, the rapid infusion of cold fluids has been reported to cause potentially lethal cardiac arrhythmias.[11]

Additional medications for treating PPH

Carboprost

If the uterus continues to relax despite initial measures, give carboprost (Hemabate; Pharmacia) 250 micrograms by deep intramuscular injection. Carboprost is a synthetic analogue of prostaglandin F2α, and can be repeated at intervals of at least 15 minutes up to a maximum of eight doses.

Carboprost can induce vomiting, diarrhoea, headache, pyrexia, hypertension and bronchospasm. Carboprost is contraindicated in mothers with cardiac or pulmonary disease, including women with severe asthma.

> **Do not give carboprost intravenously. Prostaglandins can be fatal if given intravenously.**

Misoprostol

The use of rectal or sublingual misoprostol (600–1000 micrograms) has also been described. Misoprostol is a synthetic analogue of prostaglandin E1 and has the advantage of being thermostable and inexpensive.

However, the most recent Cochrane systematic review of the prophylactic use of oral misoprostol for the management of the third stage of labour found that misoprostol was less effective than conventional uterotonics.[37] Moreover, misoprostol is no more effective at maintaining uterine tone than an oxytocin infusion when administered following primary management of PPH with a conventional uterotonic, and it causes significantly more side effects.[37] Therefore, in situations where conventional uterotonics are available these should be used in preference to misoprostol. However, misoprostol should be considered in low-resource settings where more effective (refrigerated) uterotonics are not available.[4]

Recombinant factor VIIa

Recombinant factor VIIa (rFVIIa) was originally developed for patients with haemophilia. rFVIIa induces haemostasis by enhancing thrombin generation and providing the formation of a stable fibrin clot that is resistant to premature fibrinolysis. Subsequently, it has been used for massive intraoperative haemorrhages and PPH. However, rFVIIa is associated with a high rate of thromboembolic events in patients who receive it (2.5%) and it is also extremely expensive. Therefore the current UK recommendation is that it should be used only after consultation with a consultant haematologist.[12]

The recommended dose is 40–90 micrograms/kg.[4,38] It is important to understand that rFVIIa is not effective if platelets and fibrinogen are very low, as these are essential requirements for the clot formation facilitated by rFVIIa. Therefore, before rFVIIa is given, platelets and fibrinogen must be checked: they must be above 50×10^9/L and 2 g/L, respectively.[6] It is also important that the woman is not hypothermic.

Mechanical and surgical measures

Uterine balloon tamponade

Uterine balloon tamponade (e.g. Bakri [Cook Medical] or Rusch [Teleflex Medical] balloon) can be used in preference to other mechanical or surgical management options. While evidence in this area is of poor quality, small studies suggest that the use of a balloon tamponade reduces the number of units of blood transfused per woman (3.3 fewer units per woman on average), the amount of oxytocin required to control bleeding, and the length of stay in intensive care.[39] For this reason, use of a balloon tamponade is currently recommended by NICE in preference to other surgical approaches, at least initially.[30]

To use a balloon tamponade, the balloon catheter is inserted into the uterine cavity and inflated with approximately 250–500 mL of warm 0.9% sodium chloride. An oxytocin infusion may be used to maintain uterine contraction. This method has been described as the 'tamponade test'. If the tamponade test fails to stop the bleeding (following vaginal birth), a laparotomy will be indicated. A UK review of maternal deaths states that in some cases there was an apparent tendency to continue to try an intrauterine balloon, even when the situation was extreme and definitive treatment such as hysterectomy may have been required.[3] If balloon tamponade is successful, it can be left in place for up to 24 hours and should ideally be removed in daylight hours when senior staff are available in case bleeding recurs.[4]

While conservative measures to preserve the uterus in the face of PPH are to be commended, there can be cases of major haemorrhage that require definitive treatment, i.e. hysterectomy, as the final option to control the bleeding. Such decisions should be made promptly at a senior level.[3]

Recently there has been some preliminary research that suggests that a device designed to create vacuum-induced uterine tamponade may be a reasonable alternative to other devices used to treat atonic PPH.[40] However, there were only 10 cases investigated and more research is required before they can be recommended.

Laparotomy

If the abdomen is not already opened and the bleeding is continuing, a laparotomy may be needed so that surgical methods can be used to attempt to stop the bleeding.

B-Lynch suture and other compression measures

The B-Lynch suture technique is simple and effective, with successful outcomes in a number of case reports.[4,41] However, it is not universally effective: in the UKOSS survey, 16% of peripartum hysterectomies performed in the UK were preceded by an unsuccessful B-Lynch or other brace suture.[34]

A simple diagram of the B-Lynch technique is shown in Figure 8.7. The original description of the technique requires the uterine cavity to be opened and explored and a bimanual compression test employed prior to insertion of the suture. If bimanual compression is ineffective in reducing the bleeding, the B-Lynch suture is unlikely to be successful.

A number of modifications of the B-Lynch suture have been described,[4,42] although they all follow the same principle of compressing the uterus to stop the bleeding. Some techniques do not require opening of the uterine cavity, while others describe parallel or vertical sutures that compress the anterior uterine wall against the posterior wall.[4] Most of the published series have favourable outcomes, with subsequent pregnancies reported after the procedure. However, serious complications, including uterine necrosis, pyometra[43] and uterine rupture in a subsequent pregnancy,[44] have also been reported.

Interventional radiology

Interventional radiology should be considered in high-risk cases (e.g. cases of placenta praevia with accreta) where intra-arterial balloons can be placed immediately prior to a planned caesarean section.[4] However, the technique is often difficult to perform in an emergency situation owing to the specialised equipment and personnel required. Therefore, other techniques

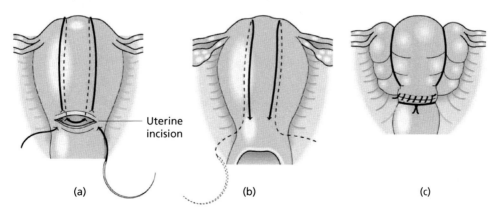

(a)   (b)   (c)

Figure 8.7 The B-Lynch suture: (a) and (b) show the anterior and posterior views of the uterus showing the application of the brace suture; (c) shows the anatomical appearance after complete application (original illustration by Mr Philip Wilson FMAA AIMI, based on the author's video record of the operation; reproduced with permission from B-Lynch C, *et al. Br J Obstet Gynaecol* 1997; 104: 372–5[41])

(e.g. uterine balloon tamponade, compression sutures or aortic compression) may be more appropriate.

Interventional radiology may be particularly useful if there is prolonged or continuous bleeding, once initial treatment has been provided and the mother is stable enough for transfer.

Women who have undergone interventional radiology to prevent or treat an obstetric haemorrhage are at risk of developing an arterial embolism, and therefore should have their pedal pulses checked every 30 minutes for 6 hours following the procedure, to ensure adequate peripheral circulation is maintained.

Uterine vessel and internal iliac artery ligation

The uterine, ovarian and internal iliac vessels can all be ligated in an attempt to stem uterine bleeding. These are potentially difficult procedures, and the assistance of a vascular surgeon should be requested by those inexperienced in the technique.[4]

It is impossible to assess which of the various 'surgical' haemostatic techniques is most effective. Nevertheless, the available observational data suggest that, on balance, balloon tamponade may be more effective than haemostatic suturing (e.g. B-Lynch) or internal iliac artery ligation and is also easier to perform.[30]

Hysterectomy

Hysterectomy may be necessary if bleeding persists. In the face of unrelenting haemorrhage, it should be performed sooner rather than later.[4] The incidence of peripartum hysterectomy in the UK in 2009–12 was 40 per 100,000 births.[3] It is good practice to involve a second senior doctor in the decision for hysterectomy;[4] however, this should not result in unnecessary delay. In addition, the procedure should not be delayed by attempts with other unfamiliar techniques.

Unrelenting haemorrhage is probably one of the most challenging situations for all professionals involved. While the decision to perform a hysterectomy is never taken lightly, it is important not to delay this course of action until the mother is moribund or the clotting has already deteriorated.

Continuing management of unrelenting haemorrhage: key points
■ Carboprost administered by deep intramuscular injection
■ Use manual holding measures while arranging further treatment
■ Invasive monitoring, regular observations and point-of-care testing
■ Early recourse to surgical intervention
■ Watch out for consumptive coagulopathy
■ Hysterectomy is life-saving and should not be delayed
■ Aftercare in maternal critical care or intensive care unit

Documentation

It is vital that all treatment and actions are documented at the time of the events. An example of a PPH documentation pro forma is shown in Figure 8.8.

It is also important that the woman's clinical response to measures to control haemorrhage and fluid replacement are regularly observed, documented and evaluated. There should be continuous monitoring of respiration rate, pulse rate, blood pressure and oxygenation. The volume and type of fluid administered should be documented so that fluid balance can be easily monitored. The maternal temperature should be regularly monitored, as hypothermia can easily develop from the administration of non-warmed blood or fluid products.

Clinical observations and fluid balance should be plotted on a maternal critical care chart that includes modified obstetric early warning scores (MOEWS) for early recognition of any deterioration in condition.[3]

Ongoing care

All women who have experienced major obstetric haemorrhage (antepartum or postpartum) that causes maternal compromise should be closely monitored after the event to ensure that any further blood loss is rapidly detected. Women who have had a massive haemorrhage are at risk of:

■ renal impairment (due to poor perfusion of the kidneys)

■ respiratory compromise (secondary to fluid overload or transfusion reactions)

■ venous thromboembolism (due to infused clotting agents and the rebound hypercoagulable state)

REMEMBER - Scan & Send a copy (2-Sided) to PostpartumHaemorrhage@nbt.nhs.uk and then file in the notes

North Bristol **NHS**
NHS Trust
OBSTETRIC HAEMORRHAGE PROFORMA
To be used for PPHs equal to or more than 1500 mls or clinical concern

Mother's Name _____
Hospital Number _____
DOB _____.
Or attach addressograph label

Date	Time	Name of person completing form	
Call for additional help (CDS)		Time called:	

CALL FOR HELP

Name	Status and Grade	Time arrived	Name	Status & Grade	Time arrived

ACTIVATE CODE RED PLAN 2222 (2000mls and ongoing haemorrhage) — TIME ACTIVATED : — NOT CLINICALLY REQUIRED □

Key staff	Name	Time informed	Time arrived
CDS co-ordinator			
Consultant Obstetrician			
Senior Anaesthetist			
Blood bank			
Clinical Site manager			
Porter			

RESUSCITATION /INITIAL MANAGEMENT

ACTION	TIME	ACTION	TIME
High flow $O_2 \geq$ 10L/min		Massage Uterus	
IV Access large bore cannula 1		Bimanual compression	
large bore cannula 2		Catheter- Foley's with hourly urine measurement	
Observations HR/BP/RR/SpO₂ Start Critical Care chart		Patient warmer/ bair hugger	
Rapid IV fluid resuscitation – detail overleaf		Arterial line	

BLOOD SAMPLES	TIME	BLOOD SAMPLES	TIME
FBC		U&Es	
Clotting		Rotem	
Group & Save (if not already taken)		Xmatch 4 units (if no code red)	

IDENTIFY CAUSE OF BLEEDING – tick cause

Atony □ | Tears □ | Retained placental tissue □ | Extension at section □ | Praevia □ | Coagulopathy □

DRUGS	Dose	Time	Order		Time
Syntometrine IM 1ˢᵗ dose					
Syntometrine IM 2ⁿᵈ dose					
IM Syntocinon (If Syntometrine contra-indicated)					
Syntocinon 40 I.U IV via pump					
Carbetocin 100mcg IM					
Haemobate 250mcg IM	1			4	
	2			5	
	3			6	
Tranexamic acid 1g IV					
IMOX study drug 1ml IM					
Misoprostol 800mcg PR					
Calcium gluconate 10% 10ml IV					
Ergometrine 500 micrograms					

REMEMBER - Scan & Send a copy (2-Sided) to PostpartumHaemorrhage@nbt.nhs.uk and then file in the notes

Figure 8.8 An example of a PPH documentation pro forma

REMEMBER - Scan & Send a copy (2-Sided) to PostpartumHaemorrhage@nbt.nhs.uk and then file in the notes

CRYSTALLOID FLUIDS GIVEN

Type	Amount Infused	Warmed?	Time Started	Time completed
		Y/N		
		Y/N		
		Y/N		

BLOOD AND BLOOD PRODUCTS GIVEN

O -ve, group specific, X-matched, FFP, cryoprecipitate, platelets, fibrinogen conc.

			Blood loss		
Type	Volume/Unit	Time Started	Time EBL measured	Swabs Weighed	EBL

Cell salvage – use and volume gained

Used from start of surgery	Commenced during surgery	No – not applicable	No – insufficient staffing		
Volume re-infused:				Total	Total

POINT OF CARE BLOOD TESTS

Haemacue / blood gas results		ROTEM result		ROTEM repeat result	
Time:	Result:	Time:		Time:	
		Suggests FFP needed	Y/N	Suggests FFP needed	Y/N
		Suggests Cryo needed	Y/N	Suggests Cryo needed	Y/N
		Suggests Platelets needed	Y/N	Suggests Platelets needed	Y/N

FURTHER MANAGEMENT

	Performed	Order Performed	Date	Time
EUA				
Manual removal of placenta				
Arterial line				
Intra-Uterine balloon tamponade				
B Lynch suture				
Bilateral ligation Of Uterine Arteries				
Resuturing Caesarean Uterine incision/ lateral extension				
Hysterectomy				
Interventional Radiology				

What went well?	What could have gone better?

Thromboprophylaxis- risk assessment and plan. ☐

REMEMBER - Scan & Send a copy (2-Sided) to PostpartumHaemorrhage@nbt.nhs.uk and then file in the notes

Figure 8.8 (cont.)

Therefore, women after APH and/or PPH should be cared for in a critical care environment, with regular senior multi-professional team review. This closely monitored period of care also provides vital opportunities for debriefing and support for both the mother and her relatives. There is further information on the provision of maternal critical care in **Module 9**.

Situational awareness

Although obstetric haemorrhage is a common and familiar event to obstetricians, anaesthetists and midwives, who have to manage it on a regular basis, this should not mean that we are in any way 'casual' in our vigilance to recognise and respond. The *Saving Lives, Improving Mothers' Care* report recommends that to improve situational awareness and prevent delays in recognising the seriousness of the problem, staff should escalate concerns to seniors at an early stage and continuously re-evaluate the woman and her treatment, rather than persisting with ineffective or inappropriate care.[3] Staff should also be aware of the effect of the haemorrhage on the emotional wellbeing of the mother and her partner. A thorough debrief should occur a few days afterwards.

References

1. Say L, Chou D, Gemmill A, *et al.* Global causes of maternal death: a WHO systematic analysis. *Lancet Glob Health* 2014; 2: e323–33.

2. Knight M, Nair M, Tuffnell D, *et al.* (eds.); MBRRACE-UK. *Saving Lives, Improving Mothers' Care: Surveillance of Maternal Deaths in the UK 2012–14 and Lessons Learned to Inform Maternity Care from the UK and Ireland Confidential Enquiries into Maternal Deaths and morbidity 2009–14.* Oxford: National Perinatal Epidemiology Unit, University of Oxford, 2016.

3. Knight M, Kenyon S, Brocklehurst P, *et al.* (eds.); MBRRACE-UK. *Saving Lives, Improving Mothers' Care: Lessons Learned to Inform Future Maternity Care from the UK and Ireland Confidential Enquiries into Maternal Deaths and Morbidity 2009–12.* Oxford: National Perinatal Epidemiology Unit, University of Oxford, 2014.

4. Royal College of Obstetricians and Gynaecologists. *Prevention and Management of Postpartum Haemorrhage.* Green-top Guideline No. 52. London: RCOG, 2016. www.rcog.org.uk/en/guidelines-research-services/guidelines/gtg52/ (accessed June 2017).

5. Bose P, Regan F, Paterson-Brown S. Improving the accuracy of estimated blood loss at obstetric haemorrhage using clinical reconstructions. *BJOG* 2006; 113: 919–24.

6. Abdul-Kadir R, McLintock C, Ducloy AS, *et al.* Evaluation and management of postpartum hemorrhage: consensus from an international expert panel. *Transfusion* 2014; 54: 1756–68.

7. Mittermayr M, Streif W, Haas T, *et al.* Hemostatic changes after crystalloid or colloid fluid administration during major orthopedic surgery: the role of fibrinogen administration. *Anesth Analg* 2007; 105: 905–17.

8. Schierhout G, Roberts I. Fluid resuscitation with colloid or crystalloid solutions in critically ill patients: a systematic review of randomised trials. *BMJ* 1998; 316: 961–4.

9. Cantwell R, Clutton-Brock T, Cooper G, *et al.* Saving Mothers' Lives: reviewing maternal deaths to make motherhood safer: 2006–2008. The Eighth Report of the Confidential Enquiries into Maternal Deaths in the United Kingdom. *BJOG* 2011; 118 (Suppl. 1): 1–203.

10. Charbit B, Mandelbrot L, Samain E, *et al.* The decrease of fibrinogen is an early predictor of the severity of postpartum hemorrhage. *J Thromb Haemost* 2007; 5: 266–73.

11. Freedman RL, Lucas DN. MBRRACE-UK: saving lives, improving mothers' care: implications for anaesthetists. *Int J Obstet Anesth* 2015; 24: 161–73.

12. Royal College of Obstetricians and Gynaecologists. *Blood Transfusion in Obstetrics.* Green-top Guideline No. 47. London: RCOG, 2015. www.rcog.org.uk/en/guidelines-research-services/guidelines/gtg47/ (accessed June 2017).

13. Kozek-Langenecker SA, Afshari A, Albaladejo P, et al, Management of severe perioperative bleeding: guidelines from the European Society of Anaesthesiology. *Eur J Anaesthesiol* 2013; 30: 270–382.

14. Esper SA, Waters JH. Intra-operative cell salvage: a fresh look at the indications and contraindications. *Blood Transfus* 2011; 9: 139–47.

15. Khan K, Moore P, Wilson MJ, *et al.*; SALVO Study Group. Cell salvage during caesarean section: a randomised controlled trial (the SALVO trial). *Am J Obstet Gynecol* 2017; 216, (1 Suppl): S559.

16. National Institute for Health and Care Excellence. *Antenatal Care for Uncomplicated Pregnancies.* NICE Clinical Guideline CG62. London: NICE, 2008. www.nice.org.uk/guidance/CG62 (accessed June 2017).

17. Blomberg M. Maternal obesity and risk of postpartum hemorrhage. *Obstet Gynecol* 2011; 118: 561–8.

18. Royal College of Obstetricians and Gynaecologists. *Placenta Praevia, Placenta Praevia Accreta and Vasa Praevia: Diagnosis and Management.* Green-top Guideline No. 27. London: RCOG, 2011. www.rcog.org.uk/en/guidelines-research-services/guidelines/gtg27/ (accessed June 2017).

19. Royal College of Obstetricians and Gynaecologists. *Antepartum Haemorrhage.* Green-top Guideline No. 63. London: RCOG, 2011. www.rcog.org.uk/en/guidelines-research-services/guidelines/gtg63/ (accessed June 2017).

20. Sheldon WR, Blum J, Vogel JP, *et al.* Postpartum haemorrhage management, risks, and maternal outcomes: findings from the World Health Organization Multicountry Survey on Maternal and Newborn Health. *BJOG* 2014; 121 (Suppl 1): 5–13.

21. Oyelese Y, Ananth CV. Postpartum hemorrhage: epidemiology, risk factors, and causes. *Clin Obstet Gynecol* 2010; 53: 147–56.

22. Knight M, Kurinczuk JJ, Spark P, *et al.* Cesarean delivery and peripartum hysterectomy. *Obstet Gynecol* 2008; 111: 97–105.

23. National Institute for Health and Care Excellence. *Intrapartum Care: Care of Healthy Women and Their Babies During Childbirth.* NICE Clinical Guideline CG55. London: NICE, 2007.

24. Oh W. Timing of umbilical cord clamping at birth in full-term infants. *JAMA* 2007; 297: 1257–8.

25. Royal College of Obstetricians and Gynaecologists. *Clamping of the Umbilical Cord and Placental Transfusion.* Scientific Impact Paper No. 14. London: RCOG, 2014. www.rcog.org.uk/en/guidelines-research-services/guidelines/sip14/ (accessed June 2017).

26. Mercer JS, Vohr BR, McGrath MM, *et al.* Delayed cord clamping in very preterm infants reduces the incidence of intraventricular hemorrhage and late-onset sepsis: a randomized, controlled trial. *Pediatrics* 2006; 117: 1235–42.

27. Andersson O, Lindquist B, Lindgren M, *et al.* Effect of delayed cord clamping on neurodevelopment at 4 years of age: a randomized clinical trial. *JAMA Pediatr* 2015; 169: 631–8.

28. Gulmezoglu AM, Lumbiganon P, Landoulsi S, *et al.* Active management of the third stage of labour with and without controlled cord traction: a randomised, controlled, non-inferiority trial. *Lancet* 2012; 379: 1721–7.

29. Begley CM, Gyte GM, Murphy DJ, *et al.* Active versus expectant management for women in third stage of labour. *Cochrane Database Syst Rev* 2010; (7): CD007412.

30. World Health Organization. *WHO Recommendations for the Prevention and Treatment of Postpartum Haemorrhage.* Geneva: WHO, 2012. www.who.int/reproductivehealth/ publications/maternal_perinatal_health/9789241548502/en/ (accessed June 2017).

31. van der Nelson H, Jones F, Siassakos D, Draycott T. Prophylactic uterotonic use in the third stage of labour to prevent PPH: Are UK obstetric units following current guidelines? Poster presentation at 2014 RCOG World Congress, Hyderabad, India. www.epostersonline.com/ rcog2014/?q=node/1507 (accessed June 2017).

32. National Institute for Health and Care Excellence. *Intrapartum Care for Healthy Women and Babies.* NICE Clinical Guideline CG190. London: NICE, 2014. www.nice.org.uk/guidance/ cg190 (accessed June 2017).

33. Royal College of Midwives. *Third Stage of Labour.* Evidence Based Guidelines for Midwifery-Led Care in Labour. London: RCM, 2012.

34. Baker K. How to promote a physiological third stage of labour. *Midwives Magazine* 2013; (5). www.rcm.org.uk/news-views-and-analysis/analysis/how-to-promote-a-physiological-third-stage-of-labour (accessed June 2017).

35. National Maternity Review. *Better Births: Improving Outcomes of Maternity Services in England.* London: NHS England, 2016.

36. WOMAN Trial Collaborators. Effect of early tranexamic acid administration on mortality, hysterectomy, and other morbidities in women with post-partum haemorrhage (WOMAN): an international, randomised, double-blind, placebo-controlled trial. *Lancet* 2017; 389: 2105–16.

37. Mousa HA, Blum J, Abou El Senoun G, Shakur H, Alfirevic Z. Treatment for primary postpartum haemorrhage. *Cochrane Database Syst Rev* 2014; (2): CD003249.

38. Franchini M, Veneri D, Lippi G. The use of recombinant activated factor VII in congenital and acquired von Willebrand disease. *Blood Coagul Fibrinolysis* 2006; 17: 615–19.

39. Soltan MH, Mohamed A, Ibrahim E, Gohar A, Ragab H. El-menia air inflated balloon in controlling atonic post partum hemorrhage. *Int J Health Sci (Qassim)* 2007; 1: 53–9.

40. Purwosunu Y, Sarkoen W, Arulkumaran S, Segnitz J. Control of postpartum hemorrhage using vacuum-induced uterine tamponade. *Obstet Gynecol* 2016; 128: 33–6.

41. B-Lynch C, Coker A, Lawal AH, Abu J, Cowen MJ. The B-Lynch surgical technique for the control of massive postpartum haemorrhage: an alternative to hysterectomy? Five cases reported. *Br J Obstet Gynaecol* 1997; 104: 372–5.

42. Matsubara S, Yano H, Kuwata T, Usui R, Ohkuchi A. Is it time to classify various uterine compression suture techniques? *Arch Gynecol Obstet* 2013; 288: 1195–6.

43. Matsubara S, Yano H, Ohkuchi A, *et al.* Uterine compression sutures for postpartum hemorrhage: an overview. *Acta Obstet Gynecol Scand* 2013; 92: 378–85.

44. Date S, Murthy B, Magdum A. Post B-lynch uterine rupture: case report and review of literature. *J Obstet Gynaecol India* 2014; 64: 362–3.

Module 9
Maternal critical care

Key learning points

- Maternal critical care is required for pregnant and postnatal women with complex medical and obstetric problems.

- There should be appropriate critical care support for the management of pregnant and postpartum women who become unwell, and this should be provided on the labour ward or a maternal critical care unit.

- Maternal critical care requires the involvement of a multi-professional team of midwives, obstetricians, neonatologists (if mother still pregnant), anaesthetists and intensive care specialists.

- Specialised maternal critical care charts should be used for documenting observations, fluid balance, ongoing clinical investigations, results and medical reviews.

- Maternal critical care structured review sheets provide a useful framework for structured multi-professional reviews.

- Women requiring critical care should receive frequent obstetric and midwifery reviews to ensure the maintenance of their usual antenatal and postnatal obstetric care.

- All carers should be aware of the potential long-term effects of a 'near-miss' incident on a mother's health, in particular her mental health.

Common difficulties observed in training drills

- Incorrect documentation of fluid balance
- Incorrect positioning of arterial line
- Not setting 'goals of the day'
- Not remembering nutrition/gastric protection
- Not prescribing thromboprophylaxis
- Not undertaking regular multi-professional reviews

Introduction

Maternal critical care is defined as the specialised care of pregnant and postpartum women whose conditions are life-threatening and require comprehensive care and close monitoring. In the UK and in many countries across the world, pregnancy care is increasing in complexity as the pregnant population becomes older and more obese, and more commonly present with significant medical comorbidities.[1] As a result of these changing demographics, women are more likely to experience pregnancy complications that may require critical care. Women aged 35 and over have a significantly higher maternal mortality rate than women aged 20–24, and 84% of women who died in the UK between 2009 and 2012 were identified as having multiple medical comorbidities and/or significant social factors.[2]

The NHS report *Providing Equity of Critical and Maternity Care for the Critically Ill Pregnant or Recently Pregnant Woman* (2011) recommended that:

> Childbirth is a major life event for women and their families. The few women who become critically ill during this time should receive the same standard of care for both their pregnancy related and critical care needs, delivered by professionals with the same level of competences irrespective of whether these are provided in a maternity or general critical care setting.[3]

Furthermore, the MBRRACE-UK report *Saving Lives, Improving Mothers' Care* (2014) report also recommended:

> There should be adequate provision of appropriate critical care support for the management of a pregnant woman who becomes unwell. Plans should be in place

for the provision of critical care on labour wards or maternity care on critical care units, depending on the most appropriate setting for a pregnant or postpartum woman to receive care.[2]

Why is 'maternal' critical care different from 'normal' critical care?

The provision of critical care for women who are pregnant or who have recently given birth provides some additional challenges to those of the general adult population.

■ The pregnant critically ill woman requires monitoring and multi-professional management, as does her unborn child. Such care will require the combined knowledge and skills of midwives, obstetricians, anaesthetists and intensive care specialists. When an urgent birth is necessary because of a deterioration in the woman's condition, there is a need for immediate access to an operating theatre, neonatal resuscitation facilities and the neonatal unit.

■ There is often no ideal venue to provide critical care for pregnant women: giving birth in the intensive care unit (ICU) is not ideal, as ICU staff may not have the skills to deal with obstetric complications, whereas labour wards often do not have the facilities to support women with multi-organ failure, or in need of mechanical ventilation. The overriding principle is that a pregnant woman must receive the correct level of care wherever she is. Often this is an adequately equipped and staffed labour ward for antenatal and intrapartum care, but this may change to ICU if there is any further deterioration in the mother's clinical condition.

■ The physiological changes of pregnancy provide an increased physiological reserve, but they also impose increased physiological demands.

   ☐ The airway can be more difficult to intubate if invasive ventilation is required.

   ☐ There is an increased oxygen demand and reduced oxygen reserve, as well as reduced lung compliance: this means hypoxia is more likely, and adequate ventilation can be harder to achieve.[4]

   ☐ Aortocaval compression needs to be taken into account after 20 weeks' gestation.

   ☐ Cardiac output increases significantly during pregnancy.

   ☐ Not all medications can be safely given in pregnancy, and those that can may have altered plasma levels.

175

☐ The immunosuppression associated with pregnancy means that infection and sepsis can be more common and more aggressive, and may be due to atypical organisms.

☐ Aspiration and venous thromboembolism (VTE) are more common, so prophylaxis should be considered for both of these complications.

■ The critically ill woman who has recently given birth should, if possible, have continued contact with her baby to support the establishment of breastfeeding and bonding.[5] Such contact can often be achieved in a maternity unit, but is much more difficult to achieve in an ICU. Separation of mother and baby can lead to maternal emotional distress, which may inhibit the establishment of breastfeeding and increase the risk of postnatal depression.

■ Caring for mother and baby in separate locations can also be stressful for the family, who are forced to divide their time between the unwell mother and her newborn baby. Care should be as holistic as possible, without compromising clinical practice.

When might critical care be required?

There are multiple conditions for which a pregnant woman, or woman who has recently given birth, may require critical care. No list will ever be comprehensive, but common conditions may include those listed in Table 9.1.

Recognition of the critically ill pregnant woman

Early detection of mothers who may require critical care can be challenging. Severe illness in pregnancy is relatively rare, and the normal physiological changes that occur with pregnancy can mask the early warning signs normally seen in a clinically deteriorating woman. Breathlessness is a common feature of pregnancy; however, persistent breathlessness when lying flat needs investigating, as it may be due to undiagnosed cardiac disease.[6]

Mothers who report feeling unwell, or who look unwell, and/or report a 'feeling that something awful is going to happen', should be thoroughly assessed. However, it is not always necessary to wait until the observations deteriorate: early recognition and early treatment saves lives. Early recognition of critical illness, and prompt involvement of senior clinical staff and the multi-professional team remain the key factors for high-quality care for sick mothers.[6]

Table 9.1 Possible conditions requiring maternal critical care

Respiratory	■ Severe community-acquired pneumonia (including influenza) ■ Pulmonary oedema ■ Severe asthma ■ Pulmonary embolism ■ Bronchospasm
Cardiovascular	■ Severe uncontrolled hypertension ■ Cardiomyopathy ■ Massive haemorrhage ■ Pulmonary embolism ■ Septic shock
Sepsis	■ Obstetric-related: e.g. chorioamnionitis, postoperative, mastitis, urinary tract infection ■ Non-obstetric: influenza, pneumonia, meningitis
Neurological	■ Status epilepticus ■ Meningitis ■ Intracerebral bleed ■ Malignancy ■ Guillain–Barré syndrome

> **As highlighted in a recently published MBRRACE-UK report, reduced or altered conscious level is not an early warning sign; it is a red flag to indicate established illness, and should be acted on immediately and appropriately.[6]**

Modified obstetric early warning score (MOEWS) charts

The MOEWS chart combines physiological parameters with a scoring system to facilitate early recognition of, and intervention in, deteriorating pregnant women. However, be aware that the physiological changes of pregnancy mean that women can mask, and can compensate for, even quite severe degrees of illness. Therefore, clinical judgement and a detailed history and examination are at least as important as completing – and acting upon – a MOEWS chart.

An example of a MOEWS chart is included in **Module 8** (Figure 8.2). This should be used when plotting any maternal observations, except in labour

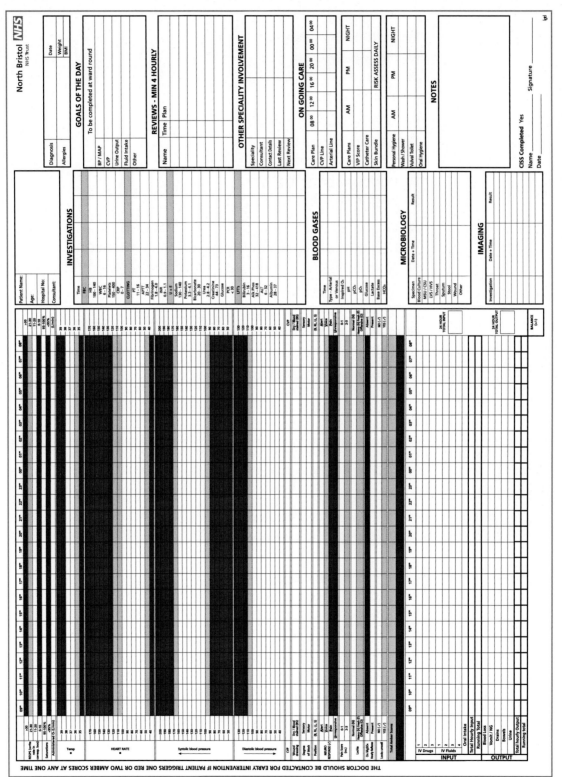

Figure 9.1 An example of a maternal critical care chart including guidance and actions

Date:

Sheet No:

North Bristol NHS

NHS Trust

OBSTETRIC CRITICAL CARE CHART

Addressograph

Obstetric Critical Care Chart

Guidance for use: The chart has pre-filled times and covers a 24 hour period from 08.00 until 08.00. The observations and fluid balance should be completed in box that corresponds with the time, even if this means only one set of observations will be completed before a new chart is started.

Respiratory rate: The single most important parameter for early detection of deterioration and should be measured at all monitoring events.

Oxygen saturation (SpO₂): The level of administered oxygen (L/min) or 'air' should be documented underneath the saturations. Oxygen is prescribed on the drug chart.

Temperature: A rise or fall in temperature may indicate sepsis. NB Septicaemic shock can be particularly difficult to recognize, if in doubt perform a venous or arterial blood gas to check pH and lactate.

Heart rate: Tachycardia may be the only sign of deterioration at an early stage and a tachycardic woman should be considered hypovolaemic until proven otherwise.

Blood pressure:
Hypertension - all pregnant women with a systolic blood pressure of 160mm/Hg or higher must be treated.
Hypotension - a late sign of deterioration and should be taken very seriously.

Central Venous Pressure: If a patient has a CVP line ensure that the transducer is correctly positioned and zeroed as per the Critical Care Guideline. Please write the CVP value in the appropriate box.

Wound: should be recorded as dry or bloodstained

Degree of block: Sensory   1 Numb to mid chest   Motor: 1 No leg or foot movement
                            2 Numb to mid abdomen   2 Slight leg or foot movement
                            3 Numb only to legs/bottom   3 Can bend knee or raise leg

Position: Regular changes (at least every 4 hours) in the patient's position is important to avoid pressure area damage. The patient's position should be documented: B – lying on back, RL - lying in right lateral, LL – lying in left lateral, S – sitting.

Pain scores: Pain levels should be recorded as follows:
                0 – No pain, 1 – Mild pain, 2 – Moderate pain, 3 – Severe pain

Neuro response: AVPU is a measure in consciousness. The best response of the following should be documented:
    A – Alert   Awake and orientated
    V – Voice   Drowsy but answers to name or some kind of response when addressed
    P – Pain   Rousable with difficulty, but makes a response when shaken or mild pain is inflicted
                       (eg rubbing sternum, pinching ears)
    U – Unresponsive   No response to voice, shaking or pain

Reflexes: If a patient is receiving intravenous Magnesium Sulphate (MgSO₄) the presence or absent of the patellar reflex should be documented hourly.

Scoring and responding: All scores for all parameters should be added up hourly and documented.

THE DOCTOR SHOULD BE CONTACTED FOR EARLY INTERVENTION IF THE PATIENT TRIGGERS
ONE RED OR TWO AMBER SCORES AT ANY ONE TIME.

Fluid Input: Fluid input is all the fluid the patient receives (eg drinking, IV fluids, IV drug infusions). Every hour the volume of each fluid type (eg oral, IV fluids, IV drugs) should be documented and added up to create an hourly total. The hourly total should then be added to the previous total input to create a running total input.
The 24-hour total input should be completed at 08.00 every day.

Fluid Output: Fluid output is all the fluid the patient looses (eg urine, blood loss, diarrhoea). Every hour the volume of each fluid type should be documented and added up to create an hourly total.
The hourly total should then be added to the previous total input to create a running total output.
The 24-hour total output should be completed at 08.00 every day.

Fluid balance: This is the 24-hour input minus the 24-hour output. This should be calculated at 08.00 every day
A new chart should be commenced at 08.00 with all fluids starting from zero.

The CISS computer system must be completed by the medical team when Obstetric Critical Care is
commenced, finished, and every 24 hours (on the 08.00 ward round) in the interim.

Figure 9.1 (cont.)

when all observations should be plotted on the partogram (which ideally should include the same parameters as on the MOEWS chart for the maternal observations section). Once critical care is indicated, a maternal critical care chart should be used (Figure 9.1).

Investigations for critically ill women

Most investigations can be carried out safely in pregnancy, and investigations to diagnose or exclude life-threatening conditions should not be denied or delayed because of pregnancy, or concerns about the risk to the fetus.[6] A multi-professional discussion between senior obstetric and radiology clinicians can be helpful in determining the most appropriate and safest investigations.

Where should critical care be provided?

Currently, most critical care is provided within intensive care units, but critical care should be a level of care provision, not a location. Most aspects of critical care can be provided outside the ICU, including on the labour ward or in an obstetric theatre.

Women who require advanced respiratory support (mechanical ventilation) or prolonged cardiovascular support with inotropes (medications that increase the force of contraction of the heart, to increase the cardiac output and maintain blood flow to vital organs and tissues) and vasopressors (medications to increase the mean arterial pressure, and therefore organ perfusion, through arterial vasoconstriction) will usually require transfer to an ICU for intensive monitoring and specialised care. However, women requiring level 2 critical care (Table 9.2) may be able to remain within the maternity unit if trained staff and suitable monitoring equipment are available. If feasible, critical care services should be brought to the woman rather than changing her location.[2] The Intensive Care Society classification of critical care (*Levels of Critical Care for Adult Patients*) focuses on the level of dependency of the individual patient, regardless of location, and is now employed in the majority of NHS institutions.[7] Examples of the different levels of care that may be required in maternity are listed in Table 9.2.

Regular structured review: ongoing assessment and management

All women receiving critical care require comprehensive, structured and regular medical review for early detection of problems and timely

Table 9.2 Examples of maternity care required at each Intensive Care Society level of support[3]

Level of care	Definition	Maternity example
Level 0	Patients whose needs can be met through normal ward care in an acute hospital	Care of low-risk mother
Level 1	Patients at risk of their condition deteriorating, or those recently relocated from higher levels of care, whose needs can be met on an acute ward with additional advice and support from the critical care team	■ Risk of haemorrhage ■ Oxytocin infusion ■ Mild pre-eclampsia on oral antihypertensives/fluid restriction ■ Woman with stable medical conditions, e.g. congenital heart disease, diabetes requiring sliding-scale insulin
Level 2	Patients requiring more detailed observation or intervention, including support for a single failing organ system or postoperative care, and those 'stepping down' from higher levels of care	Basic respiratory support ■ 50% or more oxygen via face-mask to maintain oxygen saturation ■ Continuous positive airway pressure (CPAP) ■ Bi-level positive airway pressure (BIPAP) Basic cardiovascular support ■ Intravenous antihypertensives to control blood pressure ■ Arterial line for pressure monitoring or blood sampling ■ CVP line for fluid management and CVP monitoring to guide therapy Advanced cardiovascular support ■ Simultaneous use of at least two intravenous antiarrhythmic/antihypertensive/vasoactive drugs, one of which must be a vasoactive drug ■ Need to measure and treat cardiac output Neurological support ■ Magnesium sulfate infusion to control seizures (not prophylaxis) ■ Intracranial pressure monitoring Hepatic support ■ Management of acute fulminant hepatic failure, e.g. from HELLP syndrome or acute fatty liver, such that transplantation is being considered

Table 9.2 (cont.)

Level of care	Definition	Maternity example
Level 3	Patients requiring advanced respiratory support alone, or basic respiratory support together with support of at least two organ systems. This level includes all complex patients requiring support for multi-organ failure	**Advanced respiratory support** ■ Invasive mechanical ventilation **Support of two or more organ systems** ■ Renal support and basic respiratory support ■ Basic respiratory/cardiovascular support and an additional organ supported

interventions. A systematic approach should be employed, commencing with the standard ABCDE approach, together with a regular review of medications, venous thromboembolism prophylaxis, kidney and bowel function, pain management, fluid balance and nutritional assessment.

The use of both a maternal critical care chart (Figure 9.1) and a maternal critical care structured review sheet (Figure 9.2) provides a useful framework to facilitate this regular, structured review. Staff should be given guidance and training on how to use the chart and worksheet.

A maternal critical care chart should be used to document the woman's observations, fluid balance and ongoing clinical investigations, results and medical reviews. Observations are usually performed hourly, but the frequency will depend on the clinical condition of the patient. The key observations that should be performed at least hourly are listed in Table 9.3.

The maternal critical care structured review sheet (Figure 9.2) can be laminated and placed on the ward round trolley as an aide memoire for staff conducting the multi-professional ward round. It could also be incorporated into a structured review sheet or sticker that can be used to document care, and inserted into the maternal notes each time a review occurs.

Maternal Critical Care Structured Review

This is designed to be used during the multi-professional review of a critically ill pregnant or postpartum woman.
It does not replace, nor should it repeat the observations and information recorded on the Maternal Critical Care chart.
Relevant notes can be made as each item is considered either directly into the patients notes or by annotating the pro forma which should be dated, signed and filed in the woman's maternity notes at the end of the review.

Patient ID (addressograph)

Date........................ Time....................

	Items to be considered	Notes:
A	**Airway**	
B	**Breathing** (Respiratory Rate, SpO$_2$, FiO$_2$, chest examination findings)	
C	**Circulation** (Heart rate, BP, capillary refill time, vasopressors)	
D	**Disability** (level of consciousness, pain, epidural or spinal block)	
E	**Electrolytes** (Mg^{2+}, Na$^+$, K$^+$ levels and eGFR/creatinine)	
F	**Fluids** – Review of fluid balance (input, output, blood loss, drains)	
G	**GI & glucose control** (bowel function and gastro-protection measures)	
H	**Haematology** (FBC, clotting profile, VTE prophylaxis)	
I	**Infection** (temp, inflammatory markers, cultures, antibiotics)	
M	**Maternal comorbidities** (diabetes, hypertension, asthma, epilepsy)	
N	**Neonatal considerations**	
L	**Lines** (cannulae, arterial line, central line, urinary catheter, wound drains)	
O	**Obstetric**: antenatal, intrapartum/postpartum related	
P	**Pharmacology** (review drug chart)	
Q	**Questions**	
R	**Recommendations**	
S	**Summary**	
	Signature... Print.. Date...........................	

Figure 9.2 Maternal critical care structured review

Table 9.3 Key observations when monitoring a critically ill pregnant woman on the maternity unit

Respiratory rate	This is the single most important indicator for early detection of deterioration and should be documented at all monitoring events.
Oxygen saturation	The level of administered oxygen (L/min) or 'air' should be documented, together with the oxygen saturations (SpO_2). Oxygen should be prescribed as per hospital policy.
Temperature	This is not a sensitive marker of deterioration, but a temperature rise (greater than 38 °C) or fall (less than 36 °C) may indicate sepsis.
Heart rate	This is a key indicator. Tachycardia may be the only sign of deterioration at an early stage. A woman who has a tachycardia should be considered hypovolaemic until proven otherwise.
Blood pressure (BP)	Hypotension is a late sign of deterioration, as it signifies decompensation and should be taken very seriously. Septic shock can be particularly difficult to recognise. If in doubt, perform a venous or arterial blood gas to check pH and lactate. Hypertension is equally important, and all pregnant or postpartum women with systolic BP ≥ 160 mmHg must be treated urgently.
Central venous pressure (CVP)	A CVP line is an intravenous line that measures the central venous pressure, which gives an indication of the volume status of the woman. If a woman has a CVP line, ensure the transducer is correctly positioned and zeroed as per the critical care guidelines. The CVP reading should be documented in the appropriate box.
Reflexes	If a woman is receiving IV magnesium sulfate, the presence or absence of deep tendon reflexes (usually patellar reflex) should be documented hourly.
Fluid input	This is the volume of all fluid the women receives from drinking, nasogastric fluids, IV fluids and IV drug infusions. These should be added up to create an hourly total in millilitres (mL) and a running total, and recorded on the chart. The 24-hour total input should be completed at 08.00 every day.
Urine output	This is one of the few signs of end-organ perfusion. Urine output should be recorded hourly in millilitres (mL) on the chart and contributes to fluid output in the 24-hour balance

Table 9.3 (cont.)

Fluid output	This is the volume of all fluid the woman loses from urine, blood loss, diarrhoea, vomit, nasogastric drainage, surgical drains, etc. These should be added up to create an hourly total in millilitres (mL) and a running total, and recorded on the chart. The 24-hour total output should be completed at 09.00 every day.
Fluid balance	The fluid balance must be accurate and kept up to date. It is the 24-hour input minus the 24-hour output and should be calculated at 09.00 every day. A new chart should be commenced at 09.00 with all fluids starting from zero. A positive balance means that the woman has received more fluid than she has lost in a 24-hour period. Note that there may be up to 500–800 mL of 'insensible' (i.e. unmeasurable) losses (from respiration, evaporation, etc.) per day. However, a significant and persistent positive balance is a risk factor for the development of pulmonary oedema. A negative balance means that the woman has lost more fluid than she has received in a 24-hour period. A significant and persistent negative balance is a risk factor for the development of renal failure.
Patient position	Regular changes (minimum 4-hourly) in the woman's position are essential to avoid damage to pressure areas.
Neurological response	AVPU is a measure of the woman's level of consciousness. The best descriptor should be recorded. A fall in AVPU score should always be considered significant. A score of P or below is equivalent to Glasgow Coma Score of ≤ 8. ALERT: fully awake woman VOICE: drowsy but answers to name, or some kind of response when addressed PAIN: difficult to rouse, makes a response to sternal rubbing, pinching earlobes or shaking shoulders UNRESPONSIVE: no response to voice or physical stimulus
Pain score	Pain scores guide analgesia and adequacy. Recorded as 0 (no pain), 1 (mild pain), 2 (moderate pain), 3 (severe pain).

Equipment

The RCOG's Maternal Critical Care Working Group has produced guidance on the minimum equipment required for the provision of maternity critical care.[3] This is listed in Table 9.4.

Table 9.4 Minimum equipment list for provision of maternal critical care[3]

- Monitor for HR, BP, ECG, SpO_2 and with transducer for invasive monitoring
- Piped oxygen and suction
- Intravenous fluid warmer
- Forced air warming device
- Blood gas analyser[a]
- Infusion pumps
- Emergency massive haemorrhage trolley[a]
- Emergency eclampsia box[a]
- Transfer equipment – monitor and ventilator
- Computer terminal to facilitate access to blood results, PACS system
- Copy of hospital obstetric guidelines including maternal critical care
- Resuscitation trolley with defibrillator and airway management equipment (available nearby)[a]

[a] These items may already be available in maternity theatres or on the labour ward.

Transfer of the critically ill woman to an intensive care unit

Critically ill women may need transferring from the labour ward to the ICU (or to scanners, operating theatres or another hospital). All transfers risk destabilisation and deterioration, and there is a requirement for specialised personnel and equipment. Therefore, transfers need to be timely, coordinated, smooth and well planned,[2] so that they can be safely accomplished for extremely ill women.

Senior doctors should assess the woman and, after multi-professional discussion, determine the best location for ongoing care, and there should be just a single transfer to definitive care.[6] Decisions must include the means and timing of intra- or inter-hospital transfer, to ensure that the transfer is carried out safely.[8]

Transfers should not be undertaken until the woman has been resuscitated and stabilised. In many circumstances an 'ICU outreach team' will attend to assist with both the preparation and the transfer.

- Before transfer to the ICU it may be necessary to secure the airway with an endotracheal tube (with appropriate end-tidal carbon dioxide monitoring), rather than risk deterioration en route.
- Appropriate intravenous access must be in place.
- Continuous invasive blood pressure measurement is the best technique for monitoring blood pressure during the transfer of ill women, and therefore an arterial line may need to be sited before transfer.

If a woman is transferred to an ICU for ongoing management there should be a daily consultant obstetric and midwifery review, even if only in a supportive role, until such time as she can be repatriated to the maternity unit. Regular information and neonatal updates, including photos of the baby, can be very helpful.[9]

Longer-term impacts of near-miss maternal morbidity for women, their babies and families

Community midwives and GPs should be informed when a woman is discharged from hospital after critical care. Follow-up appointments with the obstetrician and/or midwifery staff can be helpful and should be arranged for at least 6 weeks after the birth, or sometimes longer afterwards, depending on the mother's recovery. Women should be aware that their experience of a 'near-miss' incident can have long-lasting effects on their health, particularly their mental health, and may also affect their partner.[10]

References

1. Office for National Statistics. Statistical bulletin. Conceptions in England and Wales: 2015. London: ONS, 2016. www.ons.gov.uk/peoplepopulationandcommunity/birthsdeathsand marriages/conceptionandfertilityrates/bulletins/conceptionstatistics/2015 (accessed June 2017).

2. Knight M, Kenyon S, Brocklehurst P, *et al.* (eds.); MBRRACE-UK. *Saving Lives, Improving Mothers' Care: Lessons Learned to Inform Future Maternity Care from the UK and Ireland Confidential Enquiries into Maternal Deaths and Morbidity 2009–12*. Oxford: National Perinatal Epidemiology Unit, University of Oxford, 2014.

3. Maternal Critical Care Working Group. *Providing Equity of Critical and Maternal Care for the Critically Ill Pregnant or Recently Pregnant Women*. London: Royal College of Anaesthetists, 2011. www.rcog.org.uk/globalassets/documents/guidelines/prov_eq_matandcritcare.pdf (accessed June 2017).

4. Zakowski MI, Ramanathan S. CPR in pregnancy. *Curr Rev Clin Anesth* 1990; 10: 106.

5. Joint Working Party: Royal College of Obstetricians and Gynaecologists, Royal College of Midwives, Royal College of Anaesthetists, Royal College of Paediatrics and Child Health. *Safer Childbirth: Minimum Standards for the Organization and Delivery of Care in Labour*. London: RCOG, 2007. www.rcog.org.uk/en/guidelines-research-services/guidelines/safer-childbirth-minimum-standards-for-the-organisation-and-delivery-of-care-in-labour (accessed June 2017).

6. Knight M, Nair M, Tuffnell D, *et al.* (eds.); MBRRACE-UK. *Saving Lives, Improving Mothers' Care: Surveillance of Maternal Deaths in the UK 2012–14 and Lessons Learned to Inform Maternity Care from the UK and Ireland Confidential Enquiries into Maternal Deaths and morbidity 2009–14*. Oxford: National Perinatal Epidemiology Unit, University of Oxford, 2016.

7. Eddleston J, Goldhill D, Morris J. *Levels of Critical Care for Adult Patients*. London: Intensive Care Society, 2009.

8. Association of Anaesthetists of Great Britain and Ireland. *AAGBI Safety Guideline: Interhospital Transfer*. London: AAGBI, 2009. www.aagbi.org/publications/guidelines/interhospital-transfer-aagbi-safety-guideline (accessed June 2017).

9. Royal College of Obstetricians and Gynaecologists. *Bacterial Sepsis following Pregnancy*. Green-top Guideline No. 64B. London: RCOG, 2012. www.rcog.org.uk/en/guidelines-research-services/guidelines/gtg64b (accessed June 2017).

10. Knight M, Acosta C, Brocklehurst P, *et al.*; UKNeS co-applicant group. *Beyond Maternal Death: Improving the Quality of Maternal Care Through National Studies of 'Near Miss' Maternal Morbidity*. Programme Grants for Applied Research, No. 4.9. Southampton: National Institute for Health Research, 2016.

Further reading

Department of Health. *Competencies for Recognising and Responding to Acutely Ill Patients in Hospital*. London: DoH, 2008.

Intercollegiate Maternal Critical Care (MCC) Sub-Committee of the Obstetric Anaesthetists' Association. *Maternity Enhanced Care Competencies Required by Midwives Caring for Acutely Ill Women*. London: OAA, 2015.

Module 10
Shoulder dystocia

Key learning points

■ Understand that shoulder dystocia is unpredictable, and therefore difficult to prevent.

■ Understand that during shoulder dystocia, traction should only be applied in an axial direction, using the same force as for a normal birth without shoulder dystocia.

■ Be able to perform the manoeuvres required to release the shoulders during shoulder dystocia.

■ Understand the importance of clear and accurate documentation.

■ Awareness of the potential complications of shoulder dystocia, particularly that permanent brachial plexus injury is not inevitable.

Common difficulties observed in training drills

■ Not calling the neonatologist
■ Failing to state the problem clearly
■ Difficulty inserting hand into the sacral hollow
■ Confusion over internal rotational manoeuvres, particularly the use of eponyms
■ Resorting to excessive traction to release the shoulders
■ Using fundal pressure

Introduction

Shoulder dystocia is defined as a vaginal cephalic birth that requires additional obstetric manoeuvres to assist the birth of the infant after gentle traction has failed.[1] Shoulder dystocia occurs when either the anterior shoulder impacts behind the maternal symphysis pubis or, less commonly, the posterior shoulder impacts over the sacral promontory (Figure 10.1). Evidence-based algorithms for the management of shoulder dystocia recommend resolution manoeuvres designed to improve the relative dimensions of the maternal pelvis (McRoberts' position, all-fours position), reduce the diameter of the fetal shoulders (suprapubic pressure, delivery of the posterior arm) and/or move the fetal shoulders into a wider pelvic diameter (suprapubic pressure, internal rotational manoeuvres).[1]

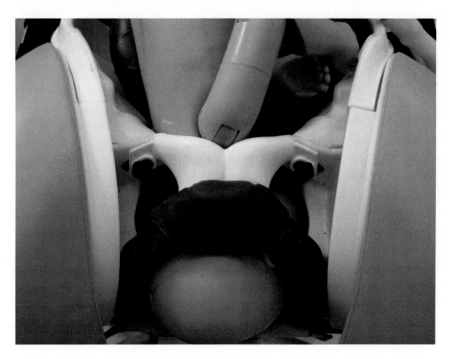

Figure 10.1 Shoulder dystocia with anterior fetal shoulder impacted on maternal symphysis pubis

Shoulder dystocia remains a largely unpredictable event and can result in serious long-term morbidity for both mother and baby. Poor outcomes can result in very significant litigation costs. In the USA, shoulder dystocia is the second most commonly litigated complication of childbirth.[2] In Saudi Arabia, it is the most commonly litigated problem.[3] In England over a decade from 2000 to 2009, the NHS Litigation Authority paid more than £100 million in legal compensation for preventable harm associated with shoulder dystocia.[4] Clearly, this is an enormous loss of resource to health care in general, notwithstanding the immediate and long-term distress to many parents and families.[5]

Recent data suggest that neonatal outcomes, including brachial plexus injury (BPI), can be improved through multi-professional simulation training.[6,7] However, not all training appears to be effective: some training has not been associated with improvement,[8,9] and, counterintuitively, some training has been associated with an increase in BPI.[10]

There appear to be important differences between effective and ineffective training in obstetrics,[11,12] and these are likely to apply in the specific case of shoulder dystocia training. Furthermore, it is now recognised that the use of eponyms and mnemonics is not as useful as previously thought.[13,14] Finally, there are likely to be differences in the mannequins used for training.[6]

The current RCOG guideline for shoulder dystocia states that:

> Shoulder dystocia training associated with improvements in clinical management and neonatal outcomes was multi-professional, with manoeuvres demonstrated and practiced on a high fidelity mannequin. Teaching used the RCOG algorithm … rather than staff being taught mnemonics (e.g. HELPERR) or eponyms (e.g. Rubin's and Woods' screw).[1]

Incidence

There is wide variation in the reported incidence of shoulder dystocia. Studies published between 1985 and 2016 reported incidences ranging from 0.1% to 3.0% of all births.[15] Recent datasets have reported that there are significant differences in rates of shoulder dystocia reported from the USA (1.4%) and outside the USA (0.6%).[16] It is unclear why the rates are different, but better awareness may increase the reported rates.[6]

Risk factors for shoulder dystocia

A number of antenatal and intrapartum characteristics are widely recognised to be associated with shoulder dystocia (Box 10.1). However, all of the characteristics are poorly predictive, and combining them is similarly poor.[1] Conventional risk factors predicted only 16% of cases of shoulder dystocia that resulted in infant morbidity. Therefore, for practical purposes, because shoulder dystocia is not clinically predictable, all staff should be prepared for its occurrence at any vaginal birth.

> ### Box 10.1 Risk factors for shoulder dystocia
>
> | Pre-labour | Intrapartum |
> | --- | --- |
> | Previous shoulder dystocia | Prolonged first stage |
> | Macrosomia | Prolonged second stage |
> | Gestational age | Labour augmentation |
> | Maternal diabetes mellitus | Operative vaginal birth (forceps or vacuum) |
> | Maternal obesity | |

Previous shoulder dystocia

Previous shoulder dystocia is a risk factor for recurrent shoulder dystocia. A prior history of a birth complicated by shoulder dystocia confers a 6-fold to nearly 30-fold increased risk of shoulder dystocia in a subsequent vaginal birth, with most reported rates between 12% and 17%.[17] Recurrence rates may however be underestimated, as caesarean section rates are higher following severe shoulder dystocia and brachial plexus injury.

Women should be informed that their birth was complicated by a shoulder dystocia and should be counselled about their options for place of birth and risks in a future pregnancy.[17]

Macrosomia

Large fetal size increases the risk of shoulder dystocia: the greater the fetal birth weight, the higher the risk of shoulder dystocia and also brachial plexus injury.[18,19] A review of 14,721 births reported rates of shoulder dystocia in non-diabetic mothers of 1% in infants weighing less than 4000 g, 10% in infants weighing 4000–4499 g, and 23% in infants weighing more than 4500 g.[20] However, macrosomia remains a weak predictor of shoulder dystocia: the large majority of infants with a birth weight greater than 4500 g do not develop shoulder dystocia, and up to 50% of cases of shoulder dystocia occur in infants with a birth weight less than 4000 g.[1]

Antenatal detection of macrosomia is also poor: third-trimester ultrasound scans have at least a 10% margin of error for actual birth weight and detect only 60% of infants weighing over 4500 g.[1] Some authors have argued that fetal biometry has no place in the decision making regarding mode of birth for possible shoulder dystocia.[21] Moreover, until recently there has been very limited evidence of benefit for interventions based on estimated fetal weight.

Gestational age

A recent study of more than two million births demonstrated that the likelihood of shoulder dystocia increases as gestational age increases, from 0.22% at 32–35 weeks, to 0.42% at 36–37 weeks, 0.57% at 38–39 weeks, 0.83% at 40–41 weeks and 0.97% at 42–43 weeks. This is likely to be related to increasing fetal size.[22]

Maternal diabetes mellitus

Maternal diabetes mellitus increases the risk of shoulder dystocia: infants of diabetic mothers have a twofold increased risk of shoulder dystocia compared with infants of the same birth weight born to non-diabetic mothers.[16] This is probably attributable to the different body shape of babies born to diabetic mothers, i.e. they are broader, not just heavier.

Operative vaginal birth

Operative vaginal birth (forceps or vacuum-assisted births) is also associated with shoulder dystocia. This is possibly because infants born operatively are more likely to be macrosomic and/or their shoulders are more likely to be brought down directly in the narrower direct anteroposterior diameter.[15] A recent systematic review identified that vacuum-assisted birth appeared to be associated with a higher risk of shoulder dystocia than normal birth in both fixed and random models (odds ratio (OR) 2.87 and 2.98 respectively). There was no difference in the rate of shoulder dystocia between vacuum and forceps ($p > 0.05$).[23]

Obesity

Women with a raised body mass index (BMI) are at higher risk of shoulder dystocia than women with a normal BMI.[1] However, women who are obese are more likely to be diabetic and tend to have larger babies. Therefore, the association between maternal obesity and shoulder dystocia is likely to be attributable to fetal macrosomia rather than the maternal obesity itself.

> **Key points**
>
> - The majority of cases of shoulder dystocia occur in women with no risk factors.
> - Shoulder dystocia is therefore an unpredictable and largely unpreventable event.
> - Clinicians should be aware of existing risk factors but must always be alert to the possibility of shoulder dystocia with any birth.

Prevention and antenatal counselling

Caesarean birth

Shoulder dystocia can only be prevented by caesarean section. However, elective caesarean section is not routinely recommended as a method of reducing potential morbidity from possible shoulder dystocia. It has been estimated that an additional 2345 caesarean births would be required to prevent one permanent injury from shoulder dystocia.[24]

The recent Montgomery judgment in the UK Supreme Court requires carers to discuss all reasonable risks for all women, including the competing risks of vaginal versus caesarean birth, in the context of shoulder dystocia.[25] The relative risks are summarised in the RCOG patient information leaflet for elective birth by caesarean section:[26]

- Risk of shoulder dystocia and permanent brachial plexus injury (BPI):[22]
  - Shoulder dystocia: 1–2% risk
  - Permanent BPI: 0.03%
- Risks arising from caesarean birth:[26]

  - Babies born by caesarean section are more likely to develop asthma in childhood and to become overweight.
  - For reasons we do not yet understand, the chances of experiencing a stillbirth in a future pregnancy are higher after a caesarean section (0.4%) compared with a vaginal birth (0.2%).
  - There is an increased risk of abnormally invasive placenta after previous caesarean section.

Therefore, an elective caesarean birth is not without consequence, and the risk of stillbirth in a future pregnancy is 10 times greater than the risk of brachial plexus injury in the index pregnancy. Clearly, there are other pros and cons that also merit discussion.

The option of birth by elective caesarean section is recognised in the RCOG guideline for shoulder dystocia,[1] and in the US equivalent,[27] for women with diabetes and an estimated fetal weight of over 4500 g, or where the estimated fetal weight is greater than 5000 g in a woman without diabetes. This is because of the higher incidence of shoulder dystocia and BPI in pregnancies affected by diabetes.

Induction of labour

Until recently there did not appear to be any benefit in pre-emptive induction of labour (IOL). However, there are now robust data supporting early IOL as a strategy to reduce the risk of shoulder dystocia in two particular circumstances: (1) maternal diabetes and (2) suspected macrosomia.

A meta-analysis of randomised controlled trials of the effect of treatment in women with gestational diabetes concluded that the incidence of shoulder dystocia is reduced by early induction of labour in those women.[28]

Furthermore, a recently reported trial randomly assigned 822 women with singleton fetuses whose estimated weight exceeded the 95th percentile, to receive induction of labour between 37^{+0} weeks and 38^{+6} weeks of gestation or expectant management.[29] Induction of labour significantly reduced the risk of shoulder dystocia and associated morbidity compared with expectant management. The likelihood of spontaneous vaginal birth was higher in women in the induction group than in those in the expectant management group, albeit the subsequent Cochrane review reported an increase in the rate of severe perineal tears in the induction group.[30]

Therefore, accurate and transparent counselling remains a priority for women and their families, to enable them to reach the right decision for them.

Management of shoulder dystocia

Current international guidance recommends four basic shoulder dystocia resolution manoeuvres: McRoberts' position/all-fours position, suprapubic pressure, delivery of the posterior arm, and internal rotation.[1,27] An algorithm for the management of shoulder dystocia is shown in Figure 10.2. This is described in detail in the following sections.

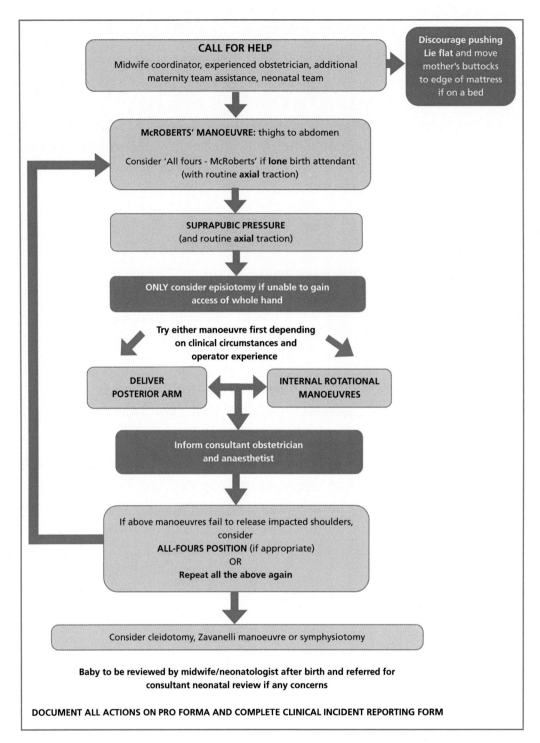

Figure 10.2 Algorithm for the management of shoulder dystocia (based on the RCOG Green-top Guideline 2012)

Recent data have identified that McRoberts' manoeuvre and/or suprapubic pressure may not be as successful as previously thought: they were successful in only 25.8% of shoulder dystocias, and the other 74.2% needed either rotational or posterior arm manoeuvres, or a combination of manoeuvres.[31] These observations have been replicated in a US dataset.[32]

Some authors have recommended employing internal manoeuvres as a first option.[33] However, internal manoeuvres are extremely invasive, and we recommend that McRoberts' and suprapubic pressure should be attempted first, with recourse to internal manoeuvres where required. Furthermore, a reduction in injury rates has been described using the RCOG algorithm.[6] Variations in the sequence of actions may be appropriate. For example, in a morbidly obese woman it may be difficult to achieve an effective McRoberts' position or perform effective suprapubic pressure, and therefore moving straight to an internal manoeuvre (e.g. delivery of the posterior arm) may be more appropriate.

Recognition of shoulder dystocia

- There may be difficulty with birth of the face and chin.
- When the head is born, it remains tightly applied to the vulva.
- The chin retracts and depresses the perineum – the 'turtle-neck' sign.
- The anterior shoulder fails to release with maternal effort and/or when routine axial traction is applied.

If a woman is giving birth in the pool, she should be asked to get out of the pool as soon as the midwife identifies a delay with the birth of the shoulders. It may not be possible to confirm if there is shoulder dystocia at this stage, but the woman should be safely moved out of the pool. No manoeuvres should be attempted in the pool.

Call for help

- Use the emergency buzzer (not the call bell) or dial 999 if in the community.
- In an obstetric unit call for:
  - ☐ senior midwife
  - ☐ additional maternity staff
  - ☐ the most experienced obstetrician available
  - ☐ neonatal team
- In the community call for:
  - ☐ paramedic ambulance
- Remember to call for the neonatologist – this is often forgotten.
- Consider calling the obstetric consultant and an anaesthetist.

Clearly state the problem. Announce 'shoulder dystocia' as help arrives.

Note the time that the head was born. Start the clock on the resuscitaire or mark the CTG, if monitoring.

Ask the mother to stop pushing. Pushing should be discouraged, as it may increase the impaction and therefore the risk of neurological and orthopaedic complications, and will not resolve the dystocia.

McRoberts' manoeuvre

The McRoberts' manoeuvre is an effective intervention with reported success rates as high as 90%, although more recent data have identified that the rate of resolution with McRoberts' is less than 50%.[32,34] McRoberts' has a low rate of complication and is one of the least invasive manoeuvres, and therefore should be employed first.

Lie the mother flat and remove any pillows from under her back. With one assistant on either side, hyperflex the mother's legs against her abdomen so that her knees are up towards her ears (Figure 10.3). If the mother is in the lithotomy position (for an operative vaginal birth), her legs will need to be removed from the supports to achieve McRoberts' positioning, unless the procedure is taking place in the maternity theatre, in which case the mother's legs may be secured in adjustable leg support boots: in this case, it may be possible to adjust the supports, to achieve McRoberts' position with mother's legs remaining safely in the boots.

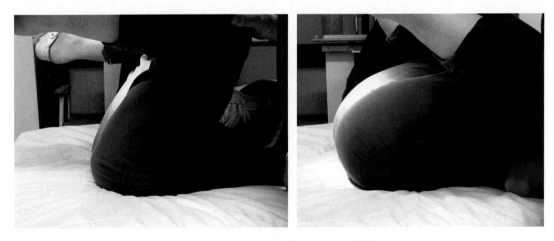

Figure 10.3 McRoberts' position

One feature of an effective McRoberts' is that the maternal buttocks are lifted off the bed during the hyperflexion of the hips, thereby rotating the pelvis.[31]

McRoberts' position increases the relative anteroposterior diameter of the pelvic inlet by rotating the maternal pelvis cephaloid and straightening the sacrum relative to the lumbar spine.

Routine axial traction – the same degree of traction as applied during a normal birth, and in an axial direction (i.e. in line with the axis of the fetal spine), should then be applied to the baby's head to assess whether the shoulders have been released (Figure 10.4).

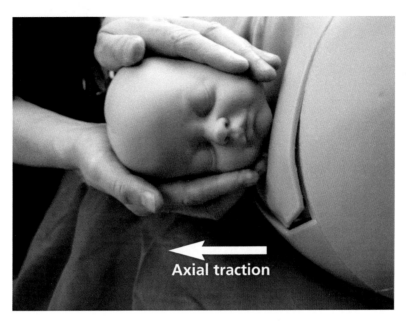

Axial traction

Figure 10.4 Routine axial traction

If the anterior shoulder is not released with McRoberts' position, move on to the next manoeuvre. Do not continue to apply traction to the baby's head.

> **Remember: shoulder dystocia is a 'bony problem' where the baby's shoulder is obstructed by the mother's pelvis. If the entrapment is not released by McRoberts' position, another manoeuvre (not traction) is required to free the shoulder and achieve birth.**

Prophylactic McRoberts' position, performed **before the birth of the baby's head**, is ineffective and therefore is not recommended.[1] Moreover, if McRoberts' position is performed in anticipation of a possible shoulder dystocia, it would not be clear as to whether there was truly a problem, and it could have implications for the mother's choice of place of birth in subsequent pregnancies.

All-fours position

The all-fours position has been described to have an 83% success rate in one small case series.[35] Positioning a woman in a flexed all-fours position with thighs against the abdomen has a similar effect on the maternal pelvis as

McRoberts': the all-fours position is essentially the McRoberts' position upside down. Individual circumstances should guide the accoucheur's decision whether to use McRoberts' or all-fours. For a slim mobile woman, with a **lone midwifery birth attendant**, the all-fours position is probably more appropriate, and clearly this may be a useful option in a home birth setting. For a less mobile woman (e.g. regional anaesthesia in place) the traditional McRoberts' position with mother lying flat will be much more appropriate.

To achieve an all-fours position, ask the mother to roll over so that she is supporting herself on her upper arms and knees, with her hips and knees flexed. This simple change of position may release the fetal shoulders. Routine axial traction should be applied to the fetal head to ascertain if the shoulder dystocia has been resolved. If dystocia remains, internal manoeuvres should be attempted (see below for more details).

> **Remember: when the woman is in an all-fours position, the maternal sacral hollow and the fetal posterior shoulder will both be uppermost.**

Suprapubic pressure

Suprapubic pressure aims to resolve shoulder dystocia by (1) reducing the fetal bisacromial (shoulder-to-shoulder) diameter and (2) rotating the anterior fetal shoulders into the wider oblique diameter of the pelvis. The anterior shoulder is freed to slip underneath the symphysis pubis with the aid of routine axial traction.

An assistant should apply suprapubic pressure from the side of the fetal back, which will reduce the diameter of the fetal shoulders by 'scrunching' (adducting) the shoulders in towards the fetal chest. Pressure should be applied just above the maternal symphysis pubis in a downward and lateral direction, to push the posterior aspect of the anterior shoulder towards the fetal chest (Figure 10.5). If there is uncertainty regarding the fetal position, suprapubic pressure should be applied from the side where it is most likely that the fetal back will be, and, if this pressure is unsuccessful at resolving the dystocia, suprapubic pressure can be attempted from the other side.

When applying suprapubic pressure, there is no evidence that rocking is better than continuous pressure, nor that pressure should be performed for 30 seconds for it to be effective. If the anterior shoulder is not released after attempting suprapubic pressure and routine axial traction, another manoeuvre should be attempted.

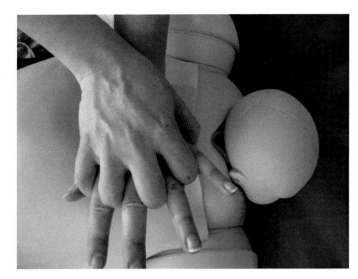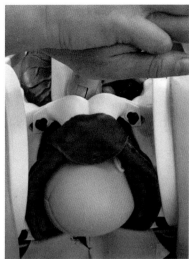

Figure 10.5 Applying suprapubic pressure

Evaluate the need for an episiotomy

An episiotomy will not relieve the bony obstruction of shoulder dystocia but may be required to allow the accoucheur more space to facilitate internal vaginal manoeuvres (delivery of the posterior arm or internal rotation of the shoulders). A recent systematic review found no evidence supporting the use of episiotomy in the prevention and management of shoulder dystocia.[36]

Often the perineum has already torn, or an episiotomy may have already been performed before birth of the head. With the correct technique, there is almost always enough room to gain internal access without performing an episiotomy.[37]

Internal manoeuvres

There are two types of internal vaginal manoeuvre that can be performed if McRoberts'/all-fours position and/or suprapubic pressure are not effective: delivery of the posterior arm and internal rotational manoeuvres. There is no evidence demonstrating that either manoeuvre is superior or that one should be attempted before the other: the decision on which manoeuvre to attempt should depend on the clinical circumstances. All internal manoeuvres start with the same action – inserting the whole hand posteriorly into the sacral hollow – and once access has been gained, a pragmatic decision can be made based on the individual set of circumstances with regard to the best manoeuvre to attempt first.

Gaining internal vaginal access

When shoulder dystocia occurs, the problem is usually at the inlet of the pelvis, with the anterior shoulder trapped above the symphysis pubis. When attempting to gain vaginal access for internal manoeuvres, the temptation is to introduce a hand anteriorly. However, if the anterior fetal shoulder is trapped because there is not enough room, there will also be insufficient room to insert a hand anteriorly to perform any manoeuvres (Figure 10.6).

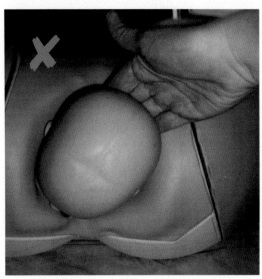
a. Attempting to gain anterior access

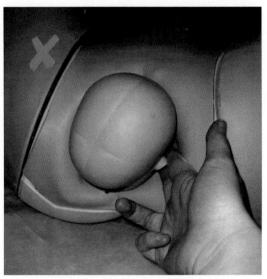
b. Attempting to gain lateral access

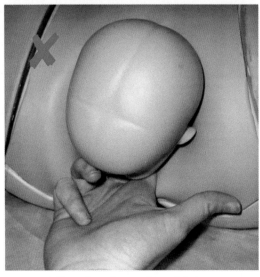
c. Entering the vagina with two fingers as if performing a routine vaginal examination

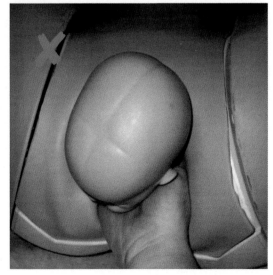
d. Leaving the thumb out of the vagina

Figure 10.6 Incorrect attempts at gaining vaginal access

The most spacious part of the pelvis is in the sacral hollow, and therefore vaginal access can be gained more easily posteriorly into the sacral hollow. If the accoucheur scrunches up her/his hand (as if putting on a tight bracelet, or reaching for the last Pringles crisp in the bottom of the container), internal rotation or delivery of the posterior arm can then be attempted using the whole hand (Figure 10.7).

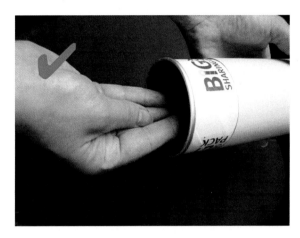 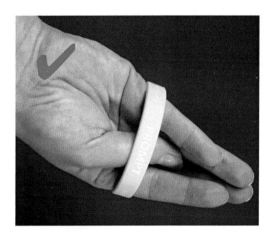

Figure 10.7 Correct vaginal access

Delivery of the posterior arm

Delivering the posterior arm will reduce the diameter of the fetal shoulders by the width of the arm. This will usually provide enough room to resolve the shoulder dystocia.

Babies will often lie with their arms flexed across their chest, and therefore, after the accoucheur places a hand into the vagina posteriorly, it is often possible to feel the hand and forearm of the posterior fetal arm (Figure 10.8). If this is the case, then the accoucheur can take hold of the fetal wrist (with fingers and thumb) and gently release the posterior arm in a straight line (Figure 10.9). This movement of the fetal arm is similar to the action of 'putting your hand up in class'. Once the posterior arm is delivered (Figure 10.10), gentle axial traction may be applied to the fetal head. If the shoulder dystocia has resolved, then the baby's body should be easily born.

If the baby is lying with its posterior arm straight and against its body (in front of the fetal abdomen), it may be possible for the accoucheur to apply pressure with a thumb to the baby's antecubital fossa and flex the posterior arm, so that the wrist can be grasped and the arm delivered as previously described. However, this is much more difficult, and it may be easier to attempt internal rotation of the fetal shoulders instead. In addition, if the accoucheur pulls on the upper arm, rather than the wrist, then this is likely to result in a humeral fracture.

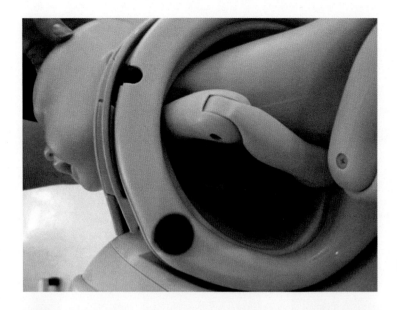

Figure 10.8 Locating the posterior arm

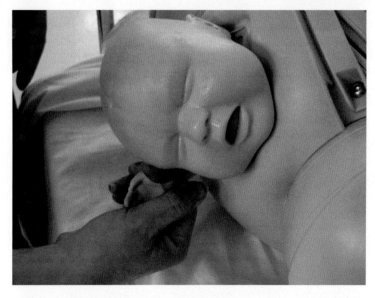

Figure 10.9 Gentle traction on the posterior arm in a straight line

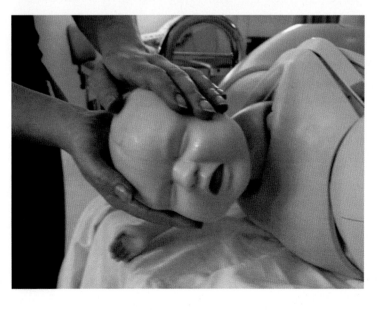

Figure 10.10 Routine axial traction to assist the rest of the body being born

Internal rotational manoeuvres

■ The aims of internal rotation are:

■ to move the fetal shoulders (the bisacromial diameter) out of the narrowest diameter of the mother's pelvis (the anterior–posterior) and into a wider pelvic diameter (the oblique or transverse).

■ to use the maternal pelvic anatomy to aid descent of the shoulders: as the fetal shoulders are rotated within the mother's pelvis, the fetal shoulder descends through the pelvis owing to the bony architecture of the pelvis.

Internal rotation of the fetal shoulders can be most easily achieved by pressing on the anterior aspect (front) or posterior aspect (back) of the posterior (lowermost) shoulder (Figure 10.11). Pressure on the posterior aspect of the posterior shoulder has the added benefit of reducing the shoulder diameter by adducting the shoulders (scrunching the shoulders together). Rotation should move the shoulders into the wider oblique diameter of the maternal pelvis, thereby resolving the shoulder dystocia and allowing release of the shoulders, aided by routine axial traction.

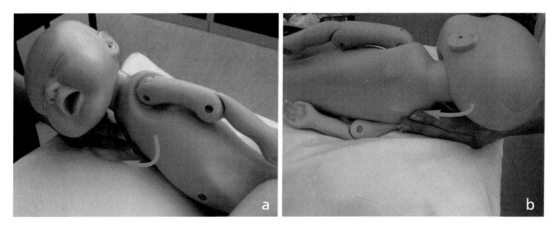

Figure 10.11 Internal rotational manoeuvres: (a) pressure on the anterior aspect (front) of the posterior shoulder to achieve rotation; (b) pressure on the posterior aspect (back) of the posterior shoulder to achieve rotation

It is not necessary to attempt to place fingers from both hands in the vagina for internal rotation, and nor is it necessary to rotate the shoulders more than 20–30°. A 180° rotation is anatomically very difficult to perform, if possible at all, and rotating the shoulders to such a degree is not usually necessary to achieve release of the shoulders.

If pressure in one direction has no effect, try to rotate the shoulders in the opposite direction by pressing on the other side of the fetal posterior shoulder (that is, change from pressing on the back of the baby's shoulder to pressing on the front of the baby's shoulder or vice versa). If you are struggling, try changing the hand that you are using.

While attempting to rotate the fetal shoulders from the inside of the pelvis, you can instruct a colleague to apply suprapubic pressure to assist your rotation, but ensure that you are pushing with, and not against, each other.

Additional manoeuvres

Several last-resort, or tertiary manoeuvres, have been described for those cases resistant to all standard measures. It is very rare that these are required if the manoeuvres described previously are performed correctly. In a recent series of more than 17,000 consecutive vaginal births with no permanent brachial plexus injuries, tertiary manoeuvres were not required.[6]

Vaginal replacement of the head (Zavanelli manoeuvre) and subsequent birth by caesarean section has been described, but success rates vary.[38] The long-term maternal consequences of this procedure are not reported, but a high proportion of fetuses have irreversible hypoxia–acidosis by the time that Zavanelli is attempted. As the uterus will have retracted following birth of the fetal head, i.e. the uterus is now smaller than when the fetal head was unborn, a tocolytic (e.g. terbutaline 0.25 mg subcutaneously or glyceryl trinitrate sublingually) should be given prior to any attempts to replace the fetal head inside the vagina, in order to reduce the risk of uterine rupture.

Symphysiotomy (partial surgical division of the maternal symphysis pubis ligament) has also been suggested as a potentially useful procedure. However, there is a high incidence of serious maternal morbidity and poor neonatal outcome.[39]

Other techniques, including the use of a posterior axillary sling,[40] have been reported, but there are few data available to recommend their use.

How much time do I have?

It is not possible to recommend an absolute time limit for the management of shoulder dystocia, as the head-to-body birth interval that each individual fetus can withstand without hypoxia occurring will vary depending on clinical circumstances and the vulnerability of the infant. Therefore, the condition of the baby at eventual birth is dependent on the head-to-body interval and the fetal condition at the start of the dystocia.

A review of fatal cases of shoulder dystocia in the UK reported that 47% of the babies that died did so within 5 minutes of the head being born; however, there was a very high proportion of cases in which the fetus had a pathological CTG prior to the shoulder dystocia.[41] Two more recent reviews reported low rates of hypoxic–ischaemic encephalopathy (HIE) if the head-to-body birth interval was less than 5 minutes.[42,43] The Hong Kong study reported that the drop in cord arterial pH observed with increasing head-to-body birth interval was mostly related to the presence of an abnormal fetal heart rate prior to birth.[42] The prolongation of the head-to-body birth interval itself was associated with a clinically insignificant drop in cord arterial pH of 0.01 per minute.

If a baby is in good condition before shoulder dystocia, the risk of HIE due to a prolonged head-to-body birth interval will be minimised. Adequate assessment of fetal wellbeing in labour is crucial (see **Module 5**).

> **Shoulder dystocia should be managed effectively (correct manoeuvres used and avoidance of excessive and/or downward traction to avert unnecessary trauma) and efficiently (recognised early and manoeuvres performed in a timely manner) to avoid hypoxia.**

What to avoid

Excessive and/or downward traction

It may be an instinctive reaction to pull on the fetal head in an attempt to assist the birth of the baby. However, traction alone will not resolve the dystocia, and **excessive traction must be avoided** because it is strongly associated with neonatal injury.[44] Traction in a downward direction is also strongly associated with obstetric brachial plexus injury.[44] **Downward traction on the fetal head** should be avoided in the management of all births.

There is also some evidence that traction applied quickly with a 'jerk', rather than applied slowly, may be more damaging to the nerves of the brachial plexus (imagine trying to snap a piece of cotton – it is much easier to break it with a quick pull than a slow pull).[45]

> **Routine traction (as for a vaginal birth without shoulder dystocia) should always be applied slowly and gently in an axial direction, and not with sudden force or in a downward direction.**
>
> **Do not pull quickly, do not pull hard, do not pull downwards.**

Fundal pressure

Fundal pressure is associated with a high rate of brachial plexus injury and rupture of the uterus. It should therefore **not be applied** during shoulder dystocia.[1]

Documentation

Accurate documentation of a difficult and potentially traumatic birth is essential. It is important to write a clear explanation of the manoeuvres that were performed, such that someone else reading it could reproduce those actions (it is not essential to use the names of manoeuvres, but better to describe the actions taken). It may be helpful to use a pro forma to aid accurate record keeping.[46] An example is provided in Figure 10.12.

It is important to record:

- time of birth of the head
- manoeuvres performed, the timing and the sequence
- traction applied
- time of birth of the body
- staff in attendance and the time they arrived
- condition of the baby
- umbilical cord blood acid–base measurements (cord pH or lactate)
- direction the baby is facing at birth, i.e. which fetal shoulder was anterior at the time of the dystocia (left or right)

After the birth

Shoulder dystocia is a frightening and potentially traumatic experience for the mother and her attending family. It is important to inform the parents at the time about what is happening and what is being done to relieve the situation, and to give the mother clear instructions during the emergency.[47] If there are sufficient staff, it is a good idea to allocate a designated team member to communicate with the woman and her relatives. By relaying the cause of the emergency, the condition of the baby and the aims of immediate and ultimate treatment, evidence suggests that this is more likely to result in a patient's perception of safety and good communication.[47] The birth and the reason for the use of manoeuvres should also be discussed afterwards.

SHOULDER DYSTOCIA DOCUMENTATION

Date .... Time ....

Person completing form ....

Designation ....

Signature ....

Mother's Name _____
Date of birth _____
Hospital Number _____
Consultant _____

Called for help at:		Emergency call via switchboard at:		
Staff present at birth of head:		**Additional staff attending for birth of shoulders**		
Name	**Role**	**Name**	**Role**	**Time arrived**

Maternal position when shoulder dystocia occurred - please circle (i.e. prior to any procedures to assist)	Semi-recumbent	Lithotomy	Side-lying	All fours	Kneeling	Standing	Squatting	Other ....

Procedures used to assist birth	**By whom**	**Time**	**Order**	**Details**	**Reason if not performed**
McRoberts' position					
Suprapubic pressure				From maternal **left / right** (circle as appropriate)	
Episiotomy				Enough access / tear present /already performed (circle as appropriate)	
Delivery of posterior arm				**Right / left** arm (circle as appropriate)	
Internal rotational manoeuvre					
Description of rotation					
Description of traction	Routine (as for normal vaginal birth)		Other -	Reason if not routine	
Other manoeuvres used					

Mode of birth of head	Spontaneous		Instrumental – vacuum / forceps	
Time of birth of head		Time of birth of baby	Head-to-body birth interval	
Fetal position during dystocia	Head facing maternal **left** / **Left** fetal shoulder anterior		Head facing maternal **right** / **Right** fetal shoulder anterior	

Birth weight		**kg**	**Apgar**	**1 min :**	**5 mins :**	**10 mins :**
Cord gases			**Art pH :**	**Art BE:**	**Venous pH :**	**Venous BE :**
Explanation to parents			Yes	By	**Risk incident form completed if clinical concerns** / Yes / N/A	

Neonatologist called: Yes / No   Time arrived: .... Neonatologists name: ....

Baby assessment at birth (maybe done by M/W):				If yes to any of these questions, for review and follow up by Consultant neonatologist
Any sign of arm weakness?		Yes	No	
Any sign of potential bony fracture?		Yes	No	
Baby admitted to Neonatal Intensive Care Unit?		Yes	No	
Assessment by				

Figure 10.12 An example of a shoulder dystocia documentation pro forma

A neonatologist should immediately review any baby with a suspected injury following shoulder dystocia. For those babies suspected of having a brachial plexus injury, early intervention is key to a good outcome. Babies should commence physiotherapy at about 5 days of age and progress should be reviewed regularly. If arm function remains unequal by 8 weeks of age a referral should be made to a specialist centre for assessment regarding future treatments. If a neonate has no active biceps movement by 12 weeks of age it is more likely the injury is severe and will be permanent, and the option of nerve graft surgery should be considered. Ideally nerve graft surgery should be performed before 9 months of age, as arm and hand function is better the earlier a nerve graft is performed.

In the UK the Erb's Palsy Group is an excellent source of information and supports families and healthcare practitioners caring for children with brachial plexus injuries (www.erbspalsygroup.co.uk).

A woman who has had a previous shoulder dystocia should be referred to a consultant-led antenatal clinic in subsequent pregnancies to discuss antenatal care and mode of birth (see previous comments about the risk of recurrence).

Consequences of shoulder dystocia

Shoulder dystocia has a high perinatal morbidity and mortality rate.[1] Maternal morbidity is also increased (Box 10.2).

Box 10.2 Perinatal morbidity and mortality associated with shoulder dystocia	
Perinatal	**Maternal**
Stillbirth	Postpartum haemorrhage
Hypoxia	Third- and fourth-degree tears
Brachial plexus injury	Uterine rupture
Fractures (humeral and clavicular)	Psychological distress

Acidosis

Shoulder dystocia is an acute life-threatening event. A healthy fetus will compensate during shoulder dystocia but only for a finite amount of time.

Babies may be born with a severe metabolic acidosis or may develop HIE, with or without long-term neurological damage (see above, under *How much time do I have?*). The necessary resuscitation equipment should therefore be prepared and neonatal staff called as soon as shoulder dystocia occurs, in case neonatal resuscitation is required.

Brachial plexus injury

The brachial plexus is one of the most complex structures in the peripheral nervous system, conveying motor, sensory and sympathetic nerve fibres to the arm and shoulder. The brachial plexus contains five roots (C5–C8, T1) that terminate in five main peripheral nerves. Sympathetic nerve fibres from the first thoracic root provide the autonomic nerve supply to the head, neck and upper limbs, and control sweat glands, pupillary dilatation and eyelid movement. Injuries can be divided into upper (Erb's palsy), lower (Klumpke's palsy) and total brachial plexus injury:

- **Erb's palsy** is the most common injury. The upper arm is flaccid and the lower arm is extended and rotated towards the body with the hand held in a classic 'waiter's tip' posture. Up to 90% of Erb's palsies recover by 12 months.

- **Klumpke's palsy** is less common. The hand is limp, with no movement of the fingers. The recovery rate is lower, with around 40% of injuries resolving by 12 months.

- **Total brachial plexus injury** occurs in approximately 20% of brachial plexus injuries. There is a total sensory and motor deficit of the entire arm, making it completely paralysed with no sensation. Horner syndrome, caused by sympathetic nerve injury resulting in contraction of the pupil and ptosis of the eyelid on the affected side, may also be present. Full functional recovery is rare without surgical intervention. The prognosis is worse if Horner syndrome is present.

The brachial plexus is vulnerable to trauma owing to its large size, superficial location and position between the neck and arm. The primary mechanism for brachial plexus injury is thought to be excessive traction on the fetal head during shoulder dystocia, although other mechanisms of injury have been proposed. The incidence of BPI in the UK and Republic of Ireland in 1998–99 was 0.43 per 1000 live births.[48] Between 8% and 12% of BPIs are reported to be permanent, i.e. an injury lasting more than 12 months.

Humeral and clavicular fractures

Humeral and clavicular fractures can also occur following shoulder dystocia and may be related to poor care and/or inaccurate execution of the release manoeuvres; the incidence of bony fractures has been reduced after training.[6,49] These fractures usually heal quickly and have a good prognosis.[50]

Shoulder dystocia is an unpredictable obstetric emergency

Problem	Clearly state the problem
Paediatrician	Immediately call the paediatrician/neonatologist
Position	McRoberts' or all-fours
Pressure	Suprapubic (*not fundal*) pressure
Posterior	Vaginal access gained posteriorly
Pringle	Get the whole hand in
Pull	Don't keep pulling if a manoeuvre has not worked
Pro forma	Documentation should be clear and concise
Parents	Communication and explanation are essential

Key points

- Shoulder dystocia is a complication of birth with potentially severe consequences for both mother and baby.

- Shoulder dystocia is unpredictable and therefore unpreventable. Therefore, all maternity carers should be ready to manage shoulder dystocia when it occurs.

- Accurate, efficient management is associated with improvements in outcome, particularly reductions in neonatal injury rates.

- Some training programmes have been associated with improvements in outcome and the RCOG currently states: *'Shoulder dystocia training associated with improvements in clinical management and neonatal outcomes was multi-professional, with manoeuvres demonstrated and practiced on a high fidelity mannequin.'*

References

1. Royal College of Obstetricians and Gynaecologists. *Shoulder Dystocia*. Green-top Guideline No. 42. London: RCOG, 2012. www.rcog.org.uk/en/guidelines-research-services/guidelines/gtg42 (accessed June 2017).

2. Angelini D, Greenwald L. Closed claims analysis of 65 medical malpractice cases involving nurse-midwives. *J Midwifery Womens Health* 2005; 50: 454–60.

3. AlDakhil LO. Obstetric and gynecologic malpractice claims in Saudi Arabia: incidence and cause. *J Forensic Leg Med* 2016; 40: 8–11.

4. NHS Litigation Authority. *Ten Years of Maternity Claims: An Analysis of NHS Litigation Authority Data*. London: NHSLA, 2012.

5. Fox R, Yelland A, Draycott T. Analysis of legal claims: informing litigation systems and quality improvement. *BJOG* 2014; 121: 6–10.

6. Crofts J, Lenguerrand E, Bentham GL, *et al.* Prevention of brachial plexus injury: 12 years of shoulder dystocia training: an interrupted time-series study. *BJOG* 2016; 123: 111–18.

7. Weiner CP, Collins L, Bentley S, Dong Y, Satterwhite CL. Multi-professional training for obstetric emergencies in a U.S. hospital over a 7-year interval: an observational study. *J Perinatol* 2016; 36: 19–24.

8. Fransen AF, van de Ven J, Schuit E, *et al.* Simulation-based team training for multi-professional obstetric care teams to improve patient outcome: a multicentre, cluster randomised controlled trial. *BJOG* 2017; 124: 641–50.

9. Walsh JM, Kandamany N, Ni Shuibhne N, *et al.* Neonatal brachial plexus injury: comparison of incidence and antecedents between 2 decades. *Am J Obstet Gynecol* 2011; 204: 324.e1–6.

10. MacKenzie I, Shah M, Lean K, *et al.* Management of shoulder dystocia: trends in incidence and maternal and neonatal morbidity. *Obstet Gynecol* 2007; 110: 1059–68.

11. Siassakos D, Crofts J, Winter C, Weiner CP, Draycott T. The active components of effective training in obstetric emergencies. *BJOG* 2009; 116: 1028–32.

12. Draycott TJ, Collins KJ, Crofts JF, *et al.* Myths and realities of training in obstetric emergencies. *Best Pract Res Clin Obstet Gynaecol* 2015; 29: 1067–76.

13. Crofts J, Fox R, Ellis D, *et al.* Observations from 450 shoulder dystocia simulations: lessons for skills training. *Obstet Gynecol* 2008; 112: 906–12.

14. Jan H, Guimicheva B, Gosh S, *et al.* Evaluation of healthcare professionals' understanding of eponymous maneuvers and mnemonics in emergency obstetric care provision. *Int J Gynaecol Obstet* 2014 125: 228–31.

15. Ouzounian JG. Shoulder dystocia: incidence and risk factors. *Clin Obstet Gynecol* 2016; 59: 791–4.

16. Hansen A, Chauhan S. Shoulder dystocia: definitions and incidence. *Semin Perinatol* 2014; 38: 184–8.

17. Gurewitsch Allen ED. Recurrent shoulder dystocia: risk factors and counseling. *Clin Obstet Gynecol* 2016; 59: 803–12.

18. Chauhan SP, Chang KW, Ankumah NE, Yang LJ. Neonatal brachial plexus palsy: obstetric factors associated with litigation. *J Matern Fetal Neonatal Med* 2016 Nov 16: 1–5. doi: 10.1080/14767058.2016.1252745.

19. Pondaag W, Allen RH, Malessy MJ. Correlating birthweight with neurological severity of obstetric brachial plexus lesions. *BJOG* 2011; 118: 1098–103.

20. Acker DB, Sachs BP, Friedman EA. Risk factors for shoulder dystocia in the average-weight infant. *Obstet Gynecol* 1986; 67: 614–18.

21. Doty MS, Al-Hafez L, Chauhan S. Sonographic examination of the fetus vis-à-vis shoulder dystocia: a vexing promise. *Clin Obstet Gynecol* 2016; 59: 795–802.

22. Chauhan S, Blackwell SB, Ananth CV. Neonatal brachial plexus palsy: incidence, prevalence, and temporal trends. *Semin Perinatol* 2014; 38: 210–18.

23. Dall'Asta A, Ghi T, Pedrazzi G, Frusca T. Does vacuum delivery carry a higher risk of shoulder dystocia? Review and meta-analysis of the literature. *Eur J Obstet Gynecol Reprod Biol* 2016; 204: 62–8.

24. Rouse DJ, Owen J. Prophylactic cesarean delivery for fetal macrosomia diagnosed by means of ultrasonography: a Faustian bargain? *Am J Obstet Gynecol* 1999; 181: 332–8.

25. Montgomery (Appellant) v Lanarkshire Health Board (Respondent) (Scotland). Supreme Court. Judgment date 11 Mar 2015. www.supremecourt.uk/decided-cases/docs/UKSC_2013_0136_Judgment.pdf (accessed June 2017).

26. Royal College of Obstetricians and Gynaecologists. *Choosing to Have a Caesarean Section*. London: RCOG, 2015. www.rcog.org.uk/en/patients/patient-leaflets/choosing-to-have-a-caesarean-section/ (accessed June 2017).

27. Chauhan S, Gherman R, Hendrix NW, Bingham JM, Hayes E. Shoulder dystocia: comparison of the ACOG Practice Bulletin with another national guideline. *Am J Perinatol* 2010; 27: 129–36.

28. Horvath K, Koch K, Jeitler K, *et al.* Effects of treatment in women with gestational diabetes mellitus: systematic review and meta-analysis. *BMJ* 2010; 340: c1395–5.

29. Boulvain M, Senat MV, Perrotin F, *et al.* Induction of labour versus expectant management for large-for-date fetuses: a randomised controlled trial. *Lancet* 2015; 385: 2600–5.

30. Boulvain M, Irion O, Dowswell T, Thornton JG. Induction of labour at or near term for suspected fetal macrosomia. *Cochrane Database Syst Rev* 2016; (5): CD000938.

31. Lok ZL, Cheng YK, Leung TY. Predictive factors for the success of McRoberts' manoeuvre and suprapubic pressure in relieving shoulder dystocia: a cross-sectional study. *BMC Pregnancy Childbirth* 2016; 16: 334.

32. Hoffman MK, Bailit JL, Branch DW, *et al.* A comparison of obstetric maneuvers for the acute management of shoulder dystocia. *Obstet Gynecol* 2011; 117: 1272–8.

33. Gurewitsch E, Allen R. Fetal manipulation for management of shoulder dystocia. *Fetal Matern Med Rev* 2006; 17: 239–80.

34. Leung T, Stuart O, Suen S, *et al.* Comparison of perinatal outcomes of shoulder dystocia alleviated by different type and sequence of manoeuvres: a retrospective review. *BJOG* 2011; 118: 985–90.

35. Bruner JP, Drummond SB, Meenan AL, Gaskin IM. All-fours maneuver for reducing shoulder dystocia during labor. *J Reprod Med* 1998; 43: 439–43.

36. Sagi-Dain L, Sagi S. The role of episiotomy in prevention and management of shoulder dystocia: a systematic review. *Obstet Gynecol Surv* 2015; 70: 354–62.

37. Johanson RB, Menon V, Burns E, *et al.* Managing Obstetric Emergencies and Trauma (MOET) structured skills training in Armenia, utilising models and reality based scenarios. *BMC Med Educ* 2002; 2: 5.

38. Vollebergh JH, van Dongen PW. The Zavanelli manoeuvre in shoulder dystocia: case report and review of published cases. *Eur J Obstet Gynecol* 2000; 89: 81–4.

39. Goodwin TM, Banks E, Millar LK, Phelan JP. Catastrophic shoulder dystocia and emergency symphysiotomy. *Am J Obstet Gynecol* 1997; 177: 463–4.

40. Cluver CA, Hofmeyr GJ. Posterior axilla sling traction for shoulder dystocia: case review and a new method of shoulder rotation with the sling. *Am J Obstet Gynecol* 2015; 212: 784.e1–7.

41. Hope P, Breslin S, Lamont L, *et al.* Fatal shoulder dystocia: a review of 56 cases reported to the Confidential Enquiry into Stillbirths and Deaths in Infancy. *Br J Obstet Gynaecol* 1998; 105: 1256–61.

42. Leung TY, Stuart O, Sahota DS, *et al.* Head-to-body delivery interval and risk of fetal acidosis and hypoxic ischaemic encephalopathy in shoulder dystocia: a retrospective review. *BJOG* 2011; 118: 474–9.

43. Lerner H, Durlacher K, Smith S, Hamilton E. Relationship between head-to-body delivery interval in shoulder dystocia and neonatal depression. *Obstet Gynecol* 2011; 118: 318–22.

44. Mollberg M, Lagerkvist AL, Johansson U, *et al.* Comparison in obstetric management on infants with transient and persistent obstetric brachial plexus palsy. *J Child Neurol* 2008; 23: 1424–32.

45. Metaizeau J, Gayet C, Plenat F. Les lesions obstetricales du plexus brachial. *Chir Pediatr* 1979; 20: 159–63.

46. Crofts J, Bartlett C, Ellis D, Fox R, Draycott T. Documentation of simulated shoulder dystocia: accurate and complete? *BJOG* 2008; 115: 1303–8.

47. Siassakos D, Bristowe K, Hambly H, *et al.* Team communication with patient actors: findings from a multisite simulation study. *Simul Healthc* 2011; 6: 143–9.

48. Evans-Jones G, Kay S, Weindling A, *et al.* Congenital brachial palsy: incidence, causes, and outcome in the United Kingdom and Republic of Ireland. *Arch Dis Child Fetal Neonatal Ed* 2003; 88: F185–9.

49. Draycott T, Crofts J, Ash JP, *et al.* Improving neonatal outcome through practical shoulder dystocia training. *Obstet Gynecol* 2008; 112: 14–20.

50. Crofts J, Bartlett C, Ellis D, *et al.* Management of shoulder dystocia: skill retention 6 and 12 months after training. *Obstet Gynecol* 2007; 110: 1069–74.

Module 11
Cord prolapse

Key learning points

- To recognise the risk factors for cord prolapse.
- To call for appropriate help.
- To be aware of the manoeuvres required to reduce cord compression.
- To communicate effectively with the woman, her partner and the multi-professional team.
- To understand the importance of appropriate documentation.

Common difficulties observed in training drills

- Difficulties in recognition of occult cord prolapse, e.g. cord trapped alongside the presenting part but not palpable or visible
- Inappropriate handling of the cord
- Delay in moving woman to an appropriate position to relieve cord compression
- Not calling for appropriate help
- Difficulties with assembling equipment for bladder filling
- Omitting to take cord gases post-birth

Introduction

Cord prolapse has been defined as the descent of the umbilical cord through the cervix, either alongside (occult) or past (overt) the presenting part, in the presence of ruptured membranes.

Cord presentation is the presence of the umbilical cord between the fetal presenting part and the maternal cervix, with or without intact membranes.

The incidence of umbilical cord prolapse ranges from 0.1% to 0.6% of all births.[1] In breech presentations the incidence is around 1%.[1]

Risk factors for cord prolapse

Cord prolapse most commonly occurs after the amniotic membranes rupture (spontaneously or artificially) and the fetal presenting part is poorly applied to the maternal cervix. The umbilical cord slips below the presenting part and may subsequently be compressed, compromising the fetal blood supply.

The presence of risk factors (Box 11.1) should raise awareness, but the occurrence of cord prolapse remains extremely unpredictable. A common feature of all the risk factors is a poorly applied fetal presenting part.

Induction of labour with prostaglandins is not associated with a higher risk of cord prolapse.[1]

Box 11.1 Risk factors for cord prolapse[1]	
Antenatal	**Intrapartum _(including procedure-related interventions)_**
■ Breech presentation ■ Multiparity ■ Fetal congenital abnormalities ■ Unstable lie ■ Oblique or transverse lie ■ Polyhydramnios ■ External cephalic version ■ Low birth weight (less than 2500 g)	Amniotomy (especially with a high presenting part) Unengaged presenting part Prematurity Breech presentation Internal podalic version Second twin Disimpaction of fetal head during rotational operative vaginal birth or other manipulation of the fetal head Fetal scalp electrode application Stabilising induction of labour Large balloon catheter induction of labour

Prevention

The RCOG recommends that women with non-cephalic presentations and preterm pre-labour rupture of membranes (PPROM) should be offered admission to hospital after 37[+0] weeks (or sooner if there are signs of labour or suspicion of ruptured membranes) before elective caesarean section at term. Elective admission will not prevent cord prolapse; however, if a cord prolapse does occur while the woman is in hospital, then immediate diagnosis and treatment is possible, resulting in improved neonatal outcome.[1]

If the umbilical cord is palpated below the presenting part on vaginal examination during labour, artificial rupture of membranes should be avoided.[1]

Any obstetric intervention (application of fetal scalp electrode, manual rotation of vertex, internal podalic version) once membranes have ruptured carries a risk of cord prolapse, and upward displacement of the presenting part should therefore be minimised.

Artificial rupture of the membranes should be avoided, when possible, if the presenting part is not engaged and/or mobile. If artificial rupture of the membranes is absolutely necessary, it should be performed with facilities to perform an immediate emergency caesarean section if required. In addition, fundal pressure and/or stabilisation of a longitudinal lie may reduce the risk of cord prolapse in these circumstances.[1]

Perinatal complications

The maternal mortality rate associated with cord prolapse has fallen over the past century. However, the perinatal mortality rate associated with umbilical cord prolapse remains high (91 per 1000),[1] and cases of cord prolapse still consistently feature in perinatal mortality enquiries.

The interval between diagnosis and birth is a contributing factor to stillbirth and perinatal death. Cord prolapse outside hospital carries a significantly worse prognosis, with the risk of perinatal death increased 10-fold. Delays associated with transfer to hospital have been identified as an important factor.[1,2,3]

Infants may suffer birth asphyxia owing to umbilical cord compression and/or arterial vasospasm of the umbilical cord. Birth asphyxia may result in hypoxic–ischaemic encephalopathy (HIE), cerebral palsy or neonatal death.[4] However, perinatal death after umbilical cord prolapse has been demonstrated to relate more to the complications of prematurity and low birth weight – the predisposing cause –than to intrapartum asphyxia.[5,6]

Initial management of cord prolapse

An outline of the management of cord prolapse is shown in Figure 11.1. This is described in detail in the following sections.

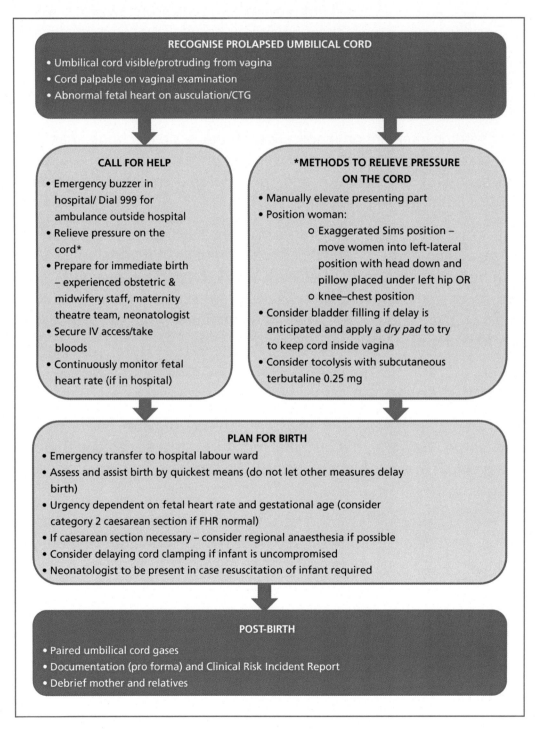

RECOGNISE PROLAPSED UMBILICAL CORD
- Umbilical cord visible/protruding from vagina
- Cord palpable on vaginal examination
- Abnormal fetal heart on ausculation/CTG

CALL FOR HELP
- Emergency buzzer in hospital/ Dial 999 for ambulance outside hospital
- Relieve pressure on the cord*
- Prepare for immediate birth – experienced obstetric & midwifery staff, maternity theatre team, neonatologist
- Secure IV access/take bloods
- Continuously monitor fetal heart rate (if in hospital)

*METHODS TO RELIEVE PRESSURE ON THE CORD
- Manually elevate presenting part
- Position woman:
    o Exaggerated Sims position – move women into left-lateral position with head down and pillow placed under left hip OR
    o knee–chest position
- Consider bladder filling if delay is anticipated and apply a *dry pad* to try to keep cord inside vagina
- Consider tocolysis with subcutaneous terbutaline 0.25 mg

PLAN FOR BIRTH
- Emergency transfer to hospital labour ward
- Assess and assist birth by quickest means (do not let other measures delay birth)
- Urgency dependent on fetal heart rate and gestational age (consider category 2 caesarean section if FHR normal)
- If caesarean section necessary – consider regional anaesthesia if possible
- Consider delaying cord clamping if infant is uncompromised
- Neonatologist to be present in case resuscitation of infant required

POST-BIRTH
- Paired umbilical cord gases
- Documentation (pro forma) and Clinical Risk Incident Report
- Debrief mother and relatives

Figure 11.1 Outline management of umbilical cord prolapse (adapted from RCOG Green-top Guideline No. 50. 2014[1])

Recognise prolapsed umbilical cord

- Early diagnosis is important. A cord prolapse may be obvious when there is a loop of umbilical cord protruding through the vulva. However, a prolapsed cord is not always apparent and may only be found on vaginal examination.

- Cord prolapse should be excluded at every vaginal examination. Auscultate the fetal heart rate, if not having continuous electronic fetal monitoring, after each vaginal examination and after spontaneous or artificial rupture of membranes.

- Cord prolapse should be suspected when there is an abnormal fetal heart rate pattern (e.g. bradycardia, decelerations) in the presence of ruptured membranes, particularly if such changes commence soon after membrane rupture.

- A speculum and/or a digital vaginal examination should be performed when cord prolapse is suspected, regardless of gestation.

- Mismanagement of abnormal fetal heart rate patterns is one aspect identified in perinatal death associated with cord prolapse.[1]

Call for help

- As soon as cord prolapse is diagnosed, urgent help should be called immediately, including (if possible) a senior midwife, additional midwifery staff, the most experienced obstetrician available, an anaesthetist, the theatre team and the neonatal team.

- If cord prolapse occurs outside hospital, an emergency ambulance should be called immediately to transfer the woman to the nearest consultant-led obstetric unit. Even if birth appears imminent, a paramedic ambulance should still be called in case of neonatal compromise at birth.

- When help arrives, state the problem – 'cord prolapse' – so that all in attendance immediately understand the emergency. Staff outside the obstetric unit (midwives, ambulance staff, general practitioners) should liaise directly with the obstetric unit, clearly stating that they are transferring a woman with a cord prolapse and giving an estimated time of arrival at hospital. This will ensure that the appropriate hospital staff are aware and preparations can be made to assist a timely birth upon arrival at hospital.

Relieve pressure on the cord

As soon as cord prolapse has been recognised, cord compression should be minimised by elevating the presenting part. This can be achieved by maternal positioning, digital elevation of the presenting part, or bladder filling. Tocolysis may also be used to reduce uterine contractions.

Maternal positioning

Traditionally, management of umbilical cord prolapse has recommended the knee–chest, face-down position. However, this position is less suitable for transportation in an ambulance or on a trolley, and therefore the exaggerated Sim's position (left-lateral with a pillow under the left hip) with or without Trendelenburg (tilted bed so that the woman's head is lower than her pelvis) may be used instead (Figure 11.2).[1] If a woman is at home in an upstairs room, it may also be quicker for her to walk down the stairs in between contractions, rather than trying to manoeuvre a trolley down narrow stairwells.

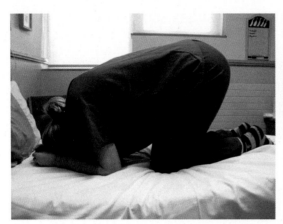 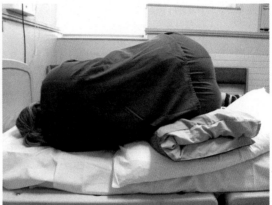

Figure 11.2 Maternal positioning to aid elevation of presenting part:
(a) knee–chest; (b) exaggerated Sim's position

Digital elevation of the presenting part

If cord prolapse is recognised at the time of rupture of membranes, the clinician's gloved fingers should be kept within the vagina to elevate the presenting part. This reduces compression of the cord, particularly during contractions. If the umbilical cord has prolapsed out from the vagina, attempt to gently replace it back into the vagina using a **dry pad**, and with minimal handling. Any handling of the umbilical cord may cause vasospasm, and therefore trying to replace the cord above the presenting part is not recommended. **There is no evidence to support the practice of covering the exposed cord with sterile gauze soaked in warmed saline.**[1]

Reduce contractions

If an oxytocin infusion is in progress, this should be stopped immediately. Tocolysis has been used to reduce contractions and improve fetal bradycardia when there is a cord prolapse. Terbutaline 0.25 mg subcutaneously has been recommended.[1]

Bladder filling

If the decision-to-birth interval is likely to be prolonged, particularly if it involves ambulance transfer into hospital, elevation of the presenting part through bladder filling may be considered.

Bladder filling was first proposed by Vago in 1970 as a method of relieving pressure on the umbilical cord. Bladder filling raises the presenting part of the fetus off the compressed cord for an extended period of time, thereby eliminating the need for an examiner's fingers to displace the presenting part.[7,8]

- ■ Insert Foley catheter into the urinary bladder.

- ■ Fill bladder via the catheter with sterile 0.9% sodium chloride, using an intravenous infusion set. The catheter should be clamped once 500 mL has been instilled.

- ■ Leave the bag of fluid attached for transfer to hospital or labour ward (this will help to remind staff to empty the bladder when the woman arrives in theatre/hospital). **NB – It is important that it has previously been checked that the IV giving set used is a good fit with the catheter, and that fluid can be effectively squeezed into the bladder via this system without undue leakage.**

- ■ It is essential to empty the bladder just before any method of birth is attempted. This can be done by detaching the giving set from the catheter and allowing the fluid from the bladder to drain out. If the catheter is to remain in situ for caesarean section, then a catheter bag may be attached. However, if vaginal birth is anticipated, then the catheter should be removed.

Any of the measures described above for relieving the pressure on the cord may be useful during preparation for assisting the birth of the fetus; however, birth should not be delayed by trying to implement these measures.[1]

Assessment of fetal wellbeing

Continuous electronic fetal monitoring should be performed. If the fetal heart is not audible, an ultrasound scan should be performed.

Plan for birth

Cord prolapse should be managed in a unit with full anaesthetic and neonatal services. If cord prolapse occurs outside of the labour ward, immediate transfer is essential.

Good communication is required so that appropriate members of staff are ready to receive the woman on arrival. Theatre staff should also be on standby.

If there is no intravenous access, site a wide-bore intravenous cannula (14/16-gauge) and take blood for full blood count and group and save.

Assessment for birth

- If the cervix is not fully dilated, caesarean section should be performed.

- A category 1 caesarean section should be performed with the aim of achieving birth within 30 minutes or less if cord prolapse is associated with a suspicious or pathological fetal heart rate pattern, but without compromising maternal safety (verbal consent is satisfactory for category 1 caesarean section).

- A category 2 caesarean section can be considered for women in whom the fetal heart rate is normal, but continuous fetal monitoring is still essential. Re-categorisation to category 1 birth should be immediately considered if there are any concerns regarding the cardiotocograph (CTG).

- If the cervix is fully dilated, consider an operative vaginal birth as long as it is anticipated that it would be accomplished quickly and safely. Ventouse or forceps should be considered only if the prerequisites for operative vaginal birth are met.

- At birth, delaying cord clamping may be considered as long as the baby is uncompromised.

- For births at the threshold of fetal viability (23^{+0} to 24^{+6} weeks), expectant management should be discussed with the parents. Women should be counselled on both continuation and termination of pregnancy following cord prolapse in these circumstances.[1]

- Breech extraction may be performed under some circumstances, for example after internal podalic version for the second twin.[1]

In general, poor fetal outcomes are associated with more difficult attempts at achieving vaginal birth. It should be remembered that any delays could be compounded by the possible need to then undertake a caesarean section if an attempt at an operative vaginal birth fails.

The use of temporary measures, as described in the previous section, to relieve pressure on the cord should enable an attempt at regional anaesthesia (spinal or epidural top-up). However, prolonged and repeated attempts at regional anaesthesia should be avoided.

The presenting part should be kept elevated while anaesthesia is undertaken. Clear communication about the urgency and timing of birth is required between the obstetric, midwifery and anaesthetic teams to ensure that the safest method of anaesthesia for both mother and fetus is chosen.

Neonatal resuscitation

An experienced neonatal team must be present at birth to ensure full cardiorespiratory support is given to the neonate, if required.

Post birth

Paired umbilical cord gases should be taken after birth to aid assessment of the neonatal condition.

Documentation

Documentation should include the time the cord prolapse occurred, the time help was called and arrived, methods used to alleviate cord compression, the time of the decision to assist the birth, and the method and time of birth. A pro forma (Figure 11.3) may aid documentation. Risk management reporting forms should also be completed.

Debrief of parents

Cord prolapse is a frightening experience for the parents. If one of the team can be allocated to communicate with the parents this can be very helpful, not only to relay specific instructions, if needed, to the mother but also to provide a running commentary of events as they happen, which may help the mother and her partner to cope with this emergency situation. An opportunity to discuss events after the birth should also be offered to the mother and relatives at a mutually convenient time.[1]

Training

All staff involved in maternity care should receive training in the management of cord prolapse. Training should be multi-professional and include team rehearsals with hospital, birth centre and community teams. With regular training, the procedures required to relieve cord compression can be conducted efficiently and without delaying birth. A retrospective

CORD PROLAPSE PROFORMA

Please tick the relevant boxes

Addressograph
or name and unit no

Diagnosed: **Home** ☐ **Birth Centre** ☐ **CDS** ☐ **Ward** ☐

Time of diagnosis:.........................

Cervical dilatation at diagnosis: .... cm

If at Home / Birth Centre

Ambulance called? Yes ☐ No ☐ Time called: .... Arrived: ....

CDS contacted? Yes ☐ No☐ Time called: .... Arrival time at Hospital: ....

If on CDS/Ward

Senior Midwife called Yes ☐ No ☐ Time............ Arrived...............

Senior Obstetrician called Yes ☐ No ☐ Time............ Arrived...............

Grade of Obstetrician: ....

Neonatologist called Yes ☐ No ☐ Time............ Arrived...............

Procedure used in managing cord prolapse				
Elevating the presenting part manually	**Yes** ☐	**No** ☐		
Filling the bladder	**Yes** ☐	**No** ☐		
Exaggerated Sims (left lateral) / Knee-Chest position / Head Tilt / Trolley / bed **(Please circle)**				
Tocolysis with sc Terbutaline 0.25mg or other	**Yes** ☐	**No** ☐		
Decision to birth interval: ....minutes				

Mode of birth		Mode of Anaesthesia	
Spontaneous vaginal	☐	GA	☐
Forceps	☐	Spinal	☐
Ventouse	☐	Epidural	☐
LSCS	☐		

Apgar Score		Baby's weight:	
:1 min		Cord pH	Base Excess:
:5 min		Venous:	
:10 min		Arterial:	
Admission to NICU? Yes ☐ No ☐			
Clinical Incident Reporting form completed? Yes ☐			
Known Risk Factor? YES ☐ NO ☐ If YES, please state:			
Mother debriefed Yes ☐ No ☐			

Signature: .... Print: ....

Designation: .... Date: ....

Figure 11.3 Example of cord prolapse documentation pro forma

study examined the effect of team training for the management of cord prolapse, and found that the introduction of regular training was associated with both more frequent actions to relieve cord compression and a shorter diagnosis-to-birth interval; crucially, it was also associated with consistently better neonatal outcomes.[9]

References

1. Royal College of Obstetricians and Gynaecologists. *Umbilical Cord Prolapse*. Green-top Guideline No. 50. London: RCOG, 2014. www.rcog.org.uk/en/guidelines-research-services/guidelines/gtg50 (accessed June 2017).

2. Confidential Enquiry into Stillbirths and Deaths in Infancy. *7th Annual Report*. London: Maternal and Child Health Research Consortium, 2000.

3. Johnson KC, Daviss BA. Outcomes of planned home births with certified professional midwives: large prospective study in North America. *BMJ* 2005; 330: 1416.

4. MacLennan A. A template for defining a causal relation between acute intrapartum events and cerebral palsy: international consensus statement. *BMJ* 1999; 319: 1054–9.

5. Murphy DJ, MacKenzie IZ. The mortality and morbidity associated with umbilical cord prolapse. *Br J Obstet Gynaecol* 1995; 102: 826–30.

6. Yla-Outinen A, Heinonen PK, Tuimala R. Predisposing and risk factors of umbilical cord prolapse. *Acta Obstet Gynecol Scand* 1985; 64: 567–70.

7. Vago T. Prolapse of the umbilical cord: a method of management. *Am J Obstet Gynecol* 1970; 107: 967–9.

8. Caspi E, Lotan Y, Schreyer P. Prolapse of the cord: reduction in perinatal mortality by bladder instillation and caesarean section. *Isr J Med Sci* 1983; 19: 541–5.

9. Siassakos D, Hasafa Z, Sibanda T, *et al.* Retrospective cohort study of diagnosis-delivery interval with umbilical cord prolapse: the effect of team training. *BJOG* 2009; 116: 1089–96.

Module 12
Vaginal breech birth

Key learning points

- Ensure that practitioners managing vaginal breech birth are trained and competent.
- Ensure that there is continuous electronic fetal monitoring during labour and birth (even if the decision is taken to perform a caesarean section), as this may lead to improved neonatal outcomes.
- Ensure full cervical dilatation before commencing pushing.
- Await visualisation of the breech at the perineum before encouraging active pushing.
- Avoid traction on the breech.
- Ensure a 'hands off' approach as much as possible.
- Understand the manoeuvres that may be required to assist a breech birth.

Common difficulties observed in training drills

- Reluctance to allow the breech to descend without intervention
- Premature commencement of assisted breech manoeuvres
- Pressure on the abdomen away from non-bony prominences during those manoeuvres
- Failing to flex knees and elbows in the correct direction during release manoeuvres
- Overextending the neck during birth of the head

Introduction

The incidence of breech presentation in the UK is 3–4% at term, although it is much higher earlier in pregnancy (20% at 28 weeks). Breech presentation is associated with a higher perinatal morbidity and mortality than cephalic presentation, particularly with vaginal birth. Prematurity, congenital malformations, birth asphyxia and trauma are all more common with breech presentations,[1] and these risks should inform antenatal, intrapartum and neonatal management.

Definition of breech presentation

Breech presentation is where the presenting part of the fetus is the buttocks or feet; the breech can be extended, flexed or footling (Figure 12.1).

Predisposing factors

Factors that predispose to a breech presentation are listed in Box 12.1.[1]

Box 12.1 Factors associated with breech presentation	
Previous breech birth	Uterine anomalies
Premature labour	Maternal pelvic tumour or fibroids
High parity	Placenta praevia
Multiple pregnancy	Hydrocephaly/anencephaly
Polyhydramnios	Fetal neuromuscular disorders
Oligohydramnios	Fetal head and neck tumours

There has been a large reduction in the incidence of vaginal breech birth since the publication of the Term Breech Trial.[2,3,4] This makes it all the more important that staff are trained and experienced in managing such births, as there will continue to be a small number due to failures to detect breech presentation prior to birth, and for reasons of maternal choice. The Term Breech Trial compared outcomes after planned vaginal and planned caesarean births for breech presentation, and demonstrated a significant reduction in perinatal morbidity and mortality in the planned caesarean group (reduction in mortality of 75%). In addition, there was no significant increase in maternal morbidity or mortality with planned caesarean births. However, the 2-year follow-up data from the trial did not demonstrate any statistically significant differences in neurodevelopment between infants born by caesarean section and those born vaginally.[5] Therefore, it is unclear whether the long-term benefits for the child of being born by planned caesarean section for breech presentation outweigh the maternal risks of the additional caesareans.

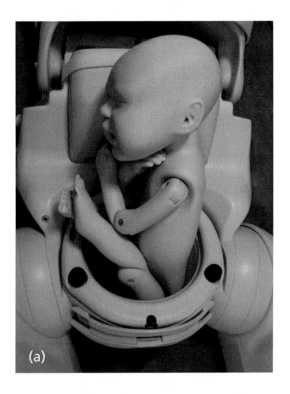

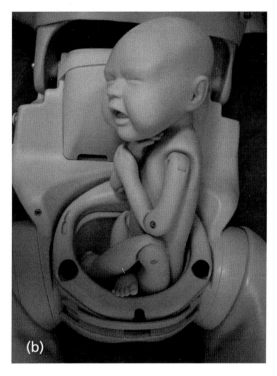

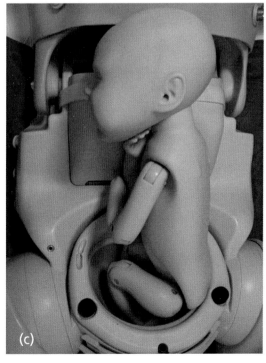

Figure 12.1 Types of breech presentation and incidence: (a) extended (65%): hips flexed, knees extended; (b) flexed (10%): hips flexed, knees flexed but feet not below the buttocks; (c) footling (25%): feet or knees are lowest (either single or double footling)

In the Netherlands, for known breech presentations at term, there was an increase in the elective caesarean section rate from 24% to 60% between 1999 and 2007, and the overall perinatal mortality decreased from 1.3 to 0.7 per 1000 births. The perinatal mortality rate remained stable in the plannel vaginal birth group (1.6 per 1000 births). The number of caesarean sections performed to prevent one perinatal death was 338.[6]

More recent data from a systematic review of breech births, including both observational and randomised studies, quantified the relative, and also the absolute, risks for both methods of birth.[7] Although the relative risks were higher for planned vaginal birth, the absolute risks for perinatal mortality, fetal neurological morbidity, birth trauma, Apgar score lower than 7 at 5 minutes and neonatal asphyxia in this group were considered small (ranging from 0.3% to 3.3%). Provided that women are informed of these risks and find them acceptable, there may be a role for planned vaginal breech birth in suitable cases. The *BJOG* editorial team observed that the risk of serious medical problems for the baby is 'within the range' for the risks quoted for home birth.[8]

The authors, and others, also argued that maintaining the clinical skills to conduct a vaginal breech birth is vital because there will always be situations where a woman presents in advanced labour with a breech presentation (and hence a caesarean section may not be possible), or women may not wish to have an elective caesarean birth.

In the UK, the Royal College of Obstetricians and Gynaecologists (RCOG) has recently released its updated Green-top Guideline on the management of breech presentation (Box 12.2).[1] The guideline states that the selection of appropriate pregnancies, together with skilled intrapartum care, may allow planned vaginal breech birth to be nearly as safe as planned vaginal cephalic birth.

Management of vaginal breech birth

Types of vaginal breech birth

- **Spontaneous breech birth** – The fetus is allowed to descend and deliver without assistance or manipulation. This accounts for a small proportion of births, most of which are preterm.

- **Assisted breech birth** – The most common method of vaginal breech birth. The fetus is allowed to descend with the accoucheur employing a 'hands-off' approach. However, recognised manoeuvres are used to assist the birth when required.

Box 12.2 Summary of national recommendations and recent evidence[1]

Mode of birth in breech presentation

■ When planning vaginal breech birth, women should be informed that the risk of perinatal mortality is approximately 0.5/1000 with caesarean section after 39 weeks of gestation and approximately 2.0/1000 with a planned vaginal breech birth.

■ Women should be informed that planned vaginal breech birth increases the risk of low Apgar scores and serious short-term complications, but has not been shown to increase the risk of long-term morbidity.

■ Planned caesarean section leads to a small reduction in perinatal mortality compared with planned vaginal breech birth. Any decision to perform a caesarean section needs to be balanced against the potential adverse consequences that may result from this.

■ The presence of a skilled birth attendant is essential for safe vaginal breech births.

Management of preterm singleton breech presentation

■ Routine caesarean section for breech presentation in *spontaneous* preterm labour is not recommended. The mode of birth should be individualised based on the gestation, stage of labour, type of breech presentation, fetal wellbeing and availability of an operator skilled in vaginal breech birth.

Management of twin pregnancy with breech presentation

■ Evidence is limited, but if the presenting twin is a breech presentation, then *planned* caesarean section is recommended.

■ Routine emergency caesarean section for a breech presentation of the first twin in *spontaneous labour* is not recommended. The mode of birth should be individualised based on cervical dilatation, station of the presenting part, type of breech presentation, fetal wellbeing of both twins and availability of an operator skilled in vaginal breech birth.

- **Breech extraction** – Mainly reserved for assisting the birth of the non-cephalic second twin. Breech extraction involves grasping one or both of the fetal feet from within the uterine cavity and bringing them down through the vagina, before continuing with the manoeuvres used in an assisted breech birth.

Management of the first stage of labour

The recent RCOG Green-top Guideline recommends that when a woman presents with an unplanned vaginal breech labour, management should depend on the gestation, stage of labour, whether factors associated with increased complications are found, the availability of appropriate clinical expertise, and informed consent from the mother. It also recommends that the birth should take place in a hospital with facilities for emergency caesarean section, but it is not routinely necessary to transfer the mother to an operating theatre for vaginal birth.[1]

Preparation

- Inform the senior midwife, senior obstetrician, anaesthetist, theatre staff and neonatologist of the mother's admission, and ensure that key members of staff are available who are skilled in managing vaginal breech birth.[1]
- Discuss the mode of birth again and ensure that the woman wishes to opt for vaginal breech birth.
- Discuss analgesia early in the process. There is no evidence to support routine epidural anaesthesia, but it may increase the risk of intervention if used; there should be a range of analgesia offered during breech labour and birth.[1] Consider a pudendal block if epidural analgesia is not used.
- Explain all birth techniques, and that a neonatologist will routinely attend a vaginal breech birth.
- Establish intravenous access and take blood for full blood count and group and save.
- Prepare the labour room and neonatal resuscitation equipment. Ensure that prerequisites for an assisted vaginal breech birth are present: operative vaginal birth pack, warm towels, obstetric forceps, lithotomy supports.

Electronic fetal monitoring

Continuous electronic fetal monitoring (EFM) should be recommended to women with a breech presentation during labour and birth, as it is likely to improve neonatal outcomes.[1] It is also vital that EFM continues right up until birth, including when the decision is made for a caesarean section during labour.

Where the CTG is considered to be pathological before the active second stage of labour, a caesarean birth is recommended, unless the buttocks are visible or progress is rapid. Fetal blood sampling is not recommended.[1]

Labour progress

Labour augmentation with oxytocin is not recommended, but the recent Green-top Guideline suggests that it may be considered if there is epidural anaesthesia in situ and the contraction frequency is less than 4:10.[1] Amniotomy for labour augmentation should be performed with caution.

Once spontaneous rupture of the membranes occurs, a vaginal examination should be performed to exclude a cord prolapse.[1]

Management of the second stage of labour

It is recommended that women presenting in labour in the near or active second stage of labour with a breech presentation should not be routinely offered a caesarean section. However, if there is delay in the descent of the breech at any point in the second stage of labour, a caesarean section should be considered, as this may be a sign of relative fetopelvic disproportion.[1]

Women undergoing a vaginal breech birth should be attended by practitioners with adequate experience and skills to conduct and assist the birth. The attendants should include a senior midwife, obstetrician and neonatologist (senior staff may have valuable experience of vaginal breech births). An anaesthetist should be present on the labour ward at the time of birth, and theatre staff should be on standby.

There are limited data in relation to position and outcome for vaginal breech birth. Some experienced obstetricians and midwives have suggested that upright maternal positioning (e.g. mother kneeling on all fours, sitting on a birthing stool, or standing upright) may confer some physiological advantages, as well as offering increased maternal choice about positioning.[9,10,11,12] Furthermore, upright positioning may lead to greater maternal satisfaction in childbirth.[11] MRI pelvimetry studies have found that upright and active positioning create greater space in the pelvis, but there are limited comparative safety data available.[12] However, an upright position for vaginal breech birth may not currently be familiar to most practitioners,[13] and it remains the responsibility of the accoucheur to practice within the limits of their own training and competencies (NMC and GMC).

The updated RCOG guideline recommends that women should be advised that either a semi-recumbent or forward-facing squatting or all-fours position may be adopted for birth, but positioning should depend on maternal preference and the experience of the attendant. If, however, a forward-facing all-fours position is adopted, then the woman should be advised that recourse to the semi-recumbent position may become necessary if manoeuvres are required, as the accoucheur may be more confident to perform manoeuvres in a dorsal recumbent position.[1]

> **Women undergoing a vaginal breech birth should be attended by practitioners with adequate experience and skills to conduct and assist the birth.**

Vaginal breech birth: assisted manoeuvres

All obstetricians and midwives should be familiar with the techniques that can be used to assist vaginal breech birth. The choice of manoeuvres used, if required, should depend on the individual experience/preference of the accoucheur.[1]

When the breech is visible at the perineum, active pushing should be encouraged. Once the buttocks have passed the perineum, significant cord compression is common. Signs that birth should be assisted include lack of fetal tone or colour, or delay commonly due to extended arms or an extended neck. In general, intervention to expedite birth is required if there is evidence of poor fetal condition or if there is a delay of 5 minutes between birth of the buttocks and birth of the fetal head (or more than 3 minutes from the umbilicus to the head).[1]

> **Aim for a 'hands-off' approach to vaginal breech birth. Keep interventions to a minimum and avoid traction. However, if progress is not made once the umbilicus is visible, or if there is poor tone, extended arms or an extended neck, then timely and appropriate intervention is necessary.**

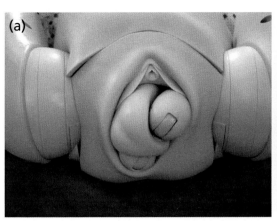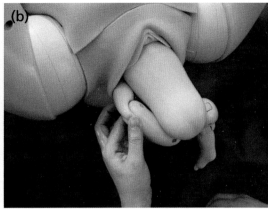

Figure 12.2 (a) Spontaneous birth of the limbs and trunk;
(b) applying pressure to popliteal fossae

- Episiotomy should be used selectively to facilitate birth.[1]
- Spontaneous birth of the limbs and trunk is preferable (Figure 12.2a), but the legs may need to be released by applying pressure to the popliteal fossae (Figure 12.2b).
- When handling the baby, it is important to ensure that support is only provided over the bony prominences of the pelvic girdle, to reduce the risk of soft-tissue internal injury.
- Ensure that the buttocks remain sacroanterior. Controlled rotation may be required if the trunk appears to be rotating to a sacroposterior position, but handling of the baby should again be only over the bony prominences
- Avoid handling the umbilical cord, as this increases vasospasm.
- Encourage spontaneous birth with maternal pushing until the scapulae are visible.
- Traction on the infant's trunk can cause nuchal arms and should therefore be avoided.
- If the arms are not released spontaneously, use the Løvsett's manoeuvre, as shown in Figure 12.3.

Engagement in the pelvis of the after-coming head

After release of the arms, support the baby until the nape of the neck becomes visible, using the weight of the baby to encourage flexion (Figure 12.4). If spontaneous birth of the head does not follow, an assistant may apply suprapubic pressure to assist flexion of the head (Figure 12.5).[1]

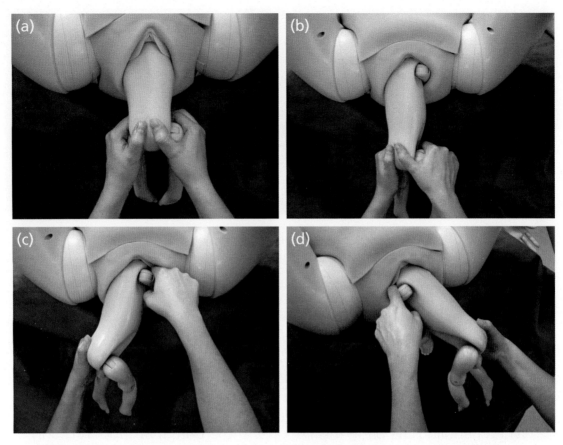

Figure 12.3 Løvsett's manoeuvre. (a) Gently hold the baby over the bony prominences of the hips and sacrum and rotate the baby so that (b) one arm is uppermost (anterior). (c) To release the uppermost arm, an index figure should be placed over the baby's shoulder and follow the infant's arm to the antecubital fossa; the arm should be flexed for delivery. (d) Following release of the first arm, rotate the baby 180 degrees, keeping the back uppermost, so that the second arm is now uppermost. Release this arm as described in (c).

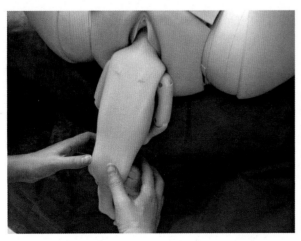

Figure 12.4 Nape of neck visible: using the weight of the baby to encourage flexion

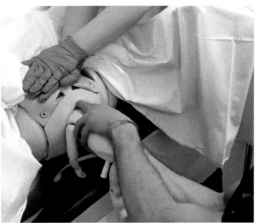

Figure 12.5 Applying suprapubic pressure to aid flexion of the head

Mauriceau–Smellie–Veit manoeuvre

The Mauriceau–Smellie–Veit manoeuvre may be required to assist birth of the after-coming head (Figure 12.6). When using this manoeuvre, the baby's body should be supported on the flexor surface of the accoucheur's forearm. The first and third finger of the accoucheur's hand should be placed on the cheekbones (note that the middle finger is no longer placed in the fetal mouth, as fetal injury has been reported). With the other hand, apply pressure to the occiput with the middle finger and place the other fingers simultaneously on the fetal shoulders to promote flexion of the fetal head (i.e. keep the chin on the chest) to reduce the fetal head diameter (Figure 12.7).

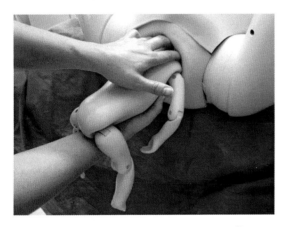

Figure 12.6 The Mauriceau–Smellie–Veit manoeuvre for birth of the after-coming head

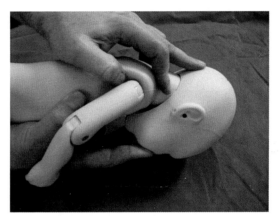

Figure 12.7 Position of fingers for the Mauriceau–Smellie–Veit manoeuvre

Burns–Marshall technique

There have been some concerns expressed about the risks of the Burns–Marshall method for assisting birth of the head, as it may lead to overextension of the baby's neck. It is therefore not advised.[1]

Forceps to assist birth of the head

Alternatively, the birth of the fetal head can be assisted with forceps. An assistant should hold the baby's body and the forceps should be applied from underneath the fetal body. The axis of traction should aim to flex the head (Figure 12.8). There is debate over which type of forceps should be used for this procedure, and Kielland's, Rhodes', Piper's and Wrigley's forceps have all been reported.[1]

There is no evidence to indicate which of the above techniques is preferable for assisting the birth of the head, and previous experience of the practitioner is a very important factor in the decision as to which method is chosen.

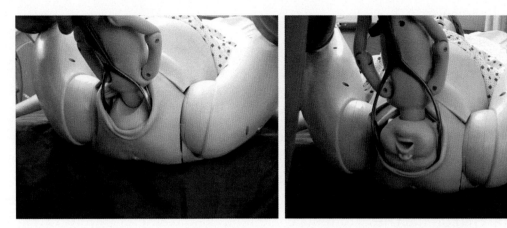

Figure 12.8 Kielland's forceps to assist birth of the head

Complications and potential solutions

Head entrapment during a preterm breech birth

The major cause of head entrapment is the passage of the preterm fetal trunk through an incompletely dilated cervix. This occurs in approximately 14% of vaginal breech births.[1] In this situation, the cervix can be incised to release the head. The RCOG recommends that incisions should be made in the cervix at the 2, 6 and 10 o'clock positions, to avoid the cervical neurovascular bundles that run in the cervix laterally, the bladder anteriorly and rectum posteriorly. Care should be taken, as extension into the lower segment of the uterus can occur.[14] For head entrapment at caesarean birth, it may be necessary to extend the uterine incision to a J shape or inverted T.[1]

Nuchal arms

This is when one or both of the arms become extended and trapped behind the fetal head (Figure 12.9). Nuchal arms complicate up to 5% of breech births and may be caused by early traction on a breech. There is high morbidity associated with nuchal arms (25% risk of neonatal trauma, e.g. brachial plexus injuries), and therefore any early traction on the breech should be avoided.

Nuchal arms can be released with rotation using the Løvsett's manoeuvre and running the accoucheur's finger along the fetal arm to the antecubital fossa, where pressure can be applied to flex the arm and achieve birth.

Cord prolapse

Cord prolapse is more common with all breech presentations, especially footling breech presentations (10–25%).[15] The most important factor with cord prolapse is prevention. Amniotomy should be undertaken with caution

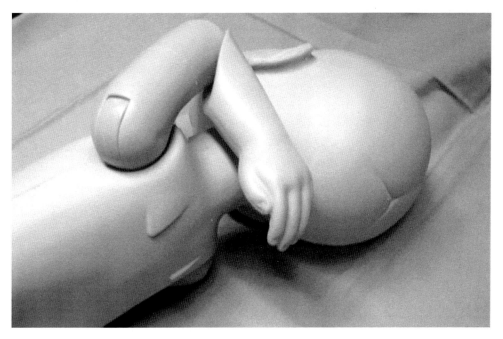

Figure 12.9 Nuchal arm

and with a presenting part filling the pelvis. The management of cord prolapse is outlined in **Module 11**.

Fetal risks associated with vaginal breech birth

Box 12.3 lists the risks associated with a vaginal breech birth. Figure 12.10 illustrates the manoeuvres that may be required to assist a vaginal breech birth.

Box 12.3 Fetal risks associated with vaginal breech birth

- Intrapartum death
- Intracranial haemorrhage
- Hypoxic–ischaemic encephalopathy
- Brachial plexus injury
- Rupture of the liver, kidney or spleen
- Dislocation of the neck, shoulder or hip
- Fractured clavicle, humerus or femur
- Cord prolapse
- Occipital diastasis and cerebellar injury

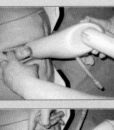
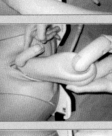
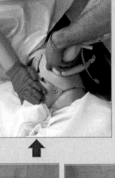
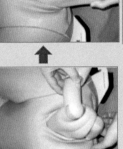
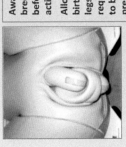

Figure 12.10 Management of vaginal breech birth (poster)

References

1. Royal College of Obstetricians and Gynaecologists. *The Management of Breech Presentation*, 4th edn. Green-top Guideline No. 20B. London: RCOG, 2017. www.rcog.org.uk/en/guidelines-research-services/guidelines/gtg20B (accessed June 2017).

2. Confidential Enquiry into Stillbirths and Deaths in Infancy. *5th Annual Report*. London: Maternal and Child Health Research Consortium, 1998.

3. Health and Social Care Information Centre. *Hospital Episode Statistics: NHS Maternity Statistics – England 2014–15*. London: HSCIC, 2015. http://content.digital.nhs.uk/catalogue/PUB19127 (accessed June 2017).

4. Hannah ME, Hannah WJ, Hewson SA, *et al.*; Term Breech Trial Collaborative Group. Planned caesarean section versus planned vaginal birth for breech presentation at term: a randomised multicentre trial. *Lancet* 2000; 356: 1375–83.

5. Whyte H, Hannah ME, Saigal S, *et al.*; Term Breech Trial Collaborative Group. Outcomes of children at 2 years after planned caesarean birth versus planned vaginal birth for breech presentation at term: the international randomized Term Breech Trial. *Am J Obstet Gynecol* 2004; 191: 864–71.

6. Vlemmix F, Bergenhenegouwen L, Schaaf JM, *et al.* Term breech deliveries in the Netherlands: did the increased cesarean rate affect neonatal outcome? A population-based cohort study. *Acta Obstet Gynecol Scand* 2014; 93: 888-96.

7. Berhan Y, Haileamlak A. The risks of planned vaginal breech delivery versus planned caesarean section for term breech birth: a meta-analysis including observational studies. *BJOG* 2016; 123: 49–57.

8. Chien, P. Editor's reply re: The risks of planned vaginal breech delivery versus planned caesarean section for term breech birth: a meta-analysis including observational studies' and accompanying editorial. *BJOG* 2016; 123: 1563–4.

9. Evans J. Understanding physiological breech birth. *Essentially MIDIRS* 2012; 3: 17–21.

10. Banks M. Breech, posterior and a deflexed head! An active birth solution? *Midwifery Today Int Midwife* 2009; 91: 22–4.

11. Thies-Lagergren L, Hildingsson I, Christensson K, Kvist LJ. Who decides the position for birth? A follow-up study of a randomised controlled trial. *Women Birth* 2013; 26: e99–104.

12. Reitter A, Daviss BA, Bisits A, *et al.* Does pregnancy and/or shifting positions create more room in a woman's pelvis? *Am J Obstet Gynecol* 2014; 211: 662.e1–9.

13. Walker S, Scamell M, Parker P. Standards for maternity care professionals attending planned upright breech births: a Delphi study. *Midwifery* 2016; 34: 7–14.

14. Robertson PA, Foran CM, Croughan-Minihane MS, Kilpatrick SJ. Head entrapment and neonatal outcome by mode of delivery in breech deliveries from 28 to 36 weeks of gestation. *Am J Obstet Gynecol* 1996; 174: 1742–7.

15. Royal College of Obstetricians and Gynaecologists. *Umbilical Cord Prolapse*. Green-top Guideline No. 50. London: RCOG, 2014. www.rcog.org.uk/en/guidelines-research-services/guidelines/gtg50 (accessed June 2017).

Module 13
Twin birth

Key learning points

- Preparation of room and equipment for twin birth.
- Intrapartum electronic fetal monitoring of both twins.
- Importance of stabilisation of the fetal lie of the second twin.
- To understand the various manoeuvres needed to facilitate birth of the second twin.
- Aim to keep twin-to-twin birth interval to less than 30 minutes.
- Justify situations in which caesarean section may be necessary.
- Recognise the increased risks of postpartum haemorrhage.
- Document details of birth accurately, clearly and legibly.

Common difficulties observed in training drills

- Not setting the room up with the necessary equipment prior to birth
- Failure to stabilise and maintain the longitudinal fetal lie of the second twin until the presenting part has engaged in the pelvis
- Premature amniotomy for the second twin

Introduction

'Non-identical' (dizygotic) twins are the most common form of twin pregnancy and result from fertilisation of two ova (eggs). Dizygotic twins are genetically no more similar than siblings, having separate placental circulations and gestational sacs (dizygotic, dichorionic, diamniotic).

'Identical' (monozygotic) twins are less common. They result from the splitting of a single developing embryo and are genetically identical. The degree of separation depends on the developmental stage at which the split takes place and can be anything from separate circulations (monozygotic, dichorionic, diamniotic) to conjoined twins.[1]

Multiple births currently account for 3% of live births. The incidence of monozygotic twins is fairly constant. The rate of dizygotic twins varies considerably, and there has recently been an increase owing to the use of fertility treatments in older mothers.[2] Up to 24% of successful IVF procedures result in multiple pregnancies. In 1980, 10 out of every 1000 women giving birth in England and Wales had a multiple birth, but by 2013 this had risen to 15.6 per 1000.[3]

All twins share increased risks of preterm birth and fetal growth restriction, but monochorionic twin pregnancies have the added risk of twin-to-twin transfusion syndrome, as they are dependent on a shared placental and umbilical circulation. They also have a higher risk of fetal loss and neurodevelopmental morbidity than dichorionic twins.[4] Around one-third of twin pregnancies in the UK have a monochorionic placenta.

Box 13.1 Risks of twin pregnancies

- Congenital abnormalities
- Gestational diabetes
- Pre-eclampsia
- Fetal growth restriction
- Twin-to-twin transfusion (in monochorionic pregnancies)
- Cord entanglement (monochorionic, monoamniotic)
- Preterm labour (50% of twins are preterm at birth)
- Malpresentation
- Cord prolapse
- Neonatal seizures
- Increased respiratory morbidity
- Increased risk of cerebral palsy (four times the risk of a singleton pregnancy)
- Postpartum haemorrhage for mother

Almost every obstetric complication (including low birth weight, preterm birth, pre-eclampsia, stillbirth and child disability) is more common with multiple pregnancy. The perinatal mortality rate of multiple births is around five times higher than that of singletons. Much of this excess perinatal mortality is attributable to antepartum factors; however, some of the mortality is related to problems during labour and birth. Furthermore, maternal mortality associated with multiple births is two and a half times that for singleton births. Box 13.1 lists some of the risks of twin pregnancies both antenatally and in labour.

As a consequence, twin pregnancies require specialist antenatal and intrapartum care in a consultant-led unit. The woman and her partner should be counselled regarding the mode and management of their twin birth prior to the onset of labour.

Presentation at birth

Approximately 30% of twins present as cephalic/cephalic (Figure 13.1),[5] 35% of twins present as cephalic/non-cephalic (Figure 13.2),[6] and the remaining 35% of twins present with the leading baby in a non-cephalic presentation at birth (Figures 13.3 and 13.4).[6]

Mode of birth

The optimal method of birth in twin pregnancies remains somewhat unclear. However, the Twin Birth Study aimed to address this question.[7] It was an international multicentre randomised controlled trial comparing planned caesarean section with planned vaginal birth for twins at 32–38 weeks of gestation when the first twin was a cephalic presentation. The study concluded that a planned caesarean section did not significantly reduce the risks of fetal or neonatal death or serious neonatal morbidity as compared with planned vaginal birth.[7] Furthermore, subgroup analysis demonstrated there was no significant benefit from planned caesarean section for any subgroup, including monochorionic twins.

Vaginal birth of the second twin is recognised as a time of high risk. A retrospective review of twin births in England, Northern Ireland and Wales between 1994 and 2003 concluded that, at term, the second twin had more than a twofold higher risk of perinatal death related to birth

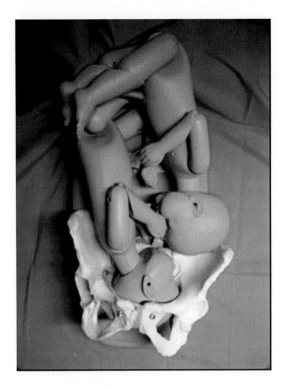

Figure 13.1 Cephalic/cephalic
presentation

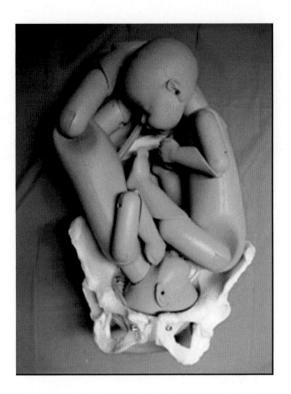

Figure 13.2 Cephalic/non-cephalic
presentation

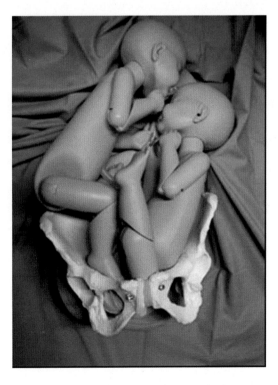

Figure 13.3 Breech/non-cephalic
presentation

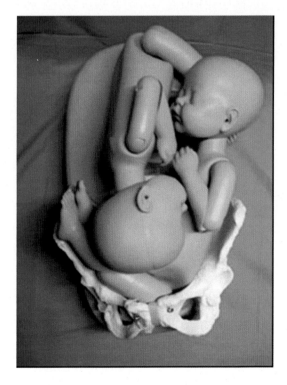

Figure 13.4 Breech/cephalic
presentation

and more than threefold higher risk of death caused by intrapartum anoxia.[6]

The planned mode of birth is dependent on presentation, amnionicity and chorionicity, predicted fetal weight, gestation and fetal and maternal wellbeing.[1]

In otherwise uncomplicated twin pregnancies at term where the first twin is cephalic, a vaginal birth should be offered (assuming there are no other relative or absolute contraindications to vaginal birth). However, it is important to emphasise to the mother that serious acute intrapartum problems can occur following the birth of the first twin (for example conversion to transverse lie of twin II, cord prolapse, prolonged time interval to birth of the second twin) which may lead to a category 1 caesarean section. In addition, perinatal death and neonatal morbidity can occur, even in cephalic/cephalic presentations.

Evidence is limited, but when the first twin is a breech presentation, a planned caesarean section should be offered.[8] Routine emergency caesarean section for a breech presentation of the first twin in *spontaneous labour* is not recommended. The mode of birth should be individualised based on cervical dilatation, station of the presenting part, type of breech, presentation, fetal wellbeing of both twins and availability of an operator skilled in vaginal breech birth.[8]

It is widely accepted that the birth of monoamniotic and conjoined twins should be by elective caesarean section.[9]

Timing of birth

The majority of women with a twin pregnancy will labour spontaneously by 37 weeks of gestation. There is no robust evidence to inform the optimal timing of birth in either identical/monochorionic or non-identical/dichorionic twin pregnancies, but the incidence of stillbirth in twins after 37–38 weeks of gestation is higher than in singleton pregnancies.[10] The NICE guideline[11] and the RCOG guideline[4] recommend that birth should be planned at 36–37 weeks of gestation in otherwise uncomplicated monochorionic twin pregnancies (following administration of antenatal corticosteroids) and at 37–38 weeks of gestation in otherwise uncomplicated dichorionic twin pregnancies.[4,11]

Management of vaginal twin birth

All women expecting twins should have a discussion by 32 weeks' gestation with a midwife and a senior obstetrician about their planned intrapartum care. These discussions should be documented in the relevant part of the women's handheld notes.

The discussion should explain:

- that there is an increased risk of morbidity for the second twin
- choices of analgesia, including advantages and disadvantages of epidural anaesthesia
- the possibility of presumed fetal compromise in the second twin
- the importance of stabilisation of the fetal lie of the second twin
- the use of oxytocin to augment contractions in the inter-twin period
- the possibility of intervention to expedite birth of the second twin
- the risk of caesarean section even after successful vaginal birth of the first twin
- the recommendation of active management of the third stage of labour and the use of an oxytocin infusion to reduce the risk of postpartum haemorrhage

First stage of labour

All women with a twin pregnancy who are in labour should be given one-to-one care by an experienced midwife and should be reviewed by the most senior obstetrician available. The anaesthetist, neonatologist and neonatal intensive care unit should be informed of the mother's admission. The midwife and obstetrician should discuss the woman's birth plan with the woman and her birth partner. A clear plan should be documented in the notes. An example of an admission checklist is given in Figure 13.5.

Fetal blood sampling of the first twin may be performed, if indicated. However, if there are concerns for the wellbeing of the second twin, birth should be expedited, as there is no access to twin II.

Oxytocin augmentation is not contraindicated for hypotonic contractions in labour but should always be discussed with a senior obstetrician.

Twin birth: Checklist on admission to labour ward		
Attach inpatient ID label:	Tick when Completed	Comments
Introduce the parents to the team.		
Review the handheld and hospital notes including the care plan to identify any antenatal risk factors.		
Explain the plan for birth.		
Establish intravenous access, take blood for full blood count (FBC) and group and save (G&S).		
Once in established labour clear fluids only and start gastric protection (e.g. oral Ranitidine 150 mg six-hourly).		
Confirm presentation of both twins with ultrasound.		
Continuous electronic fetal monitoring is recommended:		
• A scalp electrode may be used for twin I to help differentiate the fetal heart recordings.		
• Ultrasound can be used to identify the optimal location placement of the EFM transducers.		
• A suitable monitor should be used to enable the differentiation of the two fetal heart tracings.		
Discuss analgesia. An epidural is helpful as it will make any intrauterine manipulation of twin II easier and can be used for caesarean section if needed.		
Obstetrician to document a care plan for twin birth in the handheld record.		
Date: Name: Signature: Grade:		

Figure 13.5 An example of a checklist on admission to labour ward for a twin birth

Second stage of labour

A twin birth should be supervised by an experienced obstetrician. Healthcare professionals attending the birth should include:

■ at least two midwives (preferably experienced)

■ at least one experienced obstetrician

■ at least two members of the neonatal team

■ an anaesthetist and theatre team (available on the labour ward)

Prepare the labour room and required healthcare staff in advance so that there is a calm and unhurried approach at the birth.

Prepare the room and staff

Ensure prerequisites for twin birth are present. A local checklist may be helpful. A list of the equipment required is shown in Box 13.2.

Box 13.2 Equipment required for a twin birth

■ Ultrasound scanner

■ Lithotomy supports

■ Amnihook

■ Local anaesthetic (e.g. 20 mL 1% lidocaine), syringe and needle

■ Operative vaginal birth trolley

■ Forceps and ventouse

■ Birth pack

■ Additional set of cord clamps

■ Four cord blood sampling syringes

■ Two resuscitaires (labelled Twin I and Twin II)

■ Two sets of baby linen and hats

■ Oxytocin infusion for augmentation (e.g. 3 units Syntocinon in 50 mL normal saline) ready to be commenced after the birth of the first twin, if required

■ Syntocinon or Syntometrine for third stage of labour as appropriate

■ Oxytocin infusion (e.g. 40 units Syntocinon in 500 mL normal saline) for prophylactic use **after the third stage, but kept separately from the oxytocin infusion used between the first and second twin**

An oxytocin infusion should be prepared and ready to commence for augmentation after the birth of the first twin, as contractions sometimes stop or reduce in frequency at this stage.

Prepare the mother

Keep the mother and relatives informed. Explain all the staff that will be present at the twin birth and also their roles.

Twin birth – procedure

The birth of the first twin is performed as for a singleton birth. The midwife who is caring for the mother can assist the birth of the first twin (and the second twin) if there are no problems.

After the first twin is born, an assistant (preferably an experienced obstetrician) should stabilise the lie of the second twin until the presenting part descends into the pelvis. This is achieved by the assistant placing both hands on the mother's abdomen and holding the fetus in a longitudinal axis until the presenting part is fixed in the pelvis. The presentation of the second twin and also the optimal place to monitor its heart rate should be identified by ultrasound scan.

There should be continuous CTG monitoring of the second twin after the birth of the first twin. If the CTG is abnormal, the birth of the second twin should be expedited.

After the birth of twin I, the uterine contractions may stop or become irregular. Therefore, be prepared to commence an oxytocin infusion soon after the birth of the first twin; for example, an oxytocin infusion (3 units in 50 mL normal saline) started at a rate of 4 mU/minute (4 mL/hour) with the rate doubled every 5 minutes until regular contractions return, to a maximum infusion rate of 20 mU/minute (20 mL/hour). Oxytocin should only be commenced once the lie of the second twin has been confirmed as longitudinal. Once the lie is confirmed as longitudinal, await descent of the presenting part. Artificial rupture of the membranes should only be performed once the presenting part is fixed in the pelvis. This is best done during a contraction.

Provided the CTG is normal, expectant management is advisable, allowing natural progress to a vaginal birth (either cephalic or breech).

The aim should be for the second twin to be born within 30 minutes of the first twin.[12] However, if there is delay and an assisted birth is required, as long as the CTG is normal it may still be better to wait for spontaneous descent of the presenting part before performing artificial rupture of the membranes and intervening to assist the birth.

If there is delay or evidence of fetal compromise, an assisted birth is indicated. If the lie of the second twin is transverse, there are two options:

■ external cephalic version
■ internal podalic version

External cephalic version

When attempting external cephalic version (Figure 13.6), the ultrasound probe can be used as a 'hand' so that fetal lie and heart rate can be monitored simultaneously throughout.

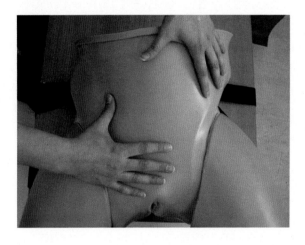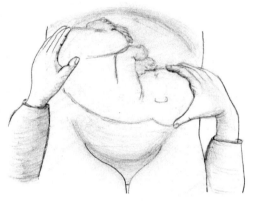

Figure 13.6 External cephalic version

Internal podalic version

With internal podalic version, one or both fetal feet are grasped inside the uterus before proceeding to a breech extraction (Figure 13.7). Before any traction is applied, the operator must confirm that she/he is holding a foot by feeling the heel (which has a 90° angle). It is important to try not to rupture the membranes too early, to reduce the risk of cord prolapse.

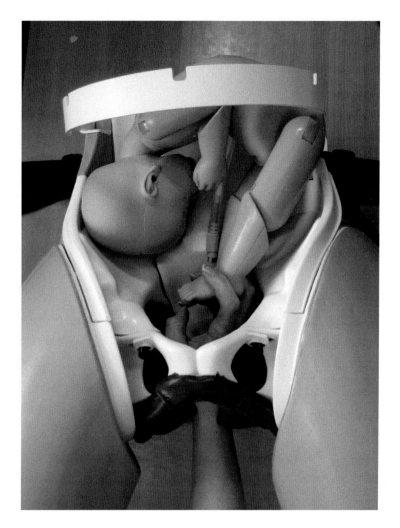

Figure 13.7 Internal podalic version

The same manoeuvres used for an assisted vaginal breech birth may be needed to assist birth of the second twin. Remember that twins are likely to be smaller than singleton fetuses. In cases of preterm twins, the cervix can close around the head of a breech baby. Sometimes the second twin may be considerably bigger than the first twin, and this too can cause problems during birth. Therefore, it is useful to check the estimated fetal weights from the last routine ultrasound scan before birth is imminent.

Several studies have reviewed outcomes after external cephalic version compared with internal podalic version, and have concluded that there were no differences in neonatal or maternal outcomes. However, internal podalic version followed by breech extraction was associated with a higher rate of success of vaginal birth and lower caesarean section rates.

Length of inter-twin birth interval

The length of the inter-twin birth interval is variable. Although a longer interval is associated with a continuous slow decline in umbilical cord pH, the small differences in pH between 15 and 30 minutes were not large enough to impact on clinical management.[12] However, it is widely accepted that the interval should ideally be no longer than 30 minutes.

Delayed cord clamping

Although it is accepted that delayed cord clamping is beneficial to the neonate during singleton births, at present there is insufficient evidence to recommend this for multiple pregnancies. In addition, there are theoretical concerns regarding the risk of acute inter-fetal transfusion in monochorionic twins following the birth of the first twin, and although these risks have not been substantiated, it may be prudent to clamp the cord of the first twin as soon as possible after its birth.

Third stage of labour

Double-clamp the umbilical cord following each birth, as usual, but also place an additional cord clamp on the placental end of the cord of the second twin so it can be identified after birth. Paired umbilical cord gas bloods should be taken from both twins.

Owing to the high risk of postpartum haemorrhage, a bolus of oxytocin should be recommended and given to the mother immediately after the birth of the second twin. A prophylactic oxytocin infusion should be commenced after the third stage and administered according to local protocol. It is very important to continue to observe the mother for signs of postpartum haemorrhage.

As with all complicated births, careful and precise documentation is paramount. Figure 13.8 is an example of a documentation pro forma that may be used to record a twin birth.

Twin birth – Documentation pro forma			
Name:	**Hospital Number:**		**Date:**
Gestation:			Comments:
Chorionicity	Dichorionic/diamniotic or Monochorionic/diamniotic		
	Twin I	**Twin II**	
Presentation at start of 2nd stage	Cephalic Breech Other	Cephalic Breech Other	
CTG	Normal Suspicious Pathological	Normal Suspicious Pathological	
Syntocinon infusion to augment labour?	Yes No	Yes No	
Analgesia	None Entonox Epidural Spinal GA	None Entonox Epidural Spinal GA	
IV access?	Yes No If no, reason for no access:		
Ranitidine?	Yes: oral IV No		
Senior midwife present?	Yes Name: No		
Obstetric registrar (ST3–5) present?	Yes Name: No		
Senior obstetric registrar (ST6–7)?	Yes Name: No		
Consultant obstetrician present?	Yes Name: No		
Experienced neonatologist present at birth?	Yes Name: No		
Mode of birth twin I **Time:**	Spontaneous vaginal Forceps Ventouse Caesarean section		
Syntocinon infusion between twins?	Yes	No	
Mode of birth twin II **Time:**	Spontaneous vaginal Caesarean section Ventouse Assisted breech Forceps Breech extraction		
	Twin I	**Twin II**	
Presentation at birth	Cephalic Breech Other	Cephalic Breech Other	
Internal or external manoeuvres performed	Yes: No	Yes: No	
Cord gases taken?	Yes No	Yes No	
Apgars (at 1, 5, 10 minutes)			
Placenta complete? (Placenta should be sent to histology)	Yes: No:	Yes: No:	
Syntocinon infusion commenced after third stage?	Yes: No:		
Date: Name:	**Signature:**		**Grade:**

Figure 13.8 Example of a documentation pro forma to record a twin birth

References

1. Hofmeyr GJ, Barrett JF, Crowther CA. Planned caesarean section for women with a twin pregnancy. *Cochrane Database Syst Rev* 2015; (12): CD006553.

2. Australian Institute of Health and Welfare, *Australia's Mothers and Babies 2014: in brief.* Perinatal Statistics Series. Canberra: AIHW, 2016. www.aihw.gov.au/publication-detail/?id=60129557656 (accessed June 2017).

3. Office for National Statistics. *Maternity Data*, 2013. London: ONS.

4. Royal College of Obstetricians and Gynaecologists. *Management of Monochorionic Twin Pregnancy*, 2nd edn. Green-top Guideline No. 51. London: RCOG, 2016. www.rcog.org.uk/en/guidelines-research-services/guidelines/gtg51 (accessed June 2017).

5. Grisaru D, Fuchs S, Kupferminc MJ, *et al.* Outcome of 306 twin deliveries according to first twin presentation and method of delivery. *Am J Perinatol* 2000; 17: 303–7.

6. Smith GC, Fleming KM, White IR. Birth order of twins and risk of perinatal death related to delivery in England, Northern Ireland, and Wales, 1994–2003: retrospective cohort study. *BMJ* 2007; 334: 576.

7. Asztalos EV, Hannah ME, Hutton EK, *et al.* Twin Birth Study: 2-year neurodevelopmental follow-up of the randomized trial of planned cesarean or planned vaginal delivery for twin pregnancy. *Am J Obstet Gynecol* 2016; 214: 371.e1–e19.

8. Royal College of Obstetricians and Gynaecologists. *The Management of Breech Presentation*, 4th edn. Green-top Guideline No. 20B. London: RCOG, 2017. www.rcog.org.uk/en/guideines-research-services/guidelines/gtg20B (accessed June 2017). .

9. Tessen JA, Zlatnik FJ. Monoamniotic twins: a retrospective controlled study. *Obstet Gynecol* 1991; 77: 832–4.

10. Hartley RS, Emanuel I, Hitti J. Perinatal mortality and neonatal morbidity rates among twin pairs at different gestational ages: optimal delivery timing at 37 to 38 weeks' gestation. *Am J Obstet Gynecol* 2001; 184: 451–8.

11. National Institute for Health and Care Excellence. *Multiple Pregnancy: Antenatal Care for Twin and Triplet Pregnancies*. NICE Clinical Guideline CG129. London: NICE, 2011. www.nice.org.uk/guidance/cg129 (accessed June 2017).

12. McGrail CD, Bryant DR. Intertwin time interval: how it affects the immediate neonatal outcome of the second twin. *Am J Obstet Gynecol* 2005; 192: 1420–2.

Module 14
Acute uterine inversion

Key learning points

- To recognise an inverted uterus and the accompanying maternal shock.
- To summon appropriate help and manage maternal shock.
- To outline mechanical manoeuvres to replace the uterus, including manually replacing the uterus as soon as possible.
- To emphasise that the placenta should not be removed, if adherent, until the uterus has been replaced.

Common difficulties observed in training drills

- Delay in recognition of uterine inversion
- Not stating the problem clearly to those first attending the emergency call
- Delay in commencing resuscitation
- Delay in manually replacing the uterus
- Not being prepared for a subsequent postpartum haemorrhage

Introduction

Uterine inversion was first described by Hippocrates (400 to 370 BC). Acute inversion of the uterus is a rare complication of childbirth. Incidence varies widely, with reported rates from 1 in 1500 births to as few as 1 in 20,000 births.[1,2] There are no randomised controlled studies to inform the best management strategies, although some successfully managed case series recommend immediate replacement of the uterus.[2]

Definition

When the uterus inverts, the fundus of the uterus descends through the genital tract, turning itself inside out. There are four grades of uterine inversion:

- grade I: fundus inverts down to the cervical canal
- grade II: fundus inverts into the vagina
- grade III: fundus is visible at the introitus
- grade IV: fundus below the level of the introitus

There are several recognised risk factors for acute uterine inversion, as described in Box 14.1.[3,4]

Box 14.1 Risk factors for uterine inversion

- Excessive traction on the umbilical cord
- Inappropriate fundal pressure
- Short umbilical cord
- Multiparity
- Abnormally adherent placenta
- Vaginal birth after caesarean (VBAC)
- Abnormalities of the uterus (e.g. unicornuate uterus)
- Previous uterine inversion
- Fetal macrosomia
- Precipitate labour
- Connective tissue disorders (e.g. Marfan syndrome, Ehlers–Danlos syndrome)

Diagnosis

Uterine inversion can be difficult to diagnose, particularly if the fundus is not visible at the introitus. Sudden maternal shock or collapse is the most common first sign of a uterine inversion, and is frequently at odds with the apparently minimal blood loss.

An abdominal and vaginal examination should be performed early. Grade IV uterine inversion is characterised by a mass (uterus) protruding through the introitus (Figure 14.1). However, there should be a high index of suspicion for uterine inversion when the uterine fundus is not palpable on abdominal examination, even where there is nothing visible at the introitus.

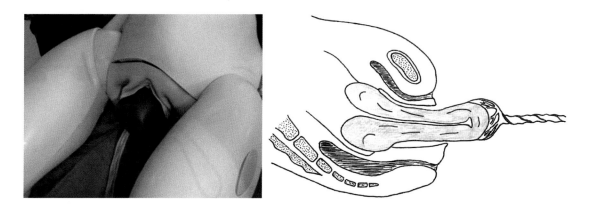

Figure 14.1 A grade IV uterine inversion

Uterine inversion is associated with vasovagal (neurogenic) shock, characterised by bradycardia[3] and hypotension.[4]

Clinically, the woman often looks as if she has fainted, but there is minimal blood loss. However, hypovolaemic shock with tachycardia and hypotension may also occur if a postpartum haemorrhage follows the uterine inversion. All women should be treated with standard initial resuscitation; however, the quickest way to resolve neurogenic shock is to replace the uterus.[3]

> **Uterine inversion is associated with atonic postpartum haemorrhage in over 90% of cases.[3,5] This occurs once the uterus has been replaced and the placenta has been removed. Care should be taken to accurately measure blood loss, as this is often underestimated.[6]**

Management

Immediate action

Figure 14.2 provides an algorithm for immediate management of an inverted uterus.

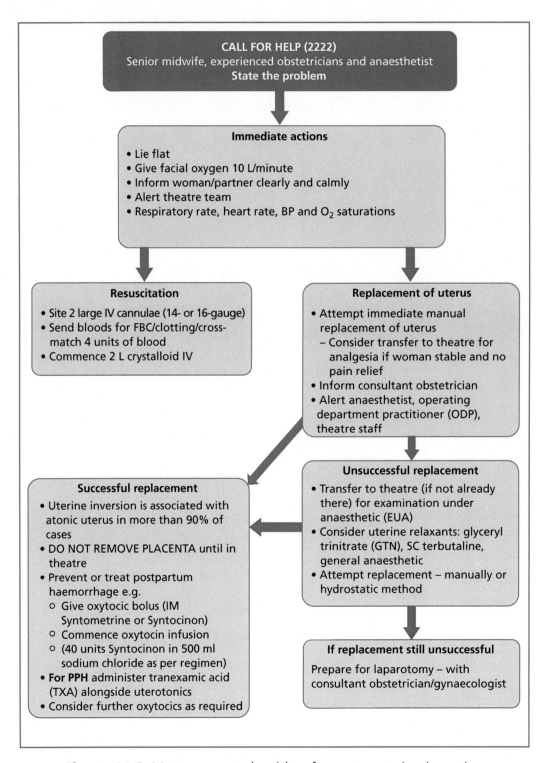

Figure 14.2 Management algorithm for acute uterine inversion

The treatment of maternal shock should be addressed immediately and appropriate assistance should be called:

■ Call for help: this should include a senior midwife, the most experienced obstetrician available and an anaesthetist.

■ Give high-flow oxygen (10 L/minute) via a non-rebreathe facemask with reservoir.

■ Clearly and calmly inform the woman of the need to immediately reposition the uterine fundus.

■ Treatment of the uterine inversion and resuscitation should take place simultaneously.

Resuscitation

■ Site two large-bore intravenous cannulae (14- or 16- gauge).

■ Commence intravenous infusion of 2 L of Hartmann's solution.

■ Take blood and send for cross-match (4 units), full blood count and clotting. (The main complication associated with uterine inversion is atonic postpartum haemorrhage.[7])

■ The quickest way to treat neurogenic shock is to replace the uterus.

Treatment

■ The uterus should be replaced as soon as possible.

■ If the woman is bleeding heavily, is haemodynamically unstable or already has effective analgesia, the accoucheur should attempt to manually replace the uterus immediately in the labour room or at home.

■ If the woman is stable and does not have adequate analgesia, prompt transfer to theatre for analgesia should be considered prior to replacement.

■ If replacement is successful, administer an intramuscular oxytocic bolus and deliver the placenta once in theatre (manual removal). This should be followed by an intravenous infusion of 40 units of oxytocin in 500 mL normal saline, administered over 4 hours.

■ If replacement is unsuccessful, transfer the patient to the operating theatre.

■ If a uterine inversion occurs outside the hospital:

   □ Immediate replacement should be attempted and an emergency ambulance should be called.

☐ If the uterus is successfully replaced, an oxytocic should be administered and the woman should still be transferred to hospital.

☐ If the uterus is not replaced, the woman should be transferred to the nearest obstetric unit as quickly as possible. The hospital should be informed so that the theatre team are ready on the woman's arrival.

Management of the inversion

The uterus can be manually replaced by putting a hand into the vagina and following the cord to the fundus. While supporting the inverted fundus in the palm of the hand, gently raise the uterus into the abdominal cavity and 'replace' it back to its anatomical position (Figure 14.3). If the placenta is still adherent, it should be removed **after** uterine replacement.[2]

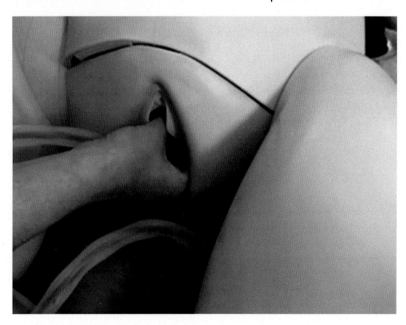

Figure 14.3 Manual replacement of the inverted uterus

The earlier the replacement of the uterus is attempted, the more likely it is to be successful.[5] As the uterus remains prolapsed it becomes more oedematous and a constriction ring may develop, making replacement more difficult.[3]

Uterine relaxants

Tocolysis can be useful to relax the uterus to assist manual correction of the inversion, particularly if a constriction ring has developed: terbutaline (0.25 mg subcutaneously) or glyceryl trinitrate spray (one metered dose sublingually). General anaesthesia may also promote uterine relaxation and can be useful if repeat attempts at uterine replacement are necessary.

> **Caution should be taken with the use of uterine relaxants, as they will exacerbate atonic postpartum haemorrhage once the uterus is replaced.**

Hydrostatic method for the management of an inverted uterus

Uterine inversion can be corrected using hydrostatic pressure to distend the vagina and push the fundus upward into its anatomical position. In the original description of this technique, the vaginal entrance was simply sealed with an assistant's hand.[8] However, a silastic ventouse cup can be used to create a better seal, thus improving the hydrostatic pressure (Figure 14.4).[9]

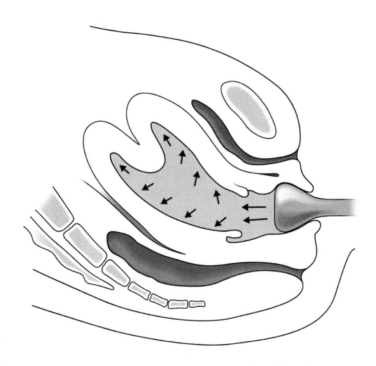

Figure 14.4 Hydrostatic method for the management of an inverted uterus

Equipment required:

- silastic vacuum cup
- wide-bore IV or blood-giving set that can be attached to the silastic cup securely
- 2 L of slightly warmed normal saline intravenous solution

The silastic vacuum cup is placed within the vagina to occlude the vaginal opening. Two litres of slightly warmed intravenous normal saline are rapidly infused through a wide-bore IV or blood-giving set which is attached directly to the end of the silastic vacuum cup. The fluid bag should be placed 100–150 cm above the level of the vagina to provide sufficient pressure for insufflation. Reduction of the inversion is usually achieved within 5–10 minutes of commencing this technique.

Continuing management

Once the uterus is successfully replaced, it should be manually held in position for a few minutes to promote uterine contraction and prevent re-inversion.[3] The use of a Bakri tamponade balloon catheter (Cook Medical Incorporated, Bloomington, IN, USA) has been described following replacement of the uterus to maintain the uterine position and prevent re-inversion, while concurrently assisting in the treatment of atony.[10] However, these are case reports only. Oxytocics should be administered at this stage, with an initial bolus dose followed by an infusion over 4 hours, in view of the risk of postpartum haemorrhage.

> **If the placenta is adherent, it should be manually removed after the uterus has been replaced.**

Antibiotics should be administered in view of the infection risk associated with manual uterine replacement. Intravenous co-amoxiclav or similar broad-spectrum antibiotics should be given at the time of the procedure and may be continued for 24 hours, in line with local guidance and the woman's allergies.

Surgical management

In rare circumstances when the above techniques are unsuccessful, laparotomy may be required. Upward traction on the uterus from the abdominal cavity can be achieved by using two Allis clamps to grasp the inferior 2 cm of the inversion ring, with sequential repositioning of the Allis clamps below the inversion ring until the correction of the inversion has been achieved (Huntington's method). If this procedure is unsuccessful, the most probable reason for failed correction of the inversion is constriction at the cervical ring. In this case, Haultain's method can be attempted, whereby a vertical incision can be made in the cervical ring posteriorly, to enable the inversion to be replaced.[3]

Finally, if abdominal correction of the uterus is not possible, a surgical vaginal technique, first described by Spinelli in 1897, may be attempted. This method involves separating the uterus into two halves by performing a vertical incision in the uterus from the vaginal route. The two separate sections of the uterine body can then be replaced into the abdominal cavity from below, and the uterus subsequently repaired abdominally.[11]

Documentation

It is important that all personnel involved, and all treatment administered, are documented in the maternal notes as soon as possible after the event.

Debriefing after the emergency

Once the woman's clinical condition is stable and she is comfortable, she needs to be debriefed about the sudden event. This is best undertaken by a member of the team that managed the clinical problem. The woman may need to be told that:

■ It is difficult to predict recurrence, as experience with uterine inversion is limited.

■ Hospital birth and active management of the third stage of labour is recommended for future pregnancies.

■ Uterine inversion can occur outside pregnancy and childbirth.

References

1. Hussain M, Jabeen T, Liaquat N, Noorani K, Bhutta SZ. Acute puerperal uterine inversion. *J Coll Physicians Surg Pak* 2004; 14: 215–17.

2. Milenkovic M, Kahn J. Inversion of the uterus: a serious complication at childbirth. *Acta Obstet Gynecol Scand* 2005; 84: 95–6.

3. Bhalla R, Wuntakal R, Odejinmi F, Khan RU. Acute inversion of the uterus. *The Obstetrician & Gynaecologist* 2009; 11: 13–18.

4. Fox KA, Belfort MA, Dildy GA. Postpartum haemorrhage and other problems of the third stage. In James D, Steer PJ, Weiner CP, Gonik B, Robson SC (eds.), *High-Risk Pregnancy: Management Options*, 5th edn. Cambridge: Cambridge University Press, 2017.

5. Watson P, Besch N, Bowes WA. Management of acute and subacute puerperal inversion of the uterus. *Obstet Gynecol* 1980; 55: 12–16.

6. Beringer RM, Patteril M. Puerperal uterine inversion and shock. *Br J Anaesth* 2004; 92: 439–41.

7. Baskett TF. Acute uterine inversion: a review of 40 cases. *J Obstet Gynaecol Can* 2002; 24: 953–6.

8. O'Sullivan JV. Acute inversion of the uterus. *Br Med J* 1945; 2: 282–3.

9. Ogueh O, Ayida G. Acute uterine inversion: a new technique of hydrostatic replacement. *Br J Obstet Gynaecol* 1997; 104: 951–2.

10. Soleymani Majd S, Pilsniak A, Reginald PW. Recurrent uterine inversion: a novel treatment approach using SOS Bakri balloon. *BJOG* 2009; 116: 999–1001.

11. Karaşahin KE, Gezginç K, Alanbay I, *et al.* A historical technique for replacement of postpartum uterine inversion: a case report. *Gynecol Obstet Reprod Med* 2008; 14: 55–7.

Module 15
Newborn resuscitation and support of transition

Key learning points

- To develop and practise a structured approach to the individual and team skills required in neonatal resuscitation.

- To understand that the primary aim of newborn resuscitation is inflation of the lungs with air or oxygen: inflation breaths followed by additional ventilations (ensuring good chest movement) should, in itself, increase the infant's heart rate.

- To understand the importance of calling for help early.

- To understand the importance of keeping the baby warm.

- To communicate effectively with all members of the maternity and neonatal team.

- To include communication with the parents during the emergency and ensure debriefing afterwards.

Difficulties observed in neonatal resuscitation drills

- Poor thermal care during resuscitation, especially in preterm infants
- Failure to open the infant's airway adequately, usually due to over-extension of the neck
- Failing to maintain an effective airway, particularly when conducting simultaneous cardiac compressions

- Performing chest compressions too slowly
- Poor communication and leadership within the multi-professional team

Introduction

This module provides an outline of the process of basic newborn resuscitation and support required until the newborn infant has successfully made the transition to air breathing. This module is not intended to be a complete guide, and further detailed information is available from the Resuscitation Council (UK) guideline on neonatal resuscitation (2015).[1]

Background

All neonates experience a degree of hypoxia during the process of labour and birth, with respiratory exchange being interrupted for as long as 50–75 seconds with each contraction throughout labour. While most healthy babies tolerate this well, some do not and may require additional help to establish normal breathing once born.[1]

The fetus is adapted to undertake the stress of labour, and the neonate's brain can withstand much longer periods without oxygen than an adult brain. In addition, a neonate's heart can continue to beat effectively for 20 minutes or more without lung aeration, even after the reserve system of gasping has ceased. Therefore, the primary aim of newborn resuscitation is inflation of the lungs with air or oxygen, so that the still-functioning circulation can then pump oxygenated blood to and from the heart to initiate recovery.[1]

Physiology of neonatal hypoxia

The neural centres in the brainstem are responsible for the control of respiration. If the hypoxic insult to the fetus is sufficient, its breathing movements in utero become deeper and more rapid, and eventually cease, as the neural centres of the brain that are responsible for controlling breathing are unable to function due to a lack of oxygen. This is known as the *primary apnoea* phase.[1]

Once the fetus enters primary apnoea, the fetal heart rate falls to about half its usual rate as the heart muscle switches from using aerobic to the less efficient anaerobic metabolism. Lactic acid build-up from anaerobic metabolism causes the fetus to become acidotic, and the circulation is diverted away from non-essential organs.

After a variable length of time of continuing hypoxia, unconscious gasping activity is initiated. The fetus produces a shuddering, whole-body gasp at an approximate rate of 12 breaths per minute.[2] If these gasps fail to aerate the fetal lungs, breathing ceases all together, leading to *secondary* or *terminal apnoea*. At this point, as the fetus becomes increasingly acidotic, the heart begins to fail. If there is no effective intervention at this stage, the baby will die (in utero if unborn or ex utero if already born) and may even die despite treatment.[1] The whole process probably takes about 20 minutes in a newborn baby.[3]

Therefore, while the heart continues to beat, the most important part of neonatal resuscitation is aerating the lungs, which will in turn oxygenate the heart, the brain and its respiratory centres. Unfortunately, it is not possible to tell at the time of birth if a baby is not breathing because of primary apnoea and is about to gasp, or if the baby is in the terminal apnoea phase. However, in most cases, once air enters the lungs, the infant will recover quickly and normal breathing will begin. A few babies may require cardiac massage, but usually only for a short period of time.[1]

Preparation of resuscitation equipment

Successful resuscitation is dependent on forward planning. Before any birth, it is the responsibility of the midwife and/or neonatologist to prepare and check resuscitation equipment.

It is important to check and prepare:

- clock and light
- air, oxygen and suction (cylinders full and suction tubing attached)
- heater (resuscitaire) and prewarmed towels and hat (and polyethylene bag if baby is less than 30 weeks' gestation)
- equipment for administering air or oxygen (bag-valve mask and appropriately sized mask, T-piece tubing) and PEEP circuit on standby
- neonatal laryngoscopes (correct size blades and light working)
- oxygen saturations monitor and probe
- notes for documentation

When preparing for birth, consider the woman's obstetric history and, if indicated, call the neonatal team and/or an additional midwife to be present in advance. It is important to explain to the parents that a neonatologist has been called, and to keep them informed of the situation.

Timely cord clamping

The 2015 Resuscitation Council (UK) guideline recommends delaying cord clamping for at least 1 minute after the complete birth of an uncompromised infant.[1] For healthy term infants, delaying cord clamping for at least 1 minute or until the cord stops pulsating following birth has been shown to improve iron status through early infancy.[1] The level at which the baby should be held in relation to the mother when delaying cord clamping in order to achieve the optimal speed and amount of placental blood transfusion is not specified in the guideline. In the study by Andersson and colleagues, the baby was held about 20 cm below the mother for approximately 30 seconds before being placed on the mother's abdomen.[4]

Taking into consideration the risk of hypothermia in the wet, newborn infant, the baby should be dried, kept warm and assessed for colour, tone, breathing and heart rate while waiting for the cord to be clamped.

There is currently insufficient evidence to recommend an appropriate time for clamping the cord in babies that are severely compromised at birth. Therefore, for asphyxiated babies requiring resuscitation, resuscitative interventions remain a priority. Stripping or 'milking' of the cord is not recommended as a routine measure except in the context of further randomised trials.[1]

Assessment and resuscitation

As with any emergency, it is important to call for help early. An outline of basic newborn resuscitation is shown in Figure 15.1. This is not intended to be a complete guide, and further information is available from the Resuscitation Council (UK).[1]

1. Warmth and assessment at birth

Newborn babies have a large body surface to mass ratio and are wet at birth. They therefore lose heat very rapidly and, if hypoxic and/or small, can quickly become hypothermic.[5] The importance of maintaining the neonate's temperature between 36.5 °C and 37.5 °C is reinforced because of the strong association with mortality and morbidity of babies who are allowed to

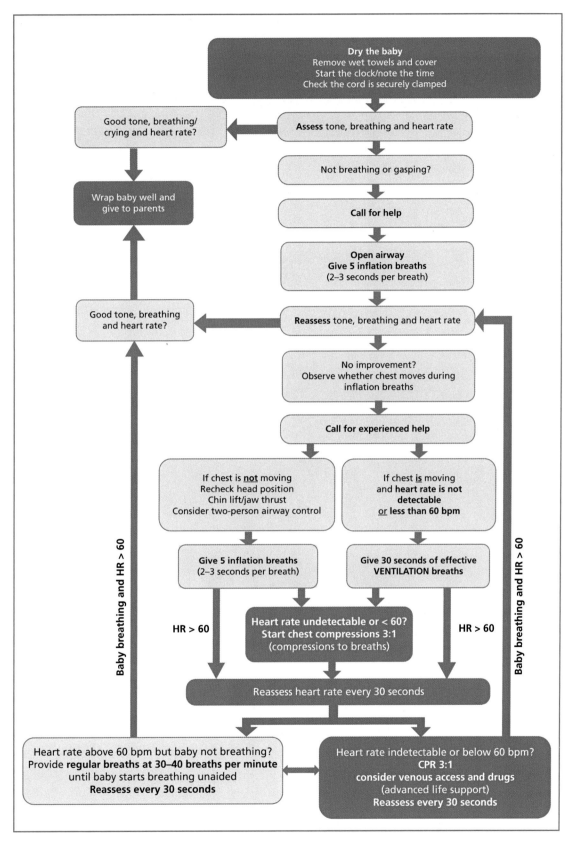

Figure 15.1 Newborn life support algorithm (adapted from UK Resuscitation Council 2015)

become hypothermic.[1] Even mild hypothermia carries a risk. See section on *Preparing for preterm birth*, for more specific information on thermal care.

At birth:

■ Start the clock and note the time of birth.

■ Dry the baby, remove any wet towels, wrap the baby in warm dry towels and put an appropriately sized hat on the baby. Drying the baby will not only stimulate the baby to breathe but will also allow time for a full assessment of colour, tone, respiratory effort and heart rate (Figures 15.2 and 15.3).

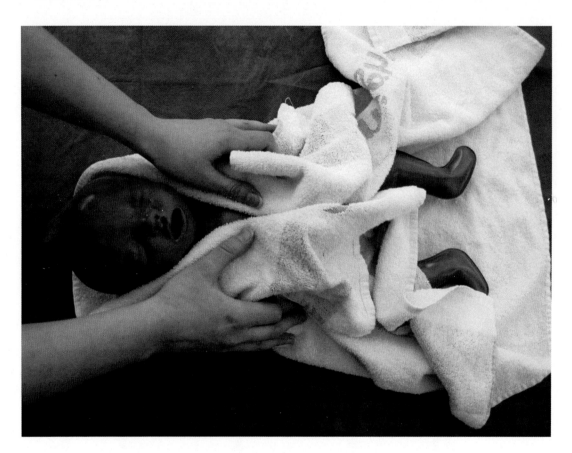

Figure 15.2 Dry the baby with a warm towel

■ For uncompromised babies, delay cord clamping for at least 1 minute from the complete birth of the infant. Then ensure that the cord is securely clamped before cutting.

> **Resuscitative intervention remains the priority in babies who require resuscitation – do not delay cord clamping if this will interfere with neonatal resuscitation.**

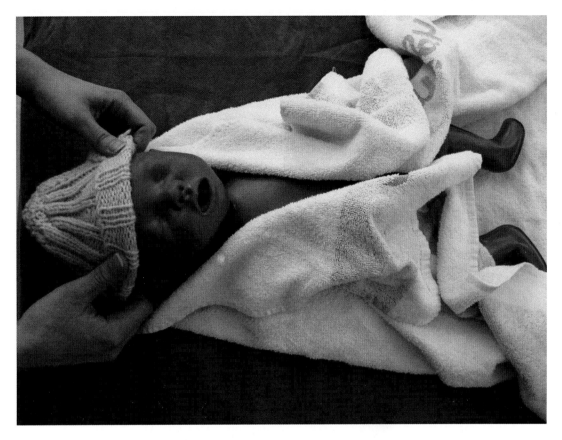

Figure 15.3 Wrap the baby in a warm dry towel and place a hat on the baby

- A healthy baby will be born blue but will have good tone, will cry within a few seconds of birth and will have a good heart rate within a few seconds of birth (the heart rate of a healthy newborn baby is about 120–150 bpm).
- A less healthy baby will be blue at birth, will have less good tone, may have a slow heart rate (less than 100 bpm) and may not establish adequate breathing by 90–120 seconds.
- An ill baby will be born pale and floppy, not breathing, and with a slow, very slow or undetectable heart rate.

2. Airway

Most babies at birth have a prominent occiput, which causes them to flex their neck if placed flat on their back; this in turn obstructs the airway (Figure 15.4).

To avoid this happening, babies should be placed on their back with their head held in a neutral position (Figure 15.5). It may help to place some support under the shoulders to maintain this position.

If the baby is very floppy, a chin lift or jaw thrust may also be necessary to keep the airway open (Figure 15.6).

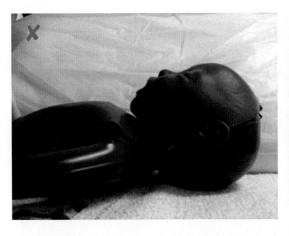 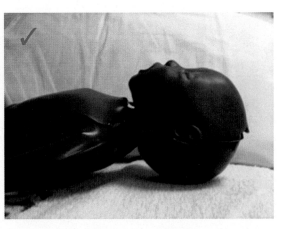

Figure 15.4 Airway obstruction caused by prominent occiput

Figure 15.5 Head in neutral position, opening airway

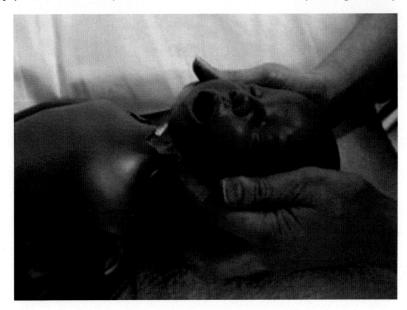

Figure 15.6 Chin lift and jaw thrust to open the airway

Airway suction immediately following birth is seldom necessary, and should be reserved for babies who have obvious airway obstruction that cannot be rectified by the appropriate head positioning outlined above. Rarely, there may be a blockage in the oropharynx or trachea. In these situations, direct visualisation and suction of the oropharynx should be performed. For tracheal obstruction, intubation and suction on withdrawal of the endotracheal tube may be effective but should only be attempted by an experienced neonatal practitioner.

3. Breathing

If the baby is not breathing adequately by about 90 seconds, five inflation breaths (of air) should be given. It is important that the correct size mask is used: covering the chin, but not over the eyes or squeezing the nose

(Figure 15.7). The baby's lungs are filled with fluid at birth, so the inflation breaths will force out the fluid and fill the lungs with air. The pressure required to initially inflate the lungs is equivalent to 30 cm of water for 2–3 seconds per breath.[1]

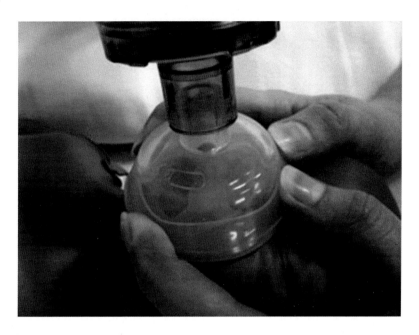

Figure 15.7 Inflation breaths using correct-sized face-mask covering the nose and mouth

If the lungs have been effectively inflated, passive movements of the chest wall will be visible, and the heart rate should also increase as oxygenated blood reaches the heart. If the heart rate increases but the baby does not start breathing on his/her own, regular ventilation breaths at a rate of 30–40 per minute should be continued until the baby begins to breathe for him/herself.

If the heart rate does not increase following inflation breaths, it may be because the baby needs more than lung aeration. However, the most likely cause is that the lungs have not been aerated effectively. Therefore, go back to the start and check the airway, making sure that the baby's head is in the neutral position, with a jaw thrust if necessary, and that there is no obstruction in the oropharynx, then attempt a further five inflation breaths. If the chest wall still does not move, request assistance in maintaining the airway and consider using a Guedel airway.

If the heart rate remains slow or is absent despite five good inflation breaths (with passive chest movement), administer 30 seconds of effective ventilation breaths (at a rate of 30 bpm).[1] If the heart rate still remains low, then chest compressions are needed and urgent senior neonatal support should be requested, if not already in attendance. If chest compressions are administered, supplemental oxygen should be increased.

Oximetry and the use of supplementary oxygen

If resources are available, pulse oximetry should be used for all births where resuscitation/assistance with transition is anticipated. Oxygen saturation can be measured reliably during the first minutes after birth with a modern pulse oximeter. In healthy term infants, oxygen saturation gradually increases from approximately 60% soon after birth to over 90% at 10 minutes of age. If, despite effective ventilation, oxygenation (ideally guided by oximetry) remains lower than the expected limits, the neonatologist may consider administering a higher concentration of oxygen. Blended oxygen and air should be given judiciously and its use guided by pulse oximetry.[1]

4. Chest compression/circulation

Almost all babies needing resuscitation at birth will respond successfully to lung inflation, with a rise in heart rate proceeding rapidly to normal breathing. However, in some cases chest compression is necessary.

It is important that chest compression should only be commenced when it is certain that the lungs have been successfully inflated. Senior neonatal support should be summoned if not already in attendance.

The most efficient way to perform chest compressions in an infant is to grip the chest with both hands, with both thumbs pressing on the lower third of the sternum, just below the nipple line, and the fingers over the spine at the back (Figure 15.8).

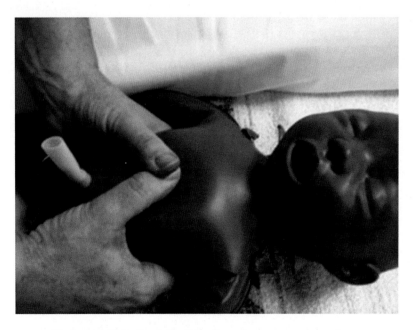

Figure 15.8 Positioning for chest compressions

Compress the chest quickly and firmly to a depth of about one-third of the distance from the chest to the spine. The ratio of compressions to breaths recommended in a newborn infant is 3:1 to achieve 90 compressions and 30 breaths in 1 minute.

Allow enough time between compressions for oxygenated blood to flow from the lungs to the heart at a rate of approximately 120 events/minute. Ensure that the chest is inflating with each ventilation breath. In a very small number of babies, lung inflation and chest compressions will not be sufficient to generate an effective circulation; in such circumstances, medication may be required.

5. Meconium at birth

There is no evidence that suctioning meconium from the nose and mouth of the infant while the head is still on the perineum prevents meconium aspiration, so this practice is not recommended.[6] Lung inflation within the first minute of life is a priority and should not be delayed. In addition, attempting to remove meconium from the airways of a vigorously crying infant has also been proved to be ineffective at preventing meconium aspiration.[7]

If a baby is born unresponsive at birth and there is thick meconium liquor present, it is reasonable to rapidly inspect the oropharynx with a view to removing any particulate matter that might obstruct the airway. However, the emphasis is on initiating ventilation within the first minute of life in the non-breathing infant, and this should not be delayed, especially if there is persistent bradycardia.[1]

6. Emergency medication

Emergency medications are needed only if there is no significant circulatory response despite effective ventilation and chest compressions. A senior neonatologist should be in attendance at this stage, and it is that person's responsibility to intubate the infant and administer medications. The outlook for these infants at this stage is poor, although a small proportion will have good outcomes after a return of spontaneous circulation followed by therapeutic hypothermia.[1]

Medications for advanced resuscitation are usually kept in a sealed 'neonatal emergency resuscitation medicines box', which may be kept in the drawer of the resuscitaire, or on the neonatal resuscitation trolley (Figure 15.9).

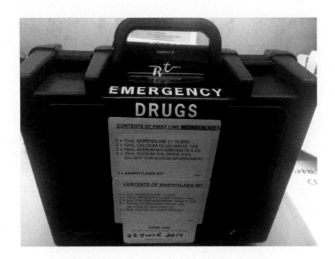

Figure 15.9 Example of a neonatal
emergency drugs box

Medications may include:

- adrenaline (epinephrine) (1:10,000)
- sodium bicarbonate (ideally 4.2% solution), only used during prolonged resuscitations
- glucose (10%)

All resuscitation medications are best delivered via an umbilical venous catheter or, if this is not possible, through an intraosseous needle.[8,9] However, any medication would only be administered by senior neonatologists and advanced neonatal nurse practitioners.

Emergency neonatal O-negative blood

Occasionally, an infant may be severely anaemic at birth (especially following abruption/vasa praevia), and a transfusion of emergency neonatal O-negative blood may be required. It is important that the obstetric/midwifery team informs the neonatal team as early as possible if an anaemic baby is anticipated, and also that the teams are aware of the location of the blood fridge and the neonatal O-negative blood (Figure 15.10).

7. Post-resuscitation care

Therapeutic hypothermia

Perinatal hypoxia severe enough to cause hypoxic–ischaemic encephalopathy (HIE) is estimated to occur in approximately 1–6 per 1000 births.[1] Targeted therapeutic hypothermia improves a range of neurodevelopmental outcomes in survivors.[10,11,12,13]

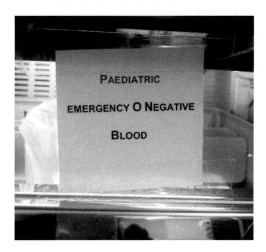

Figure 15.10 Neonatal emergency O-negative blood labelled on a specific shelf in the blood fridge

Treatment with therapeutic hypothermia should be considered in a newborn that is more than 36 completed weeks' gestation, where moderate or severe HIE is a possibility. Therapeutic hypothermia should only be instigated following a decision by a consultant neonatologist, and it must be conducted under clearly defined protocols. If therapeutic hypothermia is being considered, then the heater of the resuscitaire should be switched off.[1]

Glucose

Those infants requiring significant resuscitation, including preterm infants, should be monitored post-resuscitation and treated early to maintain their blood glucose within the normal range. Glucose levels can be documented along with other observations on the neonatal early warning score (NEWS) chart (Figure 15.11) and in the neonatal notes. Ensure that a neonatologist is informed if there are any yellow or red triggers.

Listed below are actions that may help to ensure that normal glucose levels are maintained:

■ Early skin-to-skin contact.

■ Encourage early breastfeed, or expressed breast milk if 'reluctant feeder'.

■ Prevention of hypothermia (check temperature at birth, then according to local protocols).

■ Observe for symptoms of hypoglycaemia (drowsiness, jitteriness, apnoea or seizures).

■ Monitor blood glucose levels at 3 hours old, then according to local protocols.

■ Consider administering 40% dextrose gel into the buccal mucosa and recheck blood glucose level in 30–60 minutes as per local protocols.

Name: ....

Date of Birth: .... **Ward:** ....

Hospital No: ....

Risk Factors :

PROM   Gp.B Strep   Maternal/other infection risk

Meconium staining- significant / light   Other...............

DATE																				
TIME																				Action Cues

Incubator / Hot Cot Temp																				
≥ 38.5 (Record Temp)																				Neonatal Team : infection screen
38																				Recheck <1 hr
Temperature 37.5																				
°C 37																				
36.5																				Thermal care
36																				
35.5																				Thermal care & blood glucose
35																				

< 35 (Record Temp) ≥200 (Record Rate)																				Contact neonatal team, check temp.
180																				Repeat <1 hr
160																				
Heart Rate 140																				
120																				
100																				Repeat <1 hr
80																				Contact neonatal team
60																				
<60 (Record Rate)																				
Capillary refill >3sec																				Repeat <1 hr

≥100 (Record Rate)																				Check temp., blood glucose, contact neonatal team
90																				
80																				
70																				Repeat <1 hr
Respiration Rate 60																				
50																				
40																				
30																				Check blood glucose & contact neonatal team
Cyanosis																				
Chest Recessions																				
Grunting																				
Nasal Flare																				

Alert / Normal																				
Jittery																				Check glucose
Lethargic or Drowsy																				
Irritable																				Check blood glucose & contact neonatal team
Abnormal Cry																				
Apnoea																				
Abnormal movements																				
Seizure																				

Poor feeding																				
Bilious vomit / aspirate																				Contact neonatal team
DCT+ or Jaundice <24hr																				
Blood Glucose																				Action if < 2.6

Total Yellow Observations																				
Total Red Observations																				

Reproduced by kind permission of UHBristol NHS Foundation Trust

Figure 15.11 Example of a neonatal early warning score (NEWS) chart for documenting neonatal observations

This tool is to guide midwifery staff in the relevance of observations in the newborn.
This tool does not replace clinical judgement or use of appropriate guidelines.
If the baby is unwell or you have concerns contact the neonatal team immediately.
If appropriate put out a "Neonatal Emergency" call immediately – Call 2222.

Yellow Observations

One "Yellow" observation : registered staff to assess baby and repeat observations within 1 hour. If the observation is still "Yellow" when repeated : contact neonatal team.

Two "Yellow" observations : registered staff to assess patient and then contact neonatal team.

Red Observation

Any "Red" observation: registered staff to assess baby and then contact neonatal team.

Any "Yellow", or "Red" observation: ensure full set of observations done and a blood glucose checked where appropriate.

Minimum / Routine Observations

Please see relevant NBT guidelines for frequency of observations e.g.
• Care of term infants when the mother has had prolonged rupture of membranes (PROM over 24 hours)
• Neonatal guidelines for prevention of GBS infection
• Meconium stained liquor
• Neonatal Hypoglycaemia

Alternative observation criteria

In some isolated cases (such as neonatal abstinence and pain from birth trauma) the patient may transgress some of the above criteria, the medical team responsible for the patient's care can set alternative acceptable parameters. These alternative parameters must be entered below after the baby has been reviewed by a member of the neonatal team. These parameters should be reviewed daily. The ward staff caring for the baby must know these parameters.

DATE / TIME	CONDITION / TREATMENT	Alternative Acceptable Parameter	SIGNATURE

Figure 15.11 (cont.)

Documentation

It is important that all actions are documented accurately and comprehensively in the appropriate case notes, particularly when resuscitation at birth has been necessary, as records may be carefully scrutinised many years later. Figure 15.12 is an example of a neonatal resuscitation pro forma to aid documentation.

283

Women and Children's Health	NEONATAL RESUSCITATION DOCUMENTATION	North Bristol NHS
		NHS Trust

Date .... Time ....   **Mother**

Affix small addressograph (Name, Hospital Number, DOB)

Person completing form ....

Affix small addressograph (Name, Hospital Number, DOB)

Designation .... Signature ....   **Baby**

Called for Help at:

Name of staff present	Role	Time of arrival

APGAR SCORE	1min	5min	10min	15min
Heart rate				
Respiration				
Muscle Tone				
Reflex Response				
Colour				
TOTAL				

Time of birth: ....

Mode of birth: ....

Heart Rate at Birth: ....

Time heart rate above 100 bpm: ....

Time of onset of regular respirations: ....

O2 SATS: ....

Risk factors (GBS, Prom, Mec, Maternal temp) ....

If mother transferred from the birth centre or home please complete the following:

Was an Ambulance required	Time Ambulance called	Time Ambulance arrived birth centre/ home	Time Ambulance left birth centre/home	Time arrived at Hospital

Procedure carried out	Tick	Time	By whom	Comments/ details of the baby's response (comment on changes in HR, colour or resps)
Cord clamped and cut				
Baby dried and stimulated				
5 Inflation Breaths				
Ventilation Breaths				
Cardiac compressions				
Any other procedures Intubated? Central Access?				

Figure 15.12 An example of a neonatal resuscitation pro forma

Emergency drugs (can be given in any order under the direction of a neonatologist)

Drugs are needed rarely and only if there is no significant cardiac output despite effective lung inflation and chest compression.

Adrenaline	**0.1 ml/kg of 1:10,000.** *Can go up to a dose of up to 30 mcg kg-1 (0.3 ml kg-1 of 1:10,000 solution) may be tried.*
Sodium bicarbonate 4.2%	**2-4ml/kg** *(1-2mmol/kg 4.2% bicarbonate solution).*
10% Dextrose	**2.5 ml/kg**
0.9% Sodium Chloride	**10 ml/kg** of or O negative blood

Drugs Used	Times given

O Neg blood given?	Y/N
Time	

Blood transfusion lab informed

(TICK) ☐

eAIMS completed? ....

Cord gases: Art pH.......... Art BE............   Venous pH............ Venous BE..........   Lactate...........

Figure 15.12 (cont.)

Preparing for preterm birth and optimising care on labour ward

Most preterm infants are in reasonable condition at birth and are only in need of assisted transition, not resuscitation.[14] However, babies at 30 weeks' gestation and under are fragile and require careful handling and gentle support. Senior neonatal staff with experience in dealing with preterm babies should be present at the birth.

Counselling parents for preterm birth

If possible, it is important that a senior neonatologist counsels parents prior to their preterm birth. Potential outcomes should be explained objectively and factually, without pre-judging the necessary care. It is also important to be aware of local data on outcomes. Any discussions should be documented in the medical records, and, if possible, relevant members of the midwifery and obstetric team should be present at the discussions so that they are aware of the information that has been given to the parents.

The parents should be aware of the process of placing the preterm baby into a polyethylene bag to maintain temperature, and also of the probability of their baby requiring intubation. It is also important to discuss that even with the neonatal team's best efforts to resuscitate their baby, he/she may not survive.

A visit to the neonatal unit should be arranged if appropriate, and if time permits, to prepare the parents for the appearance of the neonate at a similar gestation, and so that they can see a baby receiving intensive treatment and ventilation.

Thermal care of the preterm infant

Preterm infants are particularly vulnerable to heat loss and hypothermia, as they have immature, thin skin, reduced subcutaneous fat and poor vasomotor control, as well as an increased body surface to mass ratio. For every 1 °C below 36.5 °C, the risk of mortality increases by up to 28%.[15,16,17] Even a brief period of hypothermia is associated with impaired surfactant synthesis, pulmonary hypertension, hypoxia and coagulation defects. Hypoxia and acidosis further inhibit surfactant production.[1]

Preterm infants born in the maternity unit at less than 30 weeks of gestation should be placed in a polyethylene wrap or bag (up to the neck), without drying, immediately after birth (Figure 15.13). The head should be dried before putting on a hat, and the baby should be nursed under a radiant heater in the polyethylene bag, while being stabilised. This is a very effective method of keeping preterm infants warm. They should remain wrapped until their temperature has been checked after admission to the neonatal unit. For preterm infants, the labour room temperature should be at least 26 °C.[1]

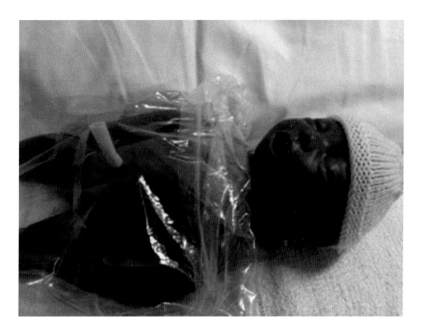

Figure 15.13 A preterm baby placed in a polyethylene bag

Timely cord clamping for the preterm infant

Provided the baby is kept warm, delaying cord clamping for at least 1 minute after birth can be considered, and gives many benefits for the preterm infant, including:

- increased circulating blood volume
- improved cardiovascular stability
- decreased risk of intraventricular haemorrhage
- decreased risk of necrotising enterocolitis

CPAP and PEEP for a preterm birth

The resuscitaire should be prepared with a positive end-expiratory pressure (PEEP) respiratory circuit and appropriately sized mask for the gestation of the baby. The lungs of a preterm baby are more fragile, and therefore continuous positive airway pressure (CPAP) will ease the effort of breathing and help to prevent alveolar collapse in expiration. Many preterm babies can be stabilised on CPAP without any need for intubation.

Oxygen saturation monitoring should be available, and an air/oxygen blender, as resuscitation may be started in air or up to 30% supplemental oxygen.

Surfactant therapy

For babies less than 30 weeks' gestation there is a serious risk of respiratory distress syndrome (RDS), and evidence shows that early prophylactic use of surfactant has advantages over rescue treatment.[1] However, this should not be considered a drug of resuscitation, as a bolus of surfactant may briefly compromise ventilation before it becomes more widely distributed.

Neuroprotection with magnesium sulfate

The incidence of cerebral palsy decreases significantly with increasing gestational age. The National Institute for Health and Care Excellence (NICE) guidance recommends that magnesium sulfate should be given to women at risk of preterm birth as a neuroprotective agent for the fetus and to improve long-term outcomes.[18]

Magnesium sulfate therapy should therefore be offered to all women in threatened preterm labour up to 30 weeks' gestation who are likely to give birth within the next 24 hours. The regimen is exactly the same as for the treatment of eclampsia. The most important factor is that it is administered up until birth (magnesium sulfate should only be continued after delivery if the mother has severe pre-eclampsia, in which case it should be continued for 24 hours post-birth). However, in time-critical situations where birth needs to be expedited for maternal or fetal wellbeing, birth should not be delayed solely for magnesium sulfate administration.

References

1. Resuscitation Council (UK). Resuscitation and support of transition of babies at birth. *Resuscitation Guidelines* 2015. www.resus.org.uk/resuscitation-guidelines/resuscitation-and-support-of-transition-of-babies-at-birth (accessed June 2017).

2. Dawes G. *Fetal and Neonatal Physiology*. Chicago, IL: Year Book, 1968, pp. 141–59.

3. Hey E, Kelly J. Gaseous exchange during endotracheal ventilation for asphyxia at birth. *J Obstet Gynaecol Br Commonw* 1968; 75: 414–23.

4. Andersson O, Hellström-Westas L, Andersson D, Domellöf M. Effect of delayed versus early umbilical cord clamping on neonatal outcomes and iron status at 4 months: a randomised controlled trial. *BMJ* 2011; 343: d7157.

5. Dahm LS, James LS. Newborn temperature and calculated heat loss in the delivery room. *Pediatrics* 1972; 49: 504–13.

6. Vain NE, Szyld EG, Prudent LM, *et al.* Oropharyngeal and nasopharyngeal suctioning of meconium-stained neonates before delivery of their shoulders: multicentre, randomised controlled trial. *Lancet* 2004; 364: 597–602.

7. Wiswell TE, Gannon CM, Jacob J, *et al.* Delivery room management of the apparently vigorous meconium-stained neonate: results of the multicenter, international collaborative trial. *Pediatrics* 2000; 105: 1–7.

8. Ellemunter H, Simma B, Trawoger R, Maurer H. Intraosseous lines in preterm and full term neonates. *Arch Dis Child Fetal Neonatal Ed* 1999; 80: F74–5

9. Engle WA. Intraosseous access for administration of medications in neonates. *Clin Perinatol* 2006; 33: 161–8.

10. Edwards AD, Brocklehurst P, Gunn AJ, *et al.* Neurological outcomes at 18 months of age after ischaemic encephalopathy: synthesis and meta-analysis of trial data. *BMJ* 2010; 340: c363.

11. Gluckman PD, Wyatt JS, Azzopardi D, *et al.* Selective head cooling with mild systemic hypothermia after neonatal encephalopathy. Multi-centre randomised trial. *Lancet* 2005; 35: 663–70.

12. Shankaran S, Laptook AR, Ehrenkranz RA, *et al.* Whole body hypothermia for neonates with hypoxic-ischaemic encephalopathy. *N Engl J Med* 2005; 353: 1574–84.

13. Azzopardi DV, Strohm B, Edwards AD, *et al.* Moderate hypothermia to treat perinatal asphyxia encephalopathy. *N Engl J Med* 2009; 361: 1349–58.

14. O'Donnell CP, Stenson BJ. Respiratory strategies for preterm infants. *Semin Fetal Neonatal Med* 2008; 13: 401–9.

15. Wyllie J, Perlman JM, Kattwinkel J, *et al.*; Neonatal Resuscitation Chapter Collaborators. Part 7: Neonatal resuscitation: 2015 international consensus on cardiopulmonary resuscitation and emergency cardiovascular care science with treatment recommendations. *Resuscitation* 2015; 95: e169–201.

16. Wyllie J, Bruinenberg J, Roerhr CC, *et al.* European Resuscitation Council Guidelines for Resuscitation 2015: Section 7. Resuscitation and support transition of babies at birth. *Resuscitation* 2015; 95: 249–63.

17. Meyer MP, Hou D, Ishrar NN, Dito I, te Pas AB. Initial respiratory support with cold, dry gas versus heated humidified gas and admission temperature of preterm infants. *J Pediatr* 2015; 166: 245–50.e1.

18. National Institute for Health and Care Excellence. *Preterm Labour and Birth*. NICE Guideline NG25. London: NICE, 2015. www.nice.org.uk/guidance/ng25 (accessed June 2017).

Module 16

Measuring quality in maternity care

Key learning points

- To understand the multifaceted nature of measurement of maternity care.
- To understand the use of process measures, clinical outcomes and other measures of care.

Common difficulties observed

- Use of arbitrary outcome measures and thresholds for action
- Failure to measure patient-reported outcome measures (PROMs)
- Problems operationalising local dashboards

Introduction

Sustainable improvement in intrapartum outcomes requires an integrated approach, combining incentivisation of best practice, training and tools to provide best care, and meaningful measurement.[1]

To achieve this, we must make measurement of care easier, more timely and more understandable to all the actors in the system, from government to women themselves. However, the measurement of quality can be difficult: quality is multifaceted and we must ensure that measurement is broad enough to include what is important to all stakeholders, not merely what can be easily measured.[2] It would also be useful to shift the focus away from 'failures', and instead investigate positive deviance, i.e. units which are performing well.[3,4] The current focus on rare, albeit tragic outcomes such as intrapartum stillbirths may provide too narrow a lens for system improvement.

Finally, we need to link measurement to operationalising improvement: we measure too much and do too little.[5] One of the most successful 'improvement' programmes is WeightWatchers, which has been demonstrated to improve weight loss more than many other programmes in a number of randomised controlled trials.[6] At its core, WeightWatchers is a framework that links measurement, interventions and support. Clearly, this model resonates with medical care that could usefully include local measurement and anonymised benchmarking, signposting to effective interventions, peer support and continual review of outcomes.

Funders also need evidence of improvement, even though incentivisation schemes based on outcomes can be fallible.[7] Training is not free and has been calculated to cost more than £120,000 per year in a unit with an annual birth rate of 6500 births.[8] Therefore, training is not cheap, but it can be cost-effective, provided that outcomes improve, and there is a parallel reduction in litigation costs.[9]

Measuring quality in maternity care is important to the health service and its staff, as well as to women and their families. The most recent NHS England National Maternity Review (*Better Births*) recommends:

> Teams should routinely collect data on the quality and outcomes of their services, measure their own performance and compare against others so that they can improve. Furthermore, there should be a nationally agreed set of indicators to help local maternity systems track, benchmark and improve the quality of maternity services.[10]

The problem is not the aim or the ambition, but the operationalisation of local measurement, particularly for smaller units that may not have the capacity to easily turn their routinely collected data into useful information.[2]

How do we define quality of care?

Quality of care has been defined across many healthcare domains and in many dimensions.[11] This is no different in maternity, where there have been many calls for a comprehensive approach to developing a system for the measurement of quality that incorporates the multiple perspectives involved in maternity care,[12,13,14] including staff[15] and women.[16]

Process and *outcomes* are two measures that are commonly deemed relevant to maternity care, but neither can provide a total picture because there is no single perfect measure of care.

Process measures

Process (e.g. caesarean birth rate) and system (e.g. size of unit) measures are commonly employed in quality measurement, at least partly because they are easy to measure. There is also an implicit assumption that the hospitals that perform best on selected process measures will have the best health outcomes.

Recently, this assumption has been challenged, and a US research group has demonstrated that although poor process measurement scores may be associated with adverse outcomes, the hospitals that performed well for those measures did not have the best risk-adjusted rates of obstetric morbidity.[17]

However, process measures can still provide valuable insight into a hospital service and could be usefully combined with clinical quality indicators (QI) to provide balance measures, i.e. the best outcomes for the least intervention.

There may also be opportunities to investigate system-level information to identify patterns and safety at a national level, e.g. staffing levels versus outcomes,[18,19] contributions of skill mix to outcomes,[20] and 'busy day' effects on perinatal outcomes.[21]

Outcome measures: clinical quality indicators (QIs)

The use of a suite of clinical indicators or outcomes is one way of measuring the quality of a clinical service. Historically, maternal mortality rate was used as the earliest measure of quality of obstetric care.[22] This remains a crude but important indicator, still employed today in international comparisons. However, the steep decline in maternal deaths over the last few decades in the UK and many other developed countries limits its value.

A number of quality measurement outcome tools have been proposed for maternity care: the Adverse Outcome Index (AOI) (the percentage of births with one or more specific adverse events), the Weighted Adverse Outcome Score (WAOS),[23] and the Severity Index (SI), which describes the severity of the outcomes.[24] However, they do not appear to have been widely implemented.

Legal claim analyses (LCAs) provide an important but limited perspective of adverse clinical outcomes and could possibly be used as part of a portfolio of indicators, but by their nature they are very narrowly focused and suffer from a significant lag time, both of which hinder useful feedback into clinical services.[25]

Clinical outcome measures are appealing but, possibly counterintuitively, patient satisfaction does not consistently correlate with clinical outcomes.[26,27] Furthermore, there can be issues with appropriate case-mix or population risk adjustment. It is widely recognised that stillbirth rates are very closely associated with maternal demographics,[28] and this makes it difficult to directly compare units in different regions.

Problems of appropriate risk adjustment notwithstanding, effective quality monitoring relies on the identification of suitable quality indicators (QIs) based on high-quality data. Ideal QIs should be:[29]

■ relevant to the area of care being monitored

■ measurable using routinely collected data

■ alterable by best practice

Although many QIs have been proposed and are in use in maternity care, there are no standardised, uniformly agreed sets of indicators. Many calls have been made for a standard set of QIs both internationally[14,30,31,32] and in the UK.[2,33] However, the current lack of structure and rigour has resulted in an enormous variation in QIs monitored and definitions used: 290 clinical indicators were identified within 96 clinical categories with up to 18 different definitions in three sets of nationally recommended intrapartum QIs from the UK.[33] Moreover, in one UK region with 10 maternity units there were 352 different QI definitions, covering 37 different QIs with up to 39 different definitions for each indicator.[34] This is clearly unnecessary variation and should be streamlined. There is an urgent requirement for a national and international core set of maternity QIs.

Suites of indicators have been developed using robust methodologies: systematic review[32] and Delphi panels.[33] In the USA, a National Quality Forum Perinatal Care Core Measure Set has been developed; this includes five very limited quality measures that would appear to be relatively unambitious in UK practice.[24]

Once a set of QIs has been selected, it is imperative that they are analysed using robust statistical methods. Unfortunately this may not always be the case, and in one review of a single UK health region the overwhelming majority of units used arbitrary thresholds for adverse outcomes and there was no benchmarking.[34] A number of researchers have recommended a cumulative sum (CUSUM) control chart as the most appropriate method to monitor the relatively low-frequency adverse outcomes in healthcare[35] and maternity care.[13,36]

Source data

Unit-based maternity databases are amongst the most accurate datasets in the NHS.[37] Since 2015, maternity units have started to submit standardised extracts from these to form a national maternity dataset that includes much of the perinatal information not currently available from routine Hospital Episode Statistics (HES) data.

Therefore, it would seem appropriate to aggregate local databases into higher-order datasets to measure and, importantly, benchmark quality measurement between units. This has been demonstrated to be feasible in the 10 maternity units across a whole NHS region.[34]

The Royal College of Obstetricians and Gynaecologists (RCOG) has established the Maternity Indicators System project, which includes detailed outcomes for mothers and babies from approximately 17 hospitals delivering 100,000 births annually, also aggregated from local databases.[38]

Insurers could also use these outcome indicators to model insurance premiums based on each individual maternity unit's current clinical performance, as well as its historical performance based on claims made, or paid.[39]

Finally, maternity units can use outcome indicators to monitor and benchmark their own clinical performance. This is supported by some preliminary work in Bristol that has demonstrated that there is a very high level of data completeness, with only 0.7% missing values.[39] Moreover, any missing data did not change their clinical relevance, as demonstrated by a sensitivity analysis, indicating that a 'first slice' of the data is accurate and further cleaning is unlikely to be necessary.

Furthermore, some important indicators have wide applicability and are therefore particularly useful for benchmarking. For instance, the Apgar score at 5 minutes, which is a good indicator for an increased risk of death in the first year of life,[40] and a reasonable predictor for perinatal brain damage related to asphyxia in labour (96% negative predictive value),[41] was independent of almost all maternal population demographics.

Overall, clinical indicators that are measurable and alterable with best practice are essential to useful measurement of quality. There is at least one example from maternity care that has demonstrated that monitoring of QIs is both feasible and beneficial: an adverse trend in infants born with a low Apgar score was identified, thereby allowing for timely corrective action and improvement in perinatal outcomes.[42]

Patient-reported outcome measures

Quality measures must also have direct relevance to patients' lives, including their experience of, and satisfaction with, the care they receive.[43]

Satisfaction depends not only on the biomedical outcome itself, but also on the values placed on different outcomes, which can vary widely between different cultures and individuals.[31] For example, caesarean birth may be the preferred mode of birth amongst a population of Brazilian women, but conversely perceived as a highly undesirable outcome in certain sub-Saharan African populations.[31]

Various surveys and tools exist to evaluate these patient perceptions of service. Since October 2013, all NHS-funded maternity services have asked women to answer a single question about how likely they would be to recommend the services they have received to friends or family (the Friends and Family Test) if they needed similar care or treatment.

The UK's Care Quality Commission (CQC) conducts triennial surveys of maternity service users in the UK. The most recent survey collated the experiences of over 20,000 women who had a live birth between January and February 2015.[44] The report measured quality issues for women-centred care around their physical care both antenatally and postnatally, care of their babies, attention to pain management and discharge arrangements, as well as the professionalism and competence of staff.

Ideally, patient-reported outcome measures (PROMs), such as results from the CQC's survey on women's experiences of maternity care, would be integrated with, and provide additional context for, a holistic interpretation of numerical indicators.[45] Other maternity PROMs have been proposed too.[46]

Culture

It is currently very fashionable to reference the 'culture' of a unit as an important predictor of good outcomes. However, culture has become a 'catch-all' word that means any number of different processes, elements or indeed anything to do with the functioning of a hospital or unit.

Safety culture refers to the way patient safety is thought about and implemented within an organisation, and the structures and processes in place to support this. Safety climate is a subset of broader culture and refers to staff attitudes about patient safety within the organisation.[47] Safety culture has been linked to improvements in process measures,[48] unit level outcomes,[49] and litigation claims.[50]

The Sexton Safety Attitudes Questionnaire is a validated tool to measure safety attitudes and/or climate that has been widely employed in maternity care,[47] and there are published data from different maternity units that permit benchmarking.[49]

However, measurements of safety culture are not routinely recommended or undertaken in maternity care.

Presenting information

Presentation of information to stakeholders is an essential part of quality measurement, but there is a dearth of data to inform best practice.

Examples of graphical displays and tools to represent health outcomes can be found as far back as the nineteenth century, when in 1858 Florence Nightingale employed a graphical display (polar-area diagram) to present her findings that the majority of deaths were due to poor sanitation in military hospitals, and not casualties in battle. This revolutionised the care provided in military hospitals in the Crimean War. The use of visual data tools and displays is equally powerful in modern healthcare systems.

Clinical dashboards are frequently proposed to facilitate this process within UK maternity settings. A maternity dashboard was first described in UK practice in 2005 for a hospital with several preventable maternal deaths, to help measure and manage what was described as serious clinical underperformance.[51]

In 2008 the RCOG recommended that all maternity units implement a dashboard to 'plan and improve their maternity services'.[52] Within this guidance the RCOG included an example dashboard which utilised a RAG (red amber green) colour coding system to alert users to monthly changes in rates or frequencies of selected events and quality indicators against locally agreed standards.

There are published examples of local dashboards,[53] but there is currently no national system, nor a national minimum dataset for intrapartum care to populate the dashboard.

The PROMPT team, particularly Thabani Sibanda and Andrea Blotkamp, have developed an Excel-based dashboard that has been successfully

NBT Maternity Dashboard 2014 -2015

	Click on each indicator below for charts and further details	Target	Previous year monthly average	Apr-14	May-14	Jun-14	Jul-14	Aug-14	Sep-14	Oct-14	Nov-14	Dec-14	Jan-15	Feb-15	Mar-15	Year to date	Trend
Activity & staffing	Number of babies born (at >= 24 weeks gestation)		518	515	552	546	570	507	571	589	531	485	515	504	553	6438	
	Number of live births (any gestation)		516	510	551	543	567	504	566	585	529	484	514	504	553	6410	
	Number of live births at term		480	471	511	512	524	455	531	537	497	433	472	475	505	5923	
	Number of women who gave birth (all gestations)		509	503	543	540	561	494	562	573	522	472	506	498	539	6313	
	Number of women who gave birth (>=24 weeks)		508	501	539	540	559	489	561	567	521	471	505	496	534	6283	
	Number of bookings for antenatal care		614	617	579	608	645	568	624	609	554	619	654	637	697	7411	
	Number of bookings for antenatal care (in area)		592	595	561	582	611	545	600	587	542	600	633	615	679	7150	
	Midwife full-time equivalent		194.0	191.9	190.0	188.9	187.9	184.2	183.8	183.8	193.2	198.5	193.9	196.8		190.3	
	Midwife to births ratio		32.2	31.4	34.3	34.3	35.8	32.2	36.7	37.4	32.4	28.5	31.3	30.4		33.2	
Place of birth	Planned homebirth rate		1.1%	0.2%	0.7%	1.1%	1.1%	1.2%	1.8%	1.2%	1.7%	1.1%	0.6%	0.8%	0.9%	1.0%	
	Freestanding MLU birth rate		8.0%	6.0%	6.6%	6.5%	6.1%	6.1%	7.5%	7.2%	7.1%	5.3%	6.7%	6.0%	7.2%	6.5%	
	Alongside MLU birth rate		12.8%	13.1%	8.7%	12.8%	8.9%	8.5%	7.7%	11.7%	12.3%	7.8%	10.3%	9.2%	9.3%	10.0%	
	Delivery Suite birth rate		76.9%	79.3%	83.1%	78.9%	83.1%	83.4%	81.9%	79.1%	77.8%	84.7%	81.2%	82.9%	79.0%	81.2%	
	Other place of birth		1.2%	1.4%	0.9%	0.7%	0.9%	0.8%	1.2%	0.9%	1.1%	1.1%	1.2%	1.0%	3.5%	1.2%	
	All midwife-led environments birth rate		21.9%	19.3%	16.0%	20.4%	16.0%	15.8%	16.9%	20.1%	21.1%	14.2%	17.6%	16.1%	17.4%	17.6%	
Mode of birth	Normal birth rate	62.5%	60.7%	62.1%	58.3%	61.7%	57.6%	59.3%	58.1%	57.8%	62.6%		60.0%	63.5%	56.9%	58.9%	
	Instrumental birth rate	12.5%	13.1%	13.6%	10.8%	12.4%	13.1%	18.0%	15.0%	14.1%	11.7%	13.2%	16.0%	11.1%	13.9%	13.5%	
	Caesarean section rate (overall)	25.0%	26.2%	24.4%		25.9%	29.3%	29.0%	26.9%	27.9%	25.7%	24.0%	24.0%	25.4%	29.2%	27.5%	
	Elective CS rate (as % of all birth episodes)		10.4%	10.8%	11.3%	11.7%	12.3%	12.1%	11.9%	12.5%	11.3%	13.6%	8.9%	11.1%	12.0%	11.6%	
	Emergency CS rate (as % of all birth episodes)		15.8%	13.6%	19.7%	14.3%	17.0%	17.0%	15.0%	15.3%	14.4%	17.6%	15.0%	14.3%	17.2%	15.9%	
	Robson group 1 (as % of all birth episodes)		3.2%	2.4%	4.1%	2.8%	3.6%	2.2%	4.1%	3.2%	3.8%	3.0%	3.8%	2.4%	3.4%	3.2%	
	Robson group 2 (as % of all birth episodes)		5.8%	6.2%	7.6%	5.6%	5.4%	7.2%	4.8%	5.8%	4.6%	7.0%	6.7%	5.2%	6.0%	6.0%	
	Robson group 5 (as % of all birth episodes)		3.0%	2.8%	2.8%	2.4%	3.2%	2.7%	3.6%	3.4%	2.5%	5.5%	2.4%	4.0%	4.5%	3.3%	
Maternal indicators	Induction of labour rate	26.0%	26.1%	30.7%	29.7%	27.6%	25.0%	29.9%	23.7%	26.1%	28.0%	28.0%	28.9%	29.0%	27.9%	27.8%	
	3rd&4th degree tear rate as % of vaginal births	3.0%	5.7%		3.0%	4.8%	4.1%	3.7%	4.3%	4.9%	4.4%	5.5%	4.0%	4.4%	4.9%	5.6%	
	3rd&4th degree tear rate in unassisted births	2.5%	4.1%		1.3%	4.2%	3.1%	3.5%	4.3%	4.9%	3.4%		4.0%	4.4%	4.9%	4.1%	
	3rd&4th degree tear rate in assisted births	4.5%	11.9%	10.8%	10.4%	6.9%	7.7%	4.3%			8.8%	12.1%				11.1%	
	PPH >=1000 ml rate	4.6%	5.0%					7.3%									9.1%	
	PPH >=1500 ml rate	1.8%	2.2%				1.8%									3.8%	
	PPH >=2000 ml rate	0.8%	0.9%	0.8%		1.5%	0.9%		1.8%	1.4%	0.6%	0.6%	2.0%			1.6%	
	Rate of women requiring level 3 care	0.12%	0.1%	0.0%	0.2%	0.2%	0.0%	0.0%	0.0%	0.0%	0.0%	0.2%	0.2%	0.2%	0.2%	0.1%	
	Preterm birth rate <37 weeks		7.2%	7.8%	6.9%	6.0%	7.9%	9.5%	6.3%	8.5%	6.0%	10.7%	8.0%	5.4%	8.1%	7.6%	
	Preterm birth rate <34 weeks		2.8%	2.5%	1.3%	1.1%	2.5%	3.4%	2.8%	4.8%	2.3%	2.7%	3.5%	2.2%	3.1%	2.7%	

Click Here For New Dashboard Explanation

Click Here For Year-On-Year Trends

Figure 16.1 North Bristol NHS Trust maternity dashboard – Excel-based

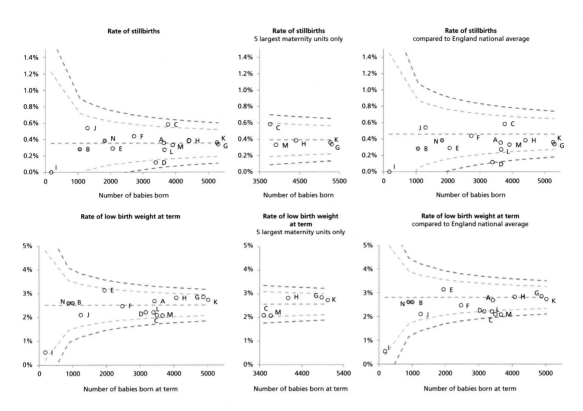

Figure 16.2 Example of anonymised regional dashboard in a funnel plot

implemented at local and regional level in the UK (Figures 16.1 and 16.2),[34] as well as in developing world settings.[54]

Summary

High-quality healthcare systems are those that produce the best outcomes with the fewest interventions, to the satisfaction of their patients, and within a cost-effective framework.

A combination of outcomes and processes is required, including, if possible, patient perception of care. There is probably a sweet spot of best care: the best outcomes, with the least intervention and the best experience.

There also needs to be less reliance on the self-assessment of risk processes and more prioritisation of what matters most: clinical outcomes, processes and patient experience. We should collect and produce a standard, relevant set of quality indicators, ideally from routinely collected data, and present these in a manner that facilitates ongoing quality improvement, just as recommended in the recent *Better Births* report.[10] Ideally, these data could then be employed to focus regulatory visits from bodies such as the CQC, as well as being used for prioritising local improvement and safety initiatives.

An Excel-based dashboard is available for units to use locally, which can then be aggregated to regional and national level. Contact the PROMPT team at info@promptmaternity.org if maternity teams would like more information.

References

1. Darzi A; Department of Health. *High Quality Care for All: NHS Next Stage Review Final Report.* London: DoH, 2008. www.gov.uk/government/publications/high-quality-care-for-all-nhs-next-stage-review-final-report (accessed June 2017).

2. Draycott T, Sibanda T, Laxton C, *et al.* Quality improvement demands quality measurement. *BJOG* 2010; 117: 1571–4.

3. Lawton R, Taylor N, Clay-Williams R, Braithwaite J. Positive deviance: a different approach to achieving patient safety. *BMJ Qual Saf* 2014; 23: 880–3.

4. Hollnagel E, Wears RL, Braithwaite J. *From Safety-I to Safety-II: A White Paper.* Resilient Health Care Net, 2015. www.england.nhs.uk/signuptosafety/wp-content/uploads/sites/16/2015/10/safety-1-safety-2-whte-papr.pdf (accessed June 2017).

5. Macrae C. The problem with incident reporting. *BMJ Qual Saf* 2016; 25: 71–5.

6. Jolly K, Lewis A, Beach J, *et al.* Comparison of range of commercial or primary care led weight reduction programmes with minimal intervention control for weight loss in obesity: lighten Up randomised controlled trial. *BMJ* 2011; 343: d6500–0.

7. Roland M, Dudley RA. How financial and reputational incentives can be used to improve medical care. *Health Serv Res* 2015; 50 (S2): 2090–115.

8. Yau CW, Pizzo E, Morris S, *et al.* The cost of local, multi-professional obstetric emergencies training. *Acta Obstet Gynecol Scand* 2016; 95: 1111–19.

9. Draycott TJ, Collins KJ, Crofts JF, *et al.* Myths and realities of training in obstetric emergencies. *Best Pract Res Clin Obstet Gynaecol* 2015; 29: 1067–76.

10. National Maternity Review. *Better Births: Improving Outcomes of Maternity Services in England.* London: NHS England, 2016.

11. Vincent C, Burnett S, Carthey J. *The Measurement and Monitoring of Safety.* London: Health Foundation, 2013. www.health.org.uk/publication/measurement-and-monitoring-safety (accessed June 2017).

12. Pettker CM, Grobman WA. Obstetric safety and quality. *Obstet Gynecol* 2015; 126:196–206.

13. Boulkedid R, Alberti C, Sibony O. Quality indicator development and implementation in maternity units. *Best Pract Res Clin Obstet Gynaecol* 2013; 27: 609–19.

14. Escuriet R, White J, Beeckman K, *et al.* Assessing the performance of maternity care in Europe: a critical exploration of tools and indicators. *BMC Health Serv Res* 2015; 15: 491.

15. Simms RA, Yelland A, Ping H, *et al.* Using data and quality monitoring to enhance maternity outcomes: a qualitative study of risk managers' perspectives. *BMJ Qual Saf* 2014; 23: 457–64.

16. Raven J, van den Broek N, Tao F, Kun H, Tolhurst R. The quality of childbirth care in China: women's voices: a qualitative study. *BMC Pregnancy Childbirth* 2015; 15: 113.

17. Grobman WA, Bailit JL, Rice MM, *et al.* Can differences in obstetric outcomes be explained by differences in the care provided? The MFMU Network APEX study. *Am J Obstet Gynecol* 2014; 211: 147.e1–e16.

18. Sandall J, Murrells T, Dodwell M, *et al.* The efficient use of the maternity workforce and the implications for safety and quality in maternity care: a population-based, cross-sectional study. Health Services and Delivery Research, No. 2.38. Southampton: National Institute for Health Research, 2014.

19. Yelland A, Winter C, Draycott T, Fox AR. Midwifery staffing: variation and mismatch in demand and capacity. *Br J Midwifery* 2013; 21: 579–89.

20. Aiken LH, Sloane D, Griffiths P, *et al.* Nursing skill mix in European hospitals: cross-sectional study of the association with mortality, patient ratings, and quality of care. *BMJ Qual Saf* 2016; 26: 525–8.

21. Snowden JM, Kozhimannil KB, Muoto I, Caughey AB, McConnell KJ. A 'busy day' effect on perinatal complications of delivery on weekends: a retrospective cohort study. *BMJ Qual Saf* 2017; 26: e1.

22. Knight M, Kenyon S, Brocklehurst P, *et al.* (eds.); MBRRACE-UK. *Saving Lives, Improving Mothers' Care: Lessons Learned to Inform Future Maternity Care from the UK and Ireland Confidential Enquiries into Maternal Deaths and Morbidity 2009–12.* Oxford: National Perinatal Epidemiology Unit, University of Oxford, 2014.

23. Mann S, Pratt S, Gluck P, *et al.* Assessing quality in obstetrical care: development of standardized measures. *Jt Comm J Qual Patient Saf* 2006; 32: 497–505.

24. Gee RE, Winkler R. Quality measurement: what it means for obstetricians and gynecologists. *Obstet Gynecol* 2013; 121: 507–10.

25. Fox R, Yelland A, Draycott T. Analysis of legal claims: informing litigation systems and quality improvement. *BJOG* 2014; 121: 6–10.

26. Kennedy GD, Tevis SE, Kent KC. Is there a relationship between patient satisfaction and favorable outcomes? *Ann Surg* 2014; 260: 592–600.

27. Howell EA, Zeitlin J, Hebert PL, Balbierz A, Egorova N. Association between hospital-level obstetric quality indicators and maternal and neonatal morbidity. *JAMA* 2014; 312: 1531–41.

28. Smith G, Fretts RC. Stillbirth. *Lancet* 2007; 370: 1715–25.

29. NHS Institute for Innovation and Improvement. *The Good Indicators Guide: Understanding How to Use and Choose Indicators.* Coventry: NHS Institute for Innovation and Improvement, 2008.

30. Boulkedid R, Sibony O, Goffinet F, *et al.* Quality indicators for continuous monitoring to improve maternal and infant health in maternity departments: a modified Delphi survey of an international multidisciplinary panel. *PLoS One* 2013; 8: e60663.

31. Pittrof R, Campbell OM, Filippi VG. What is quality in maternity care? An international perspective. *Acta Obstet Gynecol Scand* 2002; 81: 277–83.

32. Bonfill X, Roqué M, Aller MB, *et al.* Development of quality of care indicators from systematic reviews: the case of hospital delivery. *Implement Sci* 2013; 8: 42.

33. Sibanda T, Fox R, Draycott T, *et al.* Intrapartum care quality indicators: a systematic approach for achieving consensus. *Eur J Obstet Gynecol Reprod Biol* 2012; 166: 23–9.

34. Simms RA, Ping H, Yelland A, *et al.* Development of maternity dashboards across a UK health region; current practice, continuing problems. *Eur J Obstet Gynecol Reprod Biol* 2013; 170: 119–24.

35. Spiegelhalter D, Sherlaw Johnson C, Bardsley M, *et al.* Statistical methods for healthcare regulation: rating, screening and surveillance. *J R Stat Soc Ser A Stat Soc* 2012; 175: 1–47.

36. Sibanda T, Sibanda N. The CUSUM chart method as a tool for continuous monitoring of clinical outcomes using routinely collected data. *BMC Med Res Methodol* 2007; 7: 46.

37. Cleary R, Beard RW, Coles J, *et al.* The quality of routinely collected maternity data. *Br J Obstet Gynaecol* 1994; 101: 1042–7.

38. Knight HE, van der Meulen JH, Gurol-Urganci I, *et al.* Birth 'out-of-hours': an evaluation of obstetric practice and outcome according to the presence of senior obstetricians on the labour ward. *PLoS Med* 2016; 13: e1002000–15.

39. NHS Litigation Authority. *Report on the Clinical Negligence Scheme for Trusts (CNST) Consultation*. London: NHSLA, 2016.

40. Iliodromiti S, Mackay DF, Smith GC, Pell JP, Nelson SM. Apgar score and the risk of cause-specific infant mortality: a population-based cohort study. *Lancet* 2014; 384: 1749–55.

41. Ruth VJ, Raivio KO. Perinatal brain damage: predictive value of metabolic acidosis and the Apgar score. *BMJ* 1988; 297: 24–7.

42. Sibanda T, Sibanda N, Siassakos D, *et al.* Prospective evaluation of a continuous monitoring and quality-improvement system for reducing adverse neonatal outcomes. *Am J Obstet Gynecol* 2009; 201: 480.

43. Mountford J, Shojania KG. Refocusing quality measurement to best support quality improvement: local ownership of quality measurement by clinicians. *BMJ Qual Saf* 2012; 21: 519–23.

44. Care Quality Commission. *Maternity Services Survey 2015*. London: CQC, 2016. www.cqc .org.uk/publications/surveys/maternity-services-survey-2015 (accessed June 2017).

45. Chappell LC, Calderwood C, Kenyon S, Draper ES, Knight M. Understanding patterns in maternity care in the NHS and getting it right. *BMJ* 2013; 346: f2812.

46. Mahmud A, Morris E, Johnson S, Ismail KM. Developing core patient-reported outcomes in maternity: PRO-Maternity. *BJOG* 2014; 121: 15–19.

47. Health Foundation. *Measuring Safety Culture*. London: Health Foundation, 2011. www.health .org.uk/sites/health/files/MeasuringSafetyCulture.pdf (accessed June 2017).

48. van der Nelson HA, Siassakos D, Bennett J, *et al.* Multiprofessional team simulation training, based on an obstetric model, can improve teamwork in other areas of health care. *Am J Med Qual* 2014; 29: 78–82.

49. Siassakos D, Fox R, Hunt L, *et al.* Attitudes toward safety and teamwork in a maternity unit with embedded team training. *Am J Med Qual* 2011; 26: 132–7.

50. Cox L. *Towards a Safety Culture: The Relationship Between Workplace Culture and Medical Indemnity Claims in the Victorian Health Sector*. VMIA Occasional Paper. Melbourne: VMIA, 2012. www.vmia.vic.gov.au/learn/patient-safety/towards-a-safety-culture (accessed June 2012).

51. Healthcare Commission. *Investigation into 10 Maternal Deaths at, or Following Delivery at, Northwick Park Hospital, North West London Hospitals NHS Trust, Between April 2002 and April 2005*. London: Healthcare Commission, 2006.

52. Royal College of Obstetricians and Gynaecologists. *Maternity Dashboard: Clinical Performance and Governance Scorecard*. Good Practice No. 7. London: RCOG, 2008. www.rcog.org.uk/en/ guidelines-research-services/guidelines/good-practice-7 (accessed June 2017).

53. Muhammad S, Chandraharan E. The maternity dashboard: how effective is it in improving maternity care? *Obstetrics* 2016; 26: 276–9.

54. Crofts J, Moyo J, Ndebele W, *et al.* Adaptation and implementation of local maternity dashboards in a Zimbabwean hospital to drive clinical improvement. *Bull World Health Organ* 2013; 92: 146–52.

Index

acidosis, 70, 94, 131
    shoulder dystocia and, 210
Adverse Outcome Index (AOI), 293
air embolism, 27
all-fours position, 199–200
amniotic fluid embolism (AFE), 26–7
anaesthetic emergencies, 47–8
    extubation and recovery, 55
    failed tracheal intubation, 48–55
    high regional block, 56–9
    local anaesthetic toxicity, 59–63
anaphylactic reactions, 25
aneurysm rupture, 21
angina, 24
antepartum haemorrhage, 136,
        146–51, *See also* maternal
        haemorrhage
    causes, 146
    clinical presentation, 146
    major haemorrhage management,
        146–51
        actions, 149
        assessment, 150
        call for help, 149
        expediting the birth, 150
        initial management, 146
        ongoing care, 167
    situational awareness, 170
antibiotics, maternal sepsis
        management, 131
antihypertensives, 110
    choice of, 112
aortocaval compression, 30
arterial blood gas, 131

aspiration of gastric contents, 25
    difficult intubation and, 50

baseline fetal heart rate, 80
basic life support algorithm, 14
bimanual uterine compression, 160
bladder catheterisation, 160
bladder filling, 223
blood products, 141
blood tests
    arterial blood gas, 131
    clotting studies, 131
    C-reactive protein (CRP), 131
    full blood count, 130
    liver function, 131
    maternal sepsis management, 130–1
    renal function, 131
    serum lactate, 130
B-Lynch suture technique, 165
brachial plexus injury (BPI), 211
breech presentation, 230, *See also*
        vaginal breech birth
    consequences, 230–2
    definition, 230
    evidence and national
        recommendations, 233
    predisposing factors, 230
Burns–Marshall technique, 239

caesarean section
    antepartum haemorrhage
        management, 150
    general anaesthesia, 48
    perimortem caesarean pack, 36

caesarean section (cont.)
  shoulder dystocia prevention, 194
  twin births, 247
carboprost, 162
cardiac arrest, 30, *See also* maternal
    collapse
  aftermath, 44
  community setting, 32
  local anaesthetic-induced, 63
  management, 32–43
    medication, 43
    post-resuscitation care, 44
    recognition of heart rhythms,
      38–41
    team leader role, 36–7
  potentially reversible causes, 42–3
cardiac disease, 23–5
  risk factors, 23
cardiac tamponade, 43
cardiorespiratory changes during
    pregnancy, 30–2
cardiotocography (CTG), 79–92
  accelerations, 82
  antenatal, 94
    classification, 95
  baseline rate, 80
  baseline variability, 81
  decelerations, 82
  interpretation, 86–8
  normal intrapartum CTG, 79
  pathological, 88
    fetal blood sampling, 88–92
  suspicious, 88
  twin birth, 253
cell salvage, 142
cerebrovascular event (CVE), 22
chest compression, 278
chest pain, 24
clavicular fractures, 212
clotting abnormalities
  blood tests, 131
    maternal haemorrhage and, 137

with pre-eclampsia, 115
communication, 5–7
  with woman and birth partner/
      relatives, 8
continuous positive airway pressure
    (CPAP), preterm birth, 287
cord clamping, 154
  hypoxic neonate, 272
  preterm birth, 287
  twin births, 256
cord presentation, 218
cord prolapse, 218
  breech presentation, 240
  debrief of parents, 225
  documentation, 225
  management, 220–5
    assessment for birth, 224
    birth plan, 223
    bladder filling, 223
    call for help, 221
    contraction reduction, 222
    digital elevation of presenting part,
      222
    early recognition, 221
    fetal monitoring, 223
    maternal positioning, 222
    neonatal resuscitation, 225
    post birth, 225
    training, 225
  perinatal complications, 219
  prevention, 219
  risk factors, 218
cord traction, 154
C-reactive protein (CRP), 131

deep vein thrombosis (DVT), 21
  prophylaxis with maternal sepsis, 133
delayed cord clamping. *See* cord
    clamping
diabetes mellitus, 23, 193
difficult intubation, 49
  optimal positioning, 51

pre-oxygenation, 52
risk factors, 49
disseminated intravascular coagulation (DIC), 22, 131, 137
with pre-eclampsia, 115
dizygotic twins, 245, *See also* twin births
documentation
cord prolapse, 225
eclampsia, 106
newborn resuscitation, 283
postpartum haemorrhage, 167
shoulder dystocia, 208
uterine inversion, 267
drug reactions, 25, 43
eclampsia, 101
documentation, 106
incidence, 102
management, 102
basic support, 102
call for help, 102
community setting, 108–10
eclampsia box, 103
hypertension control, 110–12
magnesium sulfate emergency regimen, 105
plan for labour/birth, 116–17
post-birth care, 117
seizure control, 104–6, 112
monitoring, 112–15
presenting features, 102
seizures and coma, 22

electronic fetal monitoring (EFM), 66–8, *See also* fetal monitoring
standards, 77–8
technical considerations, 77
vaginal breech birth, 235
with cord prolapse, 223
emergency response triggers, 15, *See also* maternal collapse
episiotomy, shoulder dystocia management, 201

Erb's palsy, 211
ergometrine, 155
external cephalic version, 254
extubation, 55

failed intubation, 48–55
definition, 48
management, 50–5
algorithm, 52
fetal blood sampling (FBS), 91–2
with pathological CTG, 88–92
fetal heart rate (FHR)
accelerations, 82
baseline, 80
decelerations, 82
tachycardia, 80
variability, 81
fetal monitoring, 66–8, *See also* electronic fetal monitoring (EFM)
risk management, 68
standards and quality, 71–8
informed choice, 73
intermittent auscultation in labour, 73–6
intrapartum risk assessments, 71
training, 69
fetal oxygen supply, 70–1
hypoxia risk factors, 69
influences, 71
responses to impeded supply, 70–1
fetal scalp stimulation (FSS), 90–1
fluid balance, pre-eclampsia and, 113
fluid resuscitation, 132
major obstetric haemorrhage, 138–9
blood products, 140–1
cell salvage, 142
intravenous access, 140
point-of-care testing, 142
volume to be infused, 140
forceps use, vaginal breech birth, 239
full blood cell count, 130

general anaesthesia, 48
    indications, 48
glucose management with newborn
        resuscitation, 281
glycogenolysis, 70

haemorrhage. *See* maternal
        haemorrhage
heart disease. *See* cardiac disease
heart rate, fetal. *See* fetal heart rate
heart rhythms during cardiac arrest,
        38–41
    non-shockable rhythms, 40–1
    shockable rhythms, 39–40
high regional block, 56–9
    management, 58–9
    presentation, 56–7
    risk factors, 57
humeral fractures, 212
hydrostatic method for uterine
        inversion, 265
hyperglycaemia, 23
hyperkalaemia, 42
hypermagnesaemia, 42
hypertension, 108, *See also* eclampsia;
        pre-eclampsia
    management, 110–12
        antihypertensives, 110
hypocalcaemia, 42
hypoglycaemia, 23, 42
hypotension, fluid resuscitation, 132
hypothermia, 42
    therapeutic, 280
hypovolaemia, 21, 42, 137
hypoxia
    fetal responses to impeded oxygen
        supply, 70–1
    fetal risk factors, 69
    maternal cardiac arrest, 42
    neonatal, 270, *See also* newborn
        resuscitation

cord clamping, 272
physiology, 270–1
hysterectomy, postpartum haemorrhage
        management, 166

induction of labour, shoulder dystocia
        prevention, 195
intensive care unit transfer, 186
intermittent auscultation (IA), 73–6
    abnormal fetal heart rate guidance,
        75
    indications for changing to
        continuous EFM, 76
    optimal timing, 73–4
    practice recommendations, 74
internal iliac artery ligation, 166
internal podalic version, 254
internal rotational manoeuvres, 201,
        205
interventional radiology, postpartum
        haemorrhage, 165
intrapartum haemorrhage, 137
intravenous access, 140
intubation. *See* difficult intubation;
        failed intubation
ischaemic heart disease. *See* cardiac
        disease

Klumpke's palsy, 211

labetalol, 112
laparotomy, postpartum haemorrhage
        management, 164
leadership, 8
legal claim analyses (LCAs), 294
liver function test, 131
local anaesthetic toxicity, 59–63
    follow-up, 63
    management, 61–3
        specific treatment, 63
    signs and symptoms, 59

macrosomia, 192
magnesium sulfate, 104
    emergency regimen, 105
    neuroprotection in preterm birth, 288
    seizure prevention, 112
    toxicity, 106
        emergency protocol, 106
major obstetric haemorrhage. *See* maternal haemorrhage
maternal collapse, 14, 15, *See also* cardiac arrest
    basic life support algorithm, 14
    causes, 20–7
        air embolism, 27
        amniotic fluid embolism (AFE), 26–7
        anaphylactic or toxic reactions, 25
        cardiac disease, 23–5
        cerebrovascular event (CVE), 22
        disseminated intravascular coagulation (DIC), 22
        eclamptic seizures and coma, 22
        haemorrhage, 21
        hypo- or hyperglycaemia, 23
        pulmonary aspiration of gastric contents, 25
        pulmonary thromboembolism, 20–1
        sepsis, 22
    management, 16–19
        continuing treatment, 18–19
        initial management, 17–18
        primary obstetric survey, 18
        secondary obstetric survey, 19
maternal critical care, 174–5
    equipment, 186
    indications, 176
    investigations, 180
    long term impacts of near-miss maternal morbidity, 187
    provision location, 180

recognition of the critically ill woman, 176
        MOEWS charts, 177
    regular structured review, 180
    transfer to ICU, 186
    unique features of, 175–6
maternal critical care chart, 182
maternal critical care structured review sheet, 182
maternal death
    haemorrhage, 136
    sepsis, 120
maternal haemorrhage, 21, 136
    antenatal risk assessment, 143–4
        anaemia, 143
        haemorrhagic disorders, 143
        maternal weight, 143
        MOEWS chart use, 144
        placenta praevia and accreta, 144
        women who decline blood products, 144
    antepartum. *See* antepartum haemorrhage
    intrapartum haemorrhage, 137
    ongoing care, 167
    pathophysiology, 137
    postpartum. *See* postpartum haemorrhage
    protocol, 138–42
        blood products, 140–1
        cell salvage, 142
        fluid resuscitation, 138–9
        intravenous access, 140
        point of care testing, 142
        volume to be infused, 140
    situational awareness, 170
maternal sepsis, 22, 120–1
    imaging, 133
    management, 126–33
        actions within 1 hour, 126–9
        antibiotics, 131
        blood cultures, 129

maternal sepsis (cont.)
blood tests, 130–1
call for help, 129
clinical examination, 129
DVT prophylaxis, 133
fluid resuscitation, 132
monitoring, 132
multi-professional approach, 133
oxygen administration, 129
removal of source of infection, 133
mortality, 120
prevention, 121
recognition of, 122
risk factors, 125
signs and symptoms, 122–5
genital tract sepsis, 122–3
non-obstetric sepsis, 124–5
Mauriceau–Smellie–Veit manoeuvre, 239
McRoberts' manoeuvre, 198–9
meconium-stained liquor, 77, 279
metabolic acidosis, 70, 131
misoprostol, 163
modified obstetric early warning score (MOEWS) charts, 144, 177
monozygotic twins, 246, See also twin births

neonatal O-negative blood, 280
newborn assessment, 92–4, 272–5
newborn resuscitation, 270, 272–80
airway, 275–6
assessment at birth, 272–5
breathing, 276–7
chest compression/circulation, 278
cord clamping, 272
documentation, 283
emergency medication, 279
emergency neonatal O-negative blood, 280
equipment preparation, 271–2
meconium management, 279

oximetry and supplementary oxygen, 278
post-resuscitation care, 280–1
glucose, 281
therapeutic hypothermia, 280
warmth, 272
nifedipine, 112
non-shockable heart rhythms, 40–1
nuchal arms, 240

obesity, 193
obstetric haemorrhage. See maternal haemorrhage
oxytocin, 154, 159
twin birth, 253

patient-reported outcome measures (PROMs), 296
perimortem birth, 31, 36
caesarean pack, 36
perinatal mortality
cord prolapse, 219
multiple births, 247
placenta accreta, 144, 154
placenta praevia, 144
positive end-expiratory pressure (PEEP), preterm birth, 287
posterior arm delivery, 201, 203
postpartum haemorrhage (PPH), 137, 151–67, See also maternal haemorrhage
causes, 146–54
documentation, 167
major haemorrhage management, 155–67
bimanual uterine compression, 160
bladder catheterisation, 160
B-Lynch suture technique, 165
call for help, 157
continuing management, 167
emergency box, 157
examination under anaesthetic, 161

hysterectomy, 166
immediate actions, 157
internal iliac artery ligation, 166
interventional radiology, 165
keeping the mother warm, 162
laparotomy, 164
manual removal of retained
    products, 161
medications, 159–60, 162–3
ongoing care, 167
rapid evaluation, 158
tear repair, 161
unrelenting haemorrhage, 162
uterine balloon tamponade, 164
uterine massage, 159
uterine vessel ligation, 166
prevention, 154
    active management of third stage
        of labour, 154–5
    physiological management of third
        stage of labour, 155–4
primary, 137
risk factors, 151
    intrapartum, 152
    pre-labour, 152
secondary, 137
situational awareness, 170
with uterine inversion, 261
pre-eclampsia, 100
fetal complications, 101
management
    community setting, 108–10
    hypertension control, 110–12
    plan for labour/birth, 116–17
    post-birth care, 117
    seizure prevention, 112
    severe pre-eclampsia, 108
aternal complications, 100
onitoring, 112–15
otting abnormalities, 115
id balance, 113
lmonary oedema, 114

predisposing factors, 101
preterm birth, 286–8
    cord clamping, 287
    counselling parents, 286
    CPAP and PEEP, 287
    neuroprotection with magnesium
        sulfate, 288
    surfactant therapy, 288
    thermal care of the preterm infant,
        286
process measures, 293
pulmonary aspiration of gastric
    contents, 25
pulmonary oedema, 114
pulmonary thromboembolism, 20–1

quality indicators (QIs), 293–5
quality of care, 299
    definition, 292
    information presentation, 297
    measurement, 291–2
        clinical quality indicators (QIs),
            293–5
        culture of unit, 296
        patient reported outcome measures
            (PROMs), 296
        process measures, 293
        source data, 295–6

recombinant factor VIIa, 163
renal function test, 131
respiratory distress syndrome (RDS),
    288

safety culture, 296
Saving Babies Lives Care Bundle, 69
seizures
    eclampsia, 102
        magnesium sulfate emergency
            regimen, 105
        management, 104–6
    prevention, 112

sepsis, 121, *See also* maternal sepsis
  prevention, 121
  recognition of, 122
  signs and symptoms, 122–5
    genital tract sepsis, 122–3
    non-obstetric sepsis, 124–5
serum lactate, 130
Severity Index (SI), 293
Sexton Safety Attitudes Questionnaire,
  297
shockable heart rhythms, 39–40
shoulder dystocia, 190–1
  consequences, 210–12
    acidosis, 210
    brachial plexus injury, 211
    humeral and clavicular fractures,
    212
  documentation, 208
  incidence, 191
  management, 195–207
    after the birth, 208
    all-fours position, 199–200
    call for help, 197
    episiotomy need evaluation, 201
    gaining internal vaginal access, 202
    internal rotational manoeuvres,
    205
    McRoberts' manoeuvre, 198–9
    posterior arm delivery, 203
    suprapubic pressure, 200
    tertiary manoeuvres, 206
    time limit, 206
    what to avoid, 207–8
  prevention and antenatal counselling,
  194–5
    caesarean section, 194
    labour induction, 195
  recognition of, 197
  risk factors, 191–3
    gestational age, 193
    macrosomia, 192
    maternal diabetes, 193

    obesity, 193
    operative vaginal birth, 198
    previous occurrence, 192
situational awareness, 9–11
source data, 295–6
suprapubic pressure, 200
surfactant therapy, 288
symphysiotomy, 206
Syntometrine, 154, 159

tachycardia, fetal, 80
teamwork, 2
  communication, 5–7
  definition, 3
  high reliability and resilience, 3–4
  leadership roles and responsibilities, 8
  situational awareness, 9–11
  training, 2
    local training, 3, 4–5
  under pressure, 11
tension pneumothorax, 43
therapeutic hypothermia, 280
thromboembolism, 43, *See also*
    deep vein thrombosis (DVT);
    pulmonary thromboembolism
timely cord clamping. *See* cord clamping
tocolysis, uterine inversion
    management, 264
training
  cord prolapse management, 225
  fetal monitoring, 69
  teamwork, 2
    local training, 3, 5
tranexamic acid (TXA), 159–60
transfer or critically ill woman, 186
twin births, 245–7
  management, 250–3
    first stage of labour, 250
    preparation, 252
    second stage of labour, 252
    third stage of labour, 256
  mode of birth, 247–9